Extended Stability
for
Parenteral
Drugs

Caryn Dellamorte Bing
Anna Nowobilski-Vasilios

Donald J. Filibeck
Brenda L. Gray
J. Michael Hayes
Barbara Limburg-Mancini
Kevn M. McNamara
Diane Nitzki-George
Kevin L. Ross
Lisa Linn Siefert
Paula Zelle

American Society of Health-System Pharmacists®
Bethesda, Maryland

Any correspondence regarding this publication should be sent to the publisher, American Society of Health-System Pharmacists, 7272 Wisconsin Avenue, Bethesda, MD 20814, attention: Special Publishing.

The information presented herein reflects the opinions of the contributors and advisors. It should not be interpreted as an official policy of ASHP or as an endorsement of any product.

Because of ongoing research and improvements in technology, the information and its applications contained in this text are constantly evolving and are subject to the professional judgment and interpretation of the practitioner due to the uniqueness of a clinical situation. The editors, contributors, and ASHP have made reasonable efforts to ensure the accuracy and appropriateness of the information presented in this document. However, any user of this information is advised that the editors, contributors, and ASHP are not responsible for the continued currency of the information, for any errors or omissions, and/or for any consequences arising from the use of the information in the document in any and all practice settings. Any reader of this document is cautioned that ASHP makes no representation, guarantee, or warranty, express or implied, as to the accuracy and appropriateness of the information contained in this document and specifically disclaims any liability to any party for the accuracy and/or completeness of the material or for any damages arising out of the use or non-use of any of the information contained in this document.

Director, Acquisitions and Product Development: Jack Bruggeman
Editorial Project Manager: Ruth Bloom
Project Editor: Johnna Hershey
Cover and Page Design: David Wade

ISBN: 978-1-58528-3408

To the ever-growing network of colleagues who continue to inspire and encourage us:

It is impossible to recognize and thank you all appropriately for your continued support of this ongoing drug information project.

Acknowledgments

As with the prior editions, the preparation of this updated reference was a team effort that would not have been possible without the exceptional group of capable writers and reviewers. They spent many hours on what some might consider minutia but this team considers essential. The editors appreciate the dedication and focus that these extremely talented and very busy professionals applied to this edition.

Contents

Contents

The scarcity of published and/or labeled stability data beyond 24 hours at any temperature has been a historically complicating factor in the care of patients in the alternate care site. When home infusion practice emerged and grew in the 1980–90s, accurate information on extended parenteral stability was very limited. Independent and hospital-based home care pharmacists were challenged to find drug stability data that supported realistic and cost-effective compounding and patient delivery schedules. Some national infusion companies put considerable resources to the task of compiling drug stability information to support their operational and patient care processes and maintained full-time drug-information specialists supporting clinicians at their many national locations. The highly competitive nature of the home infusion industry also led to the development of unpublished, proprietary drug stability data based on independent studies contracted by large home infusion companies and drug product manufacturers.

The home infusion industry experienced tremendous change in the later part of the 1990s. Many formerly competing industry leaders merged or were acquired, resulting in fewer but larger national companies. A new trend includes acquisitions of home and specialty infusion providers by chain pharmacy corporations, pharmacy benefit managers, and pharmacy-by-mail companies. Hospital and health-system infusion programs expanded in number, scope, and size in many areas. Growth in the subacute care component of long-term care pharmacy continues to contribute to the increased use of infusion products outside the hospital setting. Free-standing, hospital-based, and physician-office-based ambulatory infusion programs have also increased in number and scope of services. Reduced reimbursement, increased case management, and changes in technology have reduced the typical length of service for alternate site infusion services from primarily long-term (months to years) parenteral nutrition therapy to include much more short-term (days to weeks) drug therapies such as anti-infectives. Inpatient pharmacy services increasingly rely on extended beyond-use dating to minimize the wastage of high cost parenteral medication via appropriate recycling of unused compounded sterile parenterals. Implementation of sterile compounding practices under USP <797> and other strict standards help to support extending beyond-use dating for many medications past the more traditional 24-hour post-admixture expiration date.

The extended stability monographs and parenteral nutrition monographs in this edition represent a continuing drug information project focused on identifying, reviewing, and compiling relevant available information in a concise format. Monographs selected include most of the anti-infective medications and other parenterals with useful extended stability dating. They cite the majority of extended stability data available at the time of the edition. Many of the monographs reference well-known sources, such as the *Handbook on Injectable Drugs* (a "must-have" reference for every pharmacy that compounds sterile preparations). Additional references and sources include previously unpublished data for specific types of infusion devices and containers, direct communications from drug and device manufacturers, and a focused review of previously published data from the perspective of practitioners who use this information in home and specialty infusion. The third edition included a comprehensive chapter on total parenteral nutrition; this chapter was reformatted for the fourth edition with stability and compatibility data summarized in parenteral nutrition monographs for some of the most common additives to parenteral nutrition preparations.

The practices and integrity of pharmacists and others who compound sterile preparations have been under great scrutiny in recent years. Increased awareness in the lay public, boards of pharmacy, and Federal regulators further presses us to employ the diligence and professionalism with which we are entrusted to protect the public. We strongly emphasize the importance of using the extended stability data in this compilation responsibly and as part of the overall quality and standards-focused process of preparing sterile compounds.

Preface

EXTENDED STABILITY FOR PARENTERAL DRUGS

The monographs and chapters are compiled as an easy-to-use reference on extended stability of the parenteral drugs and biologicals most common to alternate site infusion practice, including data in container types commonly used outside the acute care setting. Opportunities to obtain, review, and share unpublished or proprietary data will continue. Future editions will incorporate these data as they become available. We welcome your suggestions and pledge to review all resource material made available for future editions of this compendium.

What's New in This Edition

The 160 stability monographs in this fifth edition include updates to all but five of the monographs from the fourth edition, and 10 new stability monographs: Acetaminophen, Ceftaroline fosamil, Coagulation Factor XIII, Doripenem, Ethanol lock, Ibuprofen, Pantoprazole, Telavancin, Toclizumab, and Ziconotide acetate. The monograph updates include data revisions for a number of container types, and new information for elastomeric infusion device brands. The Parenteral Nutrition chapter includes updates to five nutrition monographs and additional considerations for calcium and phosphate solubility. The Applying Stability Data in Patient Care now includes a nursing perspective, with a primer on the types of vascular access devices used in medication administration and important considerations for pH, osmolality, concentration, and administration device. Something else is new . . . a co-editor! My long time friend and colleague Anna Nowobilski-Vasilios has been a monograph writer/reviewer since the first edition of this book over a decade ago. Her contribution as a writer and now co-editor to this edition has been invaluable. As with prior editions, the publisher, editors, and writers welcome your feedback and suggestions for continued improvement.

Caryn Dellamorte Bing, April 2013
Las Vegas, NV

Caryn Dellamorte Bing, RPh, MS, FASHP

Caryn is Senior Manager Clinical Services and PGY1 Residency Program Director for Critical Care Systems (CCS), Inc., a national home and specialty infusion provider. Her corporate responsibilities at CCS have included development of clinical standards of practice, clinician training and professional development, and leadership and management of CCS PGY1 Pharmacy Residency program at five locations. Caryn's 30-year career includes corporate leadership, general management, operations, clinical management, accreditation surveyor, consulting, training, and pharmacy practice roles in home/specialty infusion and other alternate site and acute care practice settings. Caryn holds a BS from University of Illinois College of Pharmacy and MS in Health Systems Management from Rush University. She completed her pharmacy residency at Rush-Presbyterian-St. Luke's Medical Center. She is a Rho Chi Scholar and Fellow of the American Society of Health-System Pharmacists. Caryn has been active in professional association leadership throughout her career, including terms as a presidential officer for the Illinois and Nevada ASHP state affiliates, and as an ASHP Delegate and Alternate Delegate numerous times. She served on the ASHP Home Care Section Executive Committee and was Chairperson for the ASHP Continuity of Care Task Force. Caryn received the first Distinguished Service Award from the ASHP Home Care Section. She served on editorial boards for *AJHP*, the *Journal of Pharmacy Practice*, and *Perspectives in Pharmacy*; has published a number of articles and book chapters; and has presented at many state and national meetings. Caryn has been Editor of *Extended Stability for Parenteral Drugs* since its inception.

Anna Nowobilski-Vasilios, PharmD, MBA, FASHP, CNSC, BCNSP

Anna is Principal at Anovation, Inc.; a Surveyor for the Accreditation Commission for Health Care; and Adjunct Assistant Professor at Midwestern University. Her experience includes over 30 years in pharmacy and over 25 years in home infusion and specialty pharmacy services. She served Option Care for 14 years as Senior Vice President for Care Management Services, Residency Director, Continuing Education Administrator, Vice President of Clinical Services, Senior Director of Program Development, National Director of Pharmacy, and Director of Franchise Implementation. She also held management and clinical positions with other regional and national home infusion providers and in hospital pharmacy practice. Anna holds a BS in Pharmacy from the University of Illinois, a MBA from Keller Graduate School of Management, and a PharmD from Midwestern University. She is a Rho Chi Scholar, board certified in nutrition support as well as nutrition support pharmacy, and a Fellow of the American Society of Health-System Pharmacists; she has served as Director-At-Large for ASHP's Section of Ambulatory Care Practitioners. She is an active member in the National Home Infusion Association, American Society of Health-System Pharmacists, American Society for Parenteral and Enteral Nutrition, Infusion Nurses Society, the Illinois Council of Health-System Pharmacists, and the Polish American Pharmacists' Association. Anna has delivered numerous presentations and has published articles on the subjects of home infusion therapy, specialty pharmacy, nutrition support, new drug approvals, and interdisciplinary collaboration. She is the author of the Home Infusion Chapter in the 22nd edition of *Remington: The Science and Practice of Pharmacy* and has been a contributing writer to each edition of *Extended Stability for Parenteral Drugs*.

Caryn Dellamorte Bing, RPh, MS, FASHP
Senior Manager, Clinical Services
PGY1 Residency Program Director
Critical Care Systems, Inc.
and
President
CB Healthcare Consulting
Las Vegas, Nevada

Donald J. Filibeck, PharmD, MBA
Dublin, Ohio

Brenda L. Gray, PharmD, CNSC, BCNSP
Tampa, Florida

J. Michael Hayes, PharmD, CPh
Drug Information Coordinator/Investigational
   Pharmacy Team Lead
Moffitt Cancer Center
Department of Pharmacy
Tampa, Florida

Barbara Limburg-Mancini, PharmD, BCNSP
Director of Pharmacy
Walgreens Specialty Infusion Pharmacy
Lombard, Illinois

Kevn M. McNamara, PharmD, CNSC
National Director of Clinical Pharmacy
   Operations
BioScrip Inc.
Tampa, Florida

Diane Nitzki-George, PharmD, MBA
Clinical Pharmacist
NorthShore University Health System
Pharmacy Services
Evanston, Illinois
and
Clinical Assistant Professor
Working Professional Doctor of Pharmacy
   Program
University of Florida College of Pharmacy

Anna Nowobilski-Vasilios, PharmD, MBA, FASHP, CNSC, BCNSP
Principal
Anovation, Care Management Innovation
Chicago, Illinois
and
Adjunct Assistant Professor, Pharmacy Practice
Midwestern University, Chicago College of
   Pharmacy
Downers Grove, Illinois

Kevin L. Ross, BS, RN
Nursing Consultant
Bartonville, Texas

Lisa Linn Siefert, RPh, FASHP, ASQ-CMQ/OE
Corporate Manager, Accreditation, Quality,
   and Clinical Education
Walgreens Infusion and Respiratory Services
Deerfield, Illinois

Paula Zelle, PharmD, FASHP
Health Care Consultant
Infusion Consultant Services and Accreditation
   Resources
Canton, Ohio

How to Use This Reference

Each monograph in this reference represents a drug for which some extended parenteral stability information is available from peer reviewed publications and/or drug and/or device/container manufacturers. Practitioners who are unfamiliar with this reference and the principles of extended stability should review the "Applying Stability Data in Patient Care" chapter. Selected monographs include shorter stability data that may be useful in alternate site practice. Stability monographs are alphabetical by generic drug name. Each monograph includes a compilation of drug stability data for various container systems, solutions, concentrations, and temperature storage and administration conditions. The parenteral nutrition additive monographs are only applicable to parenteral nutrition formulations.

The following temperature ranges were adapted from the USP to evaluate reported stability study conditions[1]:

Refrigerated	2°C to 8°C
Frozen	−25°C to −10°C
Room Temperature*	15°C to 30°C
Body Temperature	37°C

*See the USP definition of Controlled Room Temperature in Appendix B, Glossary of Terms.

When studied storage conditions fall outside these ranges, a monograph note will indicate the variation.

To use a stability monograph, find the desired container or material type in the first column. When a container type is not listed, then clinically useful or extended stability data were not available for the drug in that container type. Next, check the concentration, diluent, and manufacturer of the drug studied in that container type. The next column indicates the osmolality of the sample studied if it was assayed or calculated by the authors of the cited study. The pH column either includes the actual or range of pH for the specific concentration, or a note that ties to more general pH data for the drug product. Additional columns list the extended stability data that have been documented for the drug in the container and specified conditions. If frozen stability information is available, check the post-thaw stability data; this may differ from the room temperature and refrigerated stability data for the same drug in a never-frozen state. The final column indicates the reference or references used for the particular line in the monograph. When "n/a" is noted in any field, no information is available for that item.

Within the stability monograph, footnotes highlight important information. Each footnote corresponds to information in the Notes section of the monograph that is crucial to interpretation of the data. These include comments on variations from USP temperature ranges, detailed descriptions of storage conditions, and more. A Special Considerations section includes special information on drug storage, preparation, and administration.

Flush compatibility refers to the chemical compatibility of the drug with common solutions used to flush vascular access devices. Practitioners should be aware of nursing practice guidelines (such as those of the Intravenous Nurses Society), access device specifications, and drug-solution compatibility when determining the type and volume of solution(s) used for line maintenance. When a drug is incompatible with heparinized saline (i.e., heparin lock flush), it may be necessary to flush with saline before and after administration. (Commonly referred to as SASH, this stands for Saline-Administration-Saline-Heparin.) A few drugs are not compatible with saline or heparinized saline; in these cases, flushing with an alternative compatible solution, such as D5W, may be necessary. If the line flush procedures for a specific therapy vary from the organization's standard approach, the pharmacist should provide written directions to clarify the flush method used. Heparinization may not always be required to maintain line patency for some access devices (e.g., Groshong catheters) or when positive displacement catheter caps are used.

Use of Additional Resources

The information contained in these monographs is a compilation of extended stability data from multiple sources. This information is not a substitute for the official product literature. Practitioners should consult the primary literature and the product manufacturer to determine the applicability of stability data to a particular patient and practice scenario. Practitioners should maintain current drug reference resources as well as the most current edition of a comprehensive reference on drug stability and compatibility. Every pharmacy that compounds or provides sterile preparations should maintain resource files, including the phone numbers and all correspondence with the medical or clinical affairs departments of pharmaceutical manufacturers. The pharmacy should also have access to a drug information center or the expertise and ability to conduct a literature search for the most up-to-date clinical and pharmaceutical information on parenteral drugs.

General Abbreviations

d	day(s)
h	hour(s)
iso	iso-osmotic
m	month(s)
min	minute(s)
RTU	ready to use from manufacturer
unspec.	unspecified
w	week(s)
y	year(s)

Solution Abbreviations

BWFI	Bacteriostatic water for injection
D	Dextrose solution (percentage unspecified)
D2.5	Dextrose 2.5% in water
D2.5^1/$_2$S	Dextrose 2.5% in sodium chloride 0.45%
D5LR	Dextrose 5% in lactated Ringer's
D5^1/$_4$S	Dextrose 5% in sodium chloride 0.225%
D5^1/$_2$S	Dextrose 5% in sodium chloride 0.45%
D5S	Dextrose 5% in sodium chloride 0.9%
D10S	Dextrose 10% in sodium chloride 0.9%
D5W	Dextrose 5% in water
D7W	Dextrose 7% in water
D10W	Dextrose 10% in water
DXN-6	Dextran 6%
LR	Ringer's injection, lactated
M10	Mannitol 10%
NS	Sodium chloride 0.9%
R	Ringer's solution
^{1}/$_2$S	Sodium chloride 0.45%
^{1}/$_4$S	Sodium chloride 0.22%
W	Sterile water for injection

Reference

1. United States Pharmacopeial Convention. Chapter <795> Pharmaceutical Compounding—Nonsterile Preparations. Official August 1, 2008.

Part I

Applying Stability Data in Patient Care

Caryn Dellamorte Bing, Kevin L. Ross

Introduction

Alternate site pharmacists must use extended stability data to assign beyond-use dating to facilitate the cost-effective dispensing and delivery of compounded sterile preparations for multiple days of therapy. Pharmacists, regardless of practice setting, should always assign beyond-use dates that accurately represent the stability of the medication, combination of medications, or other component ingredients under the intended preparation, packing, shipping, storage, and administration conditions. To do this, the pharmacist must be familiar with the chemical and physical factors that affect the sterility, integrity, and stability of the final preparation. Additionally, environmental, operational, and personnel factors that contribute to the quality of a compound cannot be discounted. In light of very visible examples and tragic patient outcomes from contaminated preparations,[1] pharmacists and technicians must diligently ensure that their facility produces contaminant-free preparations, which can then be assigned reasonable extended stability dates that are valid for their organization. Nurses and other professionals who administer parenteral medications must understand the application of beyond-use dating and physical/chemical characteristics of compounded sterile preparations in the patient care and patient education process.

Parenteral drugs are usually compounded and/or packaged in something other than the original manufacturer's container. They are often diluted prior to administration and stored under different conditions than the bulk (source) ingredients. These factors have a direct and important impact on the stability of the final preparation.

Factors Affecting Extended Drug Stability

Key terminology, definitions, a discussion of factors affecting extended drug stability, and some considerations for alternate site practice are provided below. References 2 and 3 are additional resources on the topics of drug stability, compatibility, and beyond-use dating.[2,3]

The shelf life *stability* of a drug is the length of time that the preparation retains the labeled potency of the active ingredient(s) under the labeled storage conditions.

The *extended stability* expiration dating in the monographs contained in this reference is the maximum time in which 90% or greater of a labeled active ingredient is measurable in the solution and container specified, under the stated storage conditions. For coagulation factor products, the stability is defined as retaining at least 80% of baseline activity.

Instability refers to the chemical processes that result in drug degradation, including hydrolysis, oxidation, reduction, and photodegradation. For example, increased temperature and exposure to light can increase the likelihood of chemical instability for many drugs, particularly those that are affected by hydrolysis or oxidation reactions. Practitioners should always be aware of the basis for a preparation's instability, as the byproduct(s) of drug degradation can have therapeutic and/or toxicity implications for patient care.

Incompatibility refers to a physical or chemical phenomenon that reduces the concentration of the active ingredient. In some cases, the incompatibility is easily observed, as with a precipitate, haze, color formation, or other obvious visual change. However, many incompatibilities are not readily observed. Factors that affect drug compatibility, such as the diluent, its pH, the concentration of the drug, the component makeup of the container, and the presence of other agents and buffers, are summarized in **Table 1**.[2,4]

Table 1. Common Factors Affecting Drug Stability

Factor	Incompatibility or Instability	Common Examples
Contact with metal (e.g., needles or components of devices)	Chemical reaction	Hydralazine, metronidazole (with aluminum)
Freezing temperature	Inactivation, denaturation, emulsion cracking	Heparin, filgrastim, erythropoietin, lipid-containing TPN
Large organic anions and cations	Precipitation or formation of insoluble complex	Heparin with aminoglycosides
Light (natural and room)	Accelerated chemical degradation reactions	Dobutamine, furosemide, cisplatin, hydroxyzine, carboplatin
Low temperature (refrigerated)	Crystallization or precipitation	5-fluorouracil, furosemide, acyclovir, metronidazole
Plastic containers, sets, in-line filters	Adsorption of lipophilic agents—especially important at low concentrations	Sufentanil, filgrastim, calcitriol, lorazepam, aldesleukin, insulin
PVC or flexible plastic container permeability	Evaporation, with resultant over-concentration of solution	PVC or flexible plastic containers distributed in overwrap bags; small volume bags are most susceptible
Plasticizer content of PVC containers, sets	Leaching carcinogenic plasticizer DEHP from DEHP-containing PVC	Paclitaxel, lipid emulsion, cyclosporine
Saturation solubility exceeded	Precipitation or crystallization	Morphine sulfate, etoposide
Temperature above 8°C	Accelerated chemical degradation reactions	Ampicillin, others

Source: References 2 (Trissel) and 4 (Lima).

Combination drugs. Practitioners must establish the beyond-use date based on the least stable moiety of a combination drug. For example, with ticarcillin disodium and clavulanate potassium or piperacillin sodium and tazobactam sodium, the ticarcillin and piperacillin are the least stable components of the combinations and are the basis for determining the beyond-use dating of these combination drugs.

Concentration dependence or independence of chemical stability. Most drugs exhibit consistent chemical stabilities within the normally used clinical ranges; however, there are exceptions. For example, as the concentration of ampicillin sodium increases in solution, its stability decreases. Practitioners should verify that the drug stability is applicable to the desired concentration.

Preparation Sterility and Quality Assurance

The manufacturer-approved stability information for parenteral drugs (i.e., the information permitted by the Food and Drug Administration [FDA]) is often based on concerns for preparation *sterility* rather than chemical stability. A detailed discussion of proper aseptic technique as well as parenteral preparation quality assurance is beyond the scope of this text. Practitioners should be familiar with professional standards, including those of the American Society of Health-

System Pharmacists (ASHP) and the United States Pharmacopeia (USP), related to sterile preparation quality assurance. (See Professional, Regulatory, and Accreditation Expectations below.)

Practitioners have a responsibility to ensure that the beyond-use date assigned to a compounded parenteral preparation is consistent with the quality control practices in their parenteral preparation admixture program. Sterile preparation process validation and employee competence assessments should encompass all container systems and the longest beyond-use dating contemplated.

Professional, Regulatory, and Accreditation Expectations

Pharmacists have a professional and legal responsibility for all aspects of the medication compounding and dispensing process. In addition to any issues unique to each state's pharmacy practice act, professional standards of practice set the expectations for practitioners in alternate site care. Pharmacists should be aware of these expectations as well as any requirements that apply to their specific practice setting.

USP Standards

USP's Chapter <1206> Sterile Drug Products for Home Use outlined USP performance expectations in the provision of home-use sterile drug preparations, including stability and expiration dating.[5] However, this document only applied to one practice setting and was not considered a compendial requirement. USP published Chapter <797> Pharmaceutical Compounding—Sterile Preparations[6] in 2004 as a revision to <1206>, and further updated this compendial standard, effective June 1, 2008.[7] USP Chapter <797> is a general tests and assays chapter with regulatory weight and applicability for settings that compound sterile preparations. All practitioners involved with compounded sterile preparations (CSPs) should be familiar with the requirements set forth in USP Chapter <797>.

In the absence of sterility testing consistent with USP Chapter <71> procedures, practitioners should assign beyond-use dating that is consistent with USP Chapter <797> risk levels. **Table 2** summarizes the current guidelines for beyond-use dating and storage conditions for each risk level. The 2008 revision to USP Chapter <797> responded to requests for clarification and enhancements. One change applicable for alternate site pharmacies includes changes to the refrigerated storage beyond-use dating guidelines for medium risk level compounding; the increase to up to 9 days helps to accommodate the typical weekly compounding and delivery cycle for home parenteral nutrition services. Another significant clarification is that sterile compounding pertains to all preadministration manipulations of CSPs (including compounding, storage, and transport,) but not to the administration of CSPs to patients. Two additional risk levels accommodate the needs of immediate use and low-risk compounding where the ISO Class 5 primary engineering control (PEC) is not located in an ISO Class 7 buffer area.[7] Both of these new risk categories have implications for ambulatory infusion care. Ambulatory infusion and clinic sites with access to an ISO 5 PEC (e.g., the laminar flow hood) can prepare and administer a CSP within 12 hours without the investment in ISO 7 PEC facilities. Parenteral medications prepared outside an ISO 5 PEC must be administered within 1 hour.

ASHP Standards

ASHP's Minimum Standard for Home Care Pharmacies outlines the minimum requirements for the operation and management of pharmaceutical services provided by home care pharmacies.[8] The standards affirm the pharmacist's responsibility for sterile preparation quality and integrity, including assignment of reliable beyond-use dating. These standards should be used in conjunc-

Table 2. USP Chapter <797> Storage Conditions and Beyond-Use Dating for Compounded Sterile Preparations[7]

Condition	Controlled Room Temperature (20°C–25°C)	Cold Temperature (2°C–8°C)	Solid Frozen (−25° to −10°C)
Immediate Use	1 hour	1 hour	N/A
Low Risk	≤48 hours	≤14 days	≤45 days
Low Risk with 12 hr BUD	≤12 hours	≤12 hours	N/A
Medium Risk	≤30 hours	≤9 days	≤45 days
High Risk	≤24 hours	≤3 days	≤45 days

BUD, beyond-use dating

tion with other ASHP best practice resources that address the procedures and quality assurance for compounding sterile preparations.

ASHP developed *Guidelines on Quality Assurance for Pharmacy-Prepared Sterile Products* prior to USP Chapter <797> to assist pharmacists in establishing quality assurance procedures for sterile drug preparations based on the risk level associated with the process and preparation.[9] These professional standards of practice are now superseded by the requirements outlined in USP Chapter <797>. ASHP published a *Discussion Guide on Compounding Sterile Preparations* that recaps these requirements for CSPs.[26]

FDA Compounding Regulations

The Food and Drug Administration Modernization Act of 1997 (FDAMA) included provisions that affect pharmacy compounding activities.[10] The provisions of this act precluded pharmacies from bulk production of pharmaceuticals that are not intended for a specific or anticipated patient. In addition, pharmacists are not allowed to copy commercially available preparations (although they can modify the preparation based on patient needs, as in the removal of a dye or preservative due to patient allergy). Further, compounding pharmacists must ensure compliance with all USP standards. In 2001, however, a Federal Court of Appeals decision rendered the pharmacy compounding provisions of FDAMA to be unconstitutional. Subsequently, FDA revised its Compliance Policy Guide (CPG) related to pharmacy compounding. While jurisdiction over pharmacy practice remains within the purview of state laws, this CPG outlines criteria for potential FDA action against a pharmacy.[11]

State Laws and Regulations

Many states now have specific requirements for compounding sterile preparations. Some state boards of pharmacy have fully adopted USP Chapter <797> as the minimum standard, while others have developed state-specific provisions. These range from general guidelines to very specific facility, training, and quality assurance rules and regulations. Practitioners must be cognizant of all state requirements related to the compounding and dating of sterile preparations. However, it would be inadvisable to rely solely on the board of pharmacy or state regulations for the requirements and standards for preparing sterile compounds.

Accreditation Standards

Accreditation standards set practice and operational expectations for organizations. The Joint Commission® (TJC) has standards that apply to many types of healthcare providers. The Community Health Accreditation Program (CHAP) and the Accreditation Commission for Health Care (ACHC) have standards that apply to home care pharmacies. Although none of these accreditation standards specify beyond-use dating guidelines, they do require that accredited organizations adhere to accepted standards of practice, as well as law and regulation. Each accredited organization must establish and implement procedures that are appropriate and in compliance with legal and practice norms.

Commercial Products and Extemporaneous Compounding

Extemporaneous Compounding

A number of ready-to-use parenteral products are commercially available, and many of these have a shelf life beyond published or referenced stability data. However, practitioners should never extrapolate a commercial product's labeled shelf life stability to pharmacy-compounded sterile preparations. Commercial formulations often contain buffering systems and stabilizing agents, and use special packaging methods that allow for FDA-approved extended dating. In addition, pharmaceutical manufacturers must comply with extensive quality control standards to produce and label a sterile parenteral product.

Considerations for Nonsterile Ingredients

Because certain sterile products are not commercially available, some pharmacies have adopted the practice of compounding parenteral preparations from nonsterile ingredients, then cold sterilizing them through 0.22-micron filters. This is classified as high-risk level compounding by USP. USP Chapter <797> quality assurance measures for high-risk level compounding begins to approach the requirements applicable to parenteral manufacturers. Inadequately sterilized compounds prepared from nonsterile components have caused tragic infections and deaths of patients. Safety conscious practitioners must consider the stringent USP compendial requirements for sterilization, testing, and quality assurance as a minimum standard for compounding these types of sterile preparations from nonsterile ingredients.

Freezing Parenteral Preparations

The institutional practice of freezing extemporaneously compounded parenteral preparations set the stage for the use of frozen medications in alternate site pharmacies. However, this practice is controversial. Most of the stability studies for frozen preparations are at a very controlled −10 to −20°C; some have been conducted with a flash-freeze process in which solutions are rapidly frozen and stored in commercial freezers. These conditions cannot be replicated when compounding a large quantity of small-volume parenteral preparations and freezing them overnight in the freezer compartment of a residential-style refrigerator. Similarly, frozen stability data do not apply to scenarios in which patients are instructed to place unfrozen preparations in home freezers upon receipt. Practitioners should not extrapolate frozen or post-thaw stability data from commercial frozen product labeling to extemporaneous preparations.

Infusate Properties

Osmolarity and Osmolality

Whenever extemporaneous parenteral preparations are compounded, practitioners need to consider the osmolarity (mOsm/L of solution) or osmolality (mOsm/kg of solvent) of the final solution. In the absence of confirmed central placement of a patient's intravenous line, practitioners should prepare solutions that are within a reasonable osmotic range for peripheral infusions. Increased use of peripherally inserted central catheters has decreased concerns about peripheral vein irritation and phlebitis due to hyperosmotic/hypertonic infusions; however, hypoosmotic/hypotonic solutions can cause hemolysis, and rapid hypertonic infusions can cause a variety of clinical complications. As a general rule, the greater the volume and rate of the infusion, the closer the solution should be to isotonicity (282–288 mOsm/kg),[13] regardless of vascular access type or catheter placement.

Osmolarity is an additive figure for all of the chemical ingredients of a solution, including the diluent. Theoretical osmolar concentration of a substance or drug can be determined using a variety of equations, including the following[14]:

$$\text{Osmolar concentration (mOsm/L)} = \frac{[\text{weight of substance per liter of solution (g/L)}]}{[\text{molecular weight (g)}] \times \text{number of species} \times 1000}$$

The number of species is the number of ions formed when the drug is dissolved in solution. Drugs that are not salts produce a species number of 1; monovalent salts and electrolytes produce a species of 2; divalent salts and electrolytes produce a species number of 3. To obtain the osmolarity of the preparation, add the osmolarity of the diluent to this calculated answer.

Since various factors (including temperature, pH, and concentration) can affect dissociation in solution (species), the computed and actual measured osmolarity values may vary. Although the computation of theoretical osmolarity of complex mixtures (such as total parenteral nutrition or multiple drugs in solution) is possible, the actual measured osmolality for these mixtures is best determined experimentally if clinically significant to patient care. The monographs in this book cite the measured or calculated osmolality (mOsm/kg) when available.

Using pH Values in Practice

The pH of compounded sterile preparations will vary based on the acid-base property of the parenteral medication additives and the base solution or diluent used. The pH of the actual infusate may be important, as extremely low or high pH solutions can cause vascular irritation, phlebitis, and endothelial damage. If infiltrated, these solutions can result in further tissue damage. The normal physiologic (intravascular fluid) pH is 7.4. Some manufacturers and independent stability studies report the actual measured pH or pH range for specific CSP concentrations. However, these are often reported as a wide range and may reflect only the initial reconstituted or commercial solution pH. Practitioners should use available pH data and known pH ranges of commercial parenteral infusion solutions to determine when a preparation is suitable for infusion through peripheral-short or peripheral-midline devices. **Table 3** includes the osmolarity and pH for the some common commercial infusion solutions.

Table 3. Osmolarity and pH of Commercial Infusion Solutions

Solution	Osmolarity (calc) mOsm/L	pH	Manufacturer(s)
Sterile Water for Injection, USP	0	5.4–5.5 (5.0–7.0)	BA, BRN, HSP
Dextrose 5% in Water (D5W)	252 250 252–253	4, 4.5 (3.2–6.5) 4.4 (3.5–6.5) 4.3 (3.2–6.5)	BA BRN HSP
Normal Saline (NS) (Sodium Chloride 0.9%)	310 308 308	5.6 (4.5–7.0) 5.0, 5.5 (4.5–7.0) 5.6 (4.5–7.0)	BRN BA HSP
Sodium chloride 0.45% ($^1/_2$S)	154 154	5.5 (4.5–7.0) 5.6 (4.5–7.0)	BA HSP
Dextrose 10% in Water	505 (calculated)	4.0 (3.2–6.5)	BA
Dextrose 5% in Lactated Ringers	530 (calculated)	4.6 (4.0–6.0)	BRN

Source: NCBI PubMed/Pub Chem Substance Summary. Available at: http://pubchem.ncbi.nlm.nih.gov/.

Vascular Access Devices and Catheters Used in Medication Administration

Factors that could impact the decision to administer a medication through a type of vascular access device (VAD) include: VAD tip placement, number of lumens, catheter material, catheter size (diameter, length), and volume from hub to tip.

VAD complications can result in delays in therapy or missed doses when the VAD is not functional or must be changed. VAD complications that may be related to the drug concentration, pH, osmolality, and direct contact of irritants include:

- Infiltration (leakage of infusate into tissue surrounding a vascular access device) can occur when the VAD tip no longer resides in the blood vessel.
- Extravasation (infiltration of vesicant or irritating agents into tissue surrounding a vascular access device) can result in tissue and/or nerve damage.
- Chemical phlebitis is an inflammation of the inside of the blood vessel caused by direct contact with an irritant infusate.
- Catheter occlusion can cause a complete or partial blockage of the VAD due to incompatibility resulting in a precipitant in the line.

The clinician should be aware of the VAD type prior to selecting or recommending the medication concentration and administration method, including frequency and duration of the infusion. Peripheral short catheters and pediatric midline catheters are stated in gauge (Ga) size, whereas adult midline and central vascular access devices are stated in French (Fr) sizes.[27] Gauge refers to the diameter: the larger the gauge, the smaller the diameter. French refers to the circumference: the larger the French size, the larger the circumference.

Central Venous Access Devices

A central venous access device (CVAD) is a catheter whose tip terminates in the lower two-thirds of the superior vena cava. See **Figure 1**. CVADs have several distinct purposes in the

Figure 1. Central placement: Tip of a CVAD catheter is located in the superior vena cava

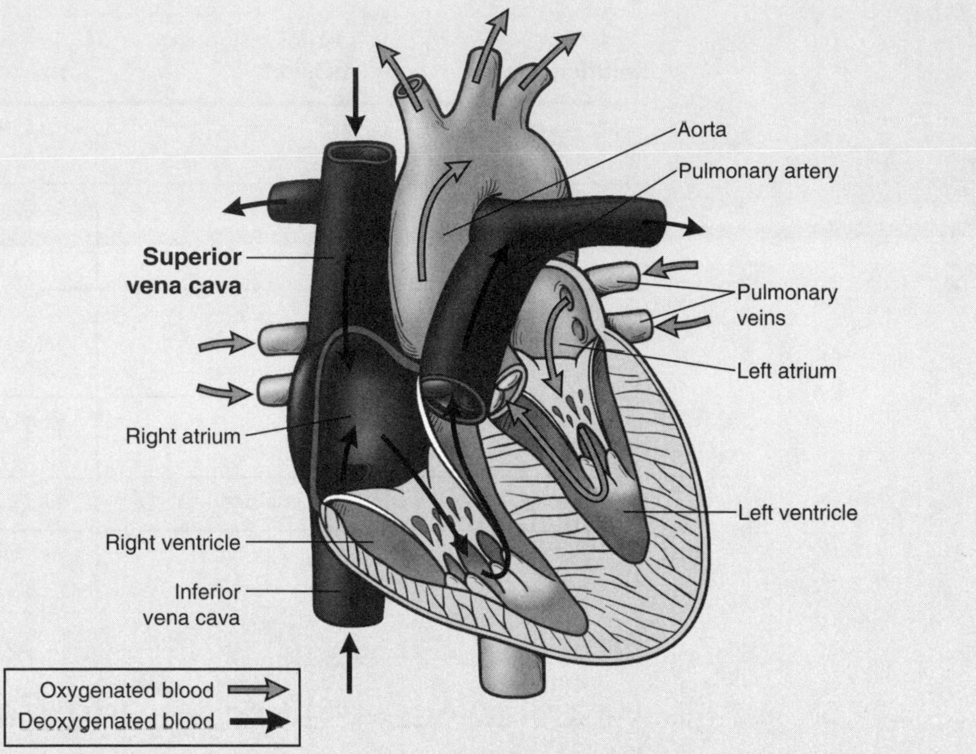

Source: Adapted with permission from Stuhan MA. *Understanding Pharmacology for Pharmacy Technicians,* Bethesda, MD: American Society of Health-System Pharmacists; 2013; 271.

clinical setting. They provide alternatives for IV administration when patients have poor peripheral venous access and also ready access for frequent blood draws. The large diameter and high flow of blood permits administration of medications with high osmolality, concentration and/or viscosity, parenteral nutrition, chemotherapy, blood products, and medications with low or high pH and other vesicant properties. CVADs may be valved or open ended. Valved catheters are designed to maintain line patency without anticoagulant flush.

There are two basic types of CVADs, tunneled and non-tunneled.

Tunneled CVADs are anchored by "tunnelling" in tissue prior to the insertion into the large blood vessel. They are generally used for permanent or long-term venous access.

Non Tunneled CVADs are placed via a percutaneous stick into the blood vessel and advanced within the blood vessel. They are not permanently placed.

A *peripherally inserted central catheter (PICC)* is a type of non tunneled CVAD which is inserted in the antecubital space into the basilic, brachial, or cephalic veins and advanced within the blood vessel to achieve central placement. See **Figure 2**.

An *implanted port* is a type of tunneled CVAD that is implanted under skin and tissue with no portion of the catheter externally exposed. Ports must be accessed using a special non-coring needle.

Non-central Vascular Access Devices

There are two types of non-central VADs, midline and peripheral short catheters. Non-central VADs should not be used for administration of continuous vesicants, total parenteral nutrition, infusates with pH less than 5 or greater than 9, or high osmolality solutions. The American Society for Parenteral and Enteral Nutrition (ASPEN) guidelines[28] recommend a CVAD for >900 mOsm/L parenteral nutrition infusates; Infusion Nurses Society (INS) standards[27] recommend a CVAD for all infusates

Figure 2. The circulatory system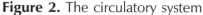

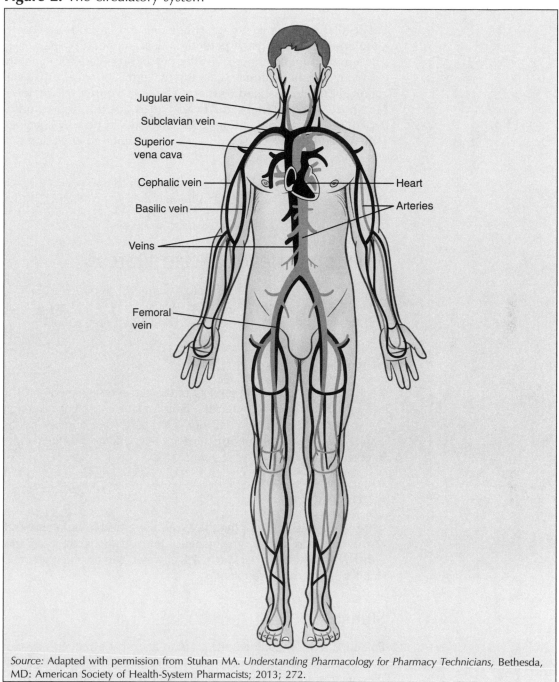

Source: Adapted with permission from Stuhan MA. *Understanding Pharmacology for Pharmacy Technicians,* Bethesda, MD: American Society of Health-System Pharmacists; 2013; 272.

>600 mOsm/L; National Home Infusion Association (NHIA) *CVAD Guidelines for the Adult Home-Based Patient*[38] recommend a CVAD for all infusates >900 mOsm/L.

Midline catheters are not CVADs. They are a type of peripherally placed VAD. A midline may be from 3 inches to 8 inches in length, with the tip terminating in the vessel between the elbow and the shoulder (the axillary region). The catheter dwell time (length of time in place) is typically two to six weeks.

Peripheral short catheters are usually 1–1.5 inches in length and are available in 14–27 gauge (Ga) sizes, with the tip terminating in the peripheral vein. These devices are used for short-term and single dose IV administration.

Labeling Instructions

Labels that specify the storage conditions and beyond-use date of compounded preparations should be placed on each parenteral dosage unit. If preparation stability varies under different temperature conditions, list the beyond-use date for each anticipated storage condition on the label; the pharmacist should make this information as clear as possible. If the preparation should be warmed to room temperature prior to administration, the label and ancillary instruction material should clearly describe this. If preparations are stable for less than 24 hours at room temperature, the label should be very specific about the end-use time. Patients and caregivers should always be trained to check preparations for current beyond-use dates prior to usage.

Practitioners should establish a standardized approach to labeling that is clear, concise, and meets all licensure and regulatory requirements, including USP Chapter <797> general labeling guidelines.[15]

Assigning Beyond-Use Dates

As noted earlier, a number of factors can affect extended stability of parenteral preparations. When assigning a beyond-use date, practitioners should consider stability, compatibility, sterility, and the final concentration of the compounded preparation.

Stability

Be aware of the chemical stability of the active drug ingredient. Is it light sensitive, heat sensitive, or likely to be pushed to the limits of labeled potency during the dispensing interval? When the contents of one drug container is infused over a number of days, be certain that the drug stability data reflect room or near body temperature conditions for the intended administration interval.

Compatibility

Note the compatibility of the drug with the available or intended diluents, as well as the most commonly used catheter maintenance flush solutions. Although many drugs are compatible with either normal saline or dextrose 5% in water, some exhibit greater compatibility and extended stability in one of these diluents.

Sterility

Possibly the most controversial point in assigning extended beyond-use dates, sterility is one of the most difficult variables to control. Pharmacy management must ensure that established sterile preparation quality control and quality assurance methods referred to earlier have been implemented and validated in their practice setting. Only with this type of risk management and quality assurance can pharmacists feel safe in assigning extended dating from any source.

Final Concentration

Pharmacists should calculate the final concentration of each compounded parenteral admixture and compare this to available stability and compatibility data. Drugs exhibit different stability at different concentrations. Whenever possible, the pharmacist should compound the parenteral preparation in a concentration within the established stability range.

Container Type and Material

The type of infusion container or device can affect extended drug stability. Practitioners should be aware of the container material for proprietary ambulatory infusion devices and administration sets. Parenteral stability data for one type of container should not be automatically extrapolated to other brands or types of containers.

Patient and Site-Specific Considerations

Home care practitioners and their patients face a number of unique and sometimes uncontrollable situations. Most home care patients do not have a nurse or other healthcare professional present for every dose, hook-up, disconnect, or parenteral route access event. Typically, the patient or caregiver is taught to administer medications that are delivered to the patient at weekly or other intervals. In addition to hooking up and infusing parenteral preparations using pumps; elastomeric devices; and intravenous push, gravity, and in-line control sets, the patients or caregivers are taught to maintain intravenous access patency with appropriate line flush and catheter care techniques. Each patient's situation is different. Practitioners must evaluate these circumstances at the start of care and reevaluate at reasonable intervals to ensure that the extended drug stability assigned is appropriate to the continuing needs of the patient.

Site of Care Considerations for Beyond-Use Dating

Practitioners must be fully aware of the circumstances in which compounded sterile preparations will be delivered, stored, and administered. As noted earlier, these circumstances may affect the integrity and stability of the compounded sterile preparations. The following are some tips for the variety of practice settings in which extended dating may be applicable.

Inpatient Acute Care

In these circumstances, the hospital may prepare large batches of specific drug admixtures in anticipation of high utilization. The internal (pharmacy) preparation and storage conditions, hospital delivery process, storage conditions on patient units, and method of handling unused medications (returns) are all factors for consideration in hospital policies regarding parenteral preparations.

Home and Hospice Infusion

Home infusion organizations often issue a weekly supply of compounded sterile preparations when documented extended stability data are available. In some cases, even longer time intervals between home deliveries may be necessary. The unpredictability of parenteral pain management for hospice and palliative care patients can pose special challenges to the preparation and delivery cycle. In addition to the pharmaceutical considerations, two key issues arise with home and hospice infusion. First, the delivery and storage methods and conditions will vary, which may affect drug stability. The pharmacy is responsible for ensuring appropriate delivery processes. Second, patient and caregiver education on proper storage conditions is a joint responsibility of the pharmacy and any home health and hospice practitioners who conduct patient training and/or make home visits.

Long-Term and Subacute Care

In many cases, these patient care facilities do not have on-site, 24-hour pharmacies to compound sterile preparations. The delivery and storage of compounded parenteral medications is similar to the circumstances for home infusion. However, a pharmacy may decide to dispense a limited number of doses due to unanticipated changes in patient status in this patient population. Any pharmacy and long-term care facility policies on the return and reuse of medications should be carefully developed to ensure that product integrity and stability are not compromised.

Ambulatory Infusion

A variety of clinical, reimbursement, and practice issues drive the administration of parenteral preparations in outpatient clinics, physician offices, or other ambulatory care settings. When the pharmacy provider is off-site from the location of the medication administration, delivery and storage factors are applicable. When the medication is started (connected) in the ambulatory care setting and the patient leaves with medication infusing, practitioners should establish the stability of the product at the ambient temperatures to which it is exposed.

Neonatal, Infant, and Pediatric Patients

The preparation and administration of injectable or infused medications and parenteral nutrition for neonatal, infant, and pediatric patients requires an understanding of the characteristics and unique needs of this patient population. The neonatal age group includes premature and term babies up to 1-month-old. Infants are from 1 month to 24 months. Children are 2- to 12-years-old, and adolescents are 12- to 18-years-old. The dosage ranges, dilutions, and complete factors for considerations are beyond the scope of this book. Practitioners providing parenteral therapy to these patients should also consult current references specific to pediatrics, such as *Pediatric Injectable Drugs*.[12]

The volume of infusion solutions administered over time to neonates, infants, and children presents challenges for healthcare professionals, especially for multiple infusion medication administrations throughout the day or over a course of treatment. The nurse or pharmacist should ensure that the volume of diluents plus medications administered does not exceed the daily fluid needs for that patient. The pharmacist may have to prepare more concentrated solutions to prevent fluid overload or to get the medication infused in reasonable time. Some medications are less stable at higher concentrations. In addition, higher concentrations increase the challenge of ensuring that the osmolarity and pH are appropriate for the type of catheter.

Another factor to consider when administering medications to younger patients is the viscosity of the solution. Viscous solutions generally require the use of infusion devices for the accurate and timely infusion of the medication. The intravenous catheters typically used in these patients may be smaller gauge (e.g., 23 or 24 gauge) so viscous solutions will infuse more slowly.

Avoid most of the preservatives used in parenteral medications (such as benzyl alcohol) in neonates. The pharmacist should ensure that the beyond-use date assigned is appropriate when utilizing products without preservatives.

Here are some additional safety considerations for young patients receiving infused medications:

1. Use standardized concentrations of medications to prevent errors.
2. The overfill in a compounded syringe or container should never be equal to or greater than the dose administered.
3. Note the potential for dosage lost in administration sets. If this amount is substantial relative to the total required dose, then provide a post dose flush bag with a compatible diluent to ensure complete and accurate dosing.

Considerations in Selecting Administration Methods and Infusion Devices

Length of Therapy

One of the most time-consuming and costly components of alternate site infusion is the start of care or admission visit. The training, assessment, and subsequent paperwork involved in a home healthcare start-up can take several hours for a typical case. However, with the increased emphasis on short hospital stays and improved treatments for many conditions, the length of many home infusion cases has also decreased. When patients are sent home for a 2- or 3-day completion of anti-infective therapy, practitioners must decide on an easy-to-teach administration method that maximizes patient compliance. In these circumstances, stability factors are not as much of an issue because the course of therapy is shorter. The more common home care scenario involves therapies expected to continue for extended periods of time with weekly delivery intervals.

Administration Method and Infusion Devices

The following factors contribute to the selection of the infusion administration method most appropriate to the patient's circumstances:

- Patient mobility
- Presence of willing and trainable caregiver(s)
- Home environmental factors (including safety and security)
- Patient functional limitations (e.g., visual abilities and manual dexterity)
- Language barriers (i.e., difficulty speaking or understanding English)
- Reimbursement for devices and home care nursing visits
- Patient proximity to the infusion provider site
- Patient risk factors for infection (e.g., immune-compromised and/or underlying illness)

Keep in mind that the choice of administration method and device may be the main determinant of extended drug stability for a CSP.

An old method of drug administration has reemerged in the alternate site care setting. Patients, caregivers, physicians, and practitioners have increasingly accepted patient- or caregiver-administered intravenous push, primarily for anti-infective therapy. Studies showing positive clinical outcomes and high satisfaction levels are expected to spur the continued growth of this practice.[16] Another positive benefit of intravenous push is that stability data for many of the anti-infective agents in syringes are readily available and easily adopted for home care and alternate site applications.

A number of infusion devices are marketed for the ambulatory and home care population. The list of electronic and disposable devices seems almost endless and continues to grow. With the increased incidence of latex allergies, most companies have converted some or all of their infusion containers to latex-free products. Practitioners should consult the product literature to ensure that latex-free products are used whenever latex allergies are a risk factor.

Specific Drug Delivery Systems

The available stability data for a given container may affect the selection of the drug delivery system for a particular patient. As noted above, the myriad of infusion devices challenge the practitioner to determine whether the available stability data are applicable to the container closure system selected. In the absence of studies of a specific container, the pharmacist should consider the component materials and compare information from similar container systems that have been evaluated. Pharmacists should be aware of manufacturer guidelines for the use of specific containers.

Flexible plastic containers. The most common parenteral container system in use today continues to be the flexible plastic container, commonly referred to as the *IV bag*. This type of container can be used with or without an infusion device, depending on the requirements for rate control, IV line pressure, and compliance with organizational policies. Many infusion solutions are available in single chamber, flexible plastic containers. Empty containers are also available and used for specialized preparations.

Polyvinyl chloride (PVC) containers. Most PVC containers (and other medical devices) are prepared using the plasticizer DEHP, which can be leached from the PVC material by some lipophilic medications, lipids, and blood products.[24] July 2002 guidelines from the FDA caution against the use of PVC in selected specialty clinical applications.[17] Practitioners should review these guidelines and establish policies that are appropriate for their patient populations and therapies provided.[18] In November 2006, the Department of Health and Human Services recommended exposure to DEHP be minimized in male infants and female patients that are pregnant with a male fetus.[25] Various manufacturers now offer lines of DEHP-free solution bags, infusion sets, and devices.

Manufacturers of parenteral products packaged in PVC and other nonrigid plastic containers recommend maximum usage times after removal from the overwrap. This time varies with the container type, volume, and solution and/or drug. **Table 4** summarizes several manufacturers' maximum out-of-overwrap storage times for plain solution container storage at room temperature. Once additives are placed in these containers, the beyond-use date changes to the shorter of the drug stability dating or the solution manufacturer's maximum recommended time for use after removal from the overwrap and storage. Always consult product labeling for commercial premixed and frozen medications for recommended storage time and conditions.

Ethyl vinyl acetate (EVA) containers. EVA containers are made of a flexible plastic that does not require phthalate plasticizers such as DEHP in the manufacturing process. An increasing number of the manufacturers of plastic medical products now make their bags and devices from ethyl vinyl acetate. EVA bags can serve as a DEHP-free alternative for preparation of medications when that choice is appropriate for the patient or therapy.

Newer types of flexible containers. Some of the newer types of flexible and semirigid plastic containers now on the market are made up of multilayers (laminates) with non-PVC fluid pathways and/or completely new types of plastic, including polyethylene, polyester, and polyolefin. Some of these newer container types no longer require an overwrap as a moisture barrier, which can reduce the amount of plastic waste and environmental consideration.

Published and available container-compatibility and stability studies in these newest types of containers are not yet available for all of the medications that had previously been studied in PVC. Those studies that have been conducted are designed to demonstrate drug compatibility with the newer containers when PVC adsorption and/or DEHP leaching was an issue with the PVC.[29]

Syringes. Plastic syringes have been increasingly used as the primary drug delivery system for alternate site use. This growth is due to several factors, including an increased awareness and acceptance of administering a number of different medications by the IV push route when it is clinically appropriate. Practitioners should consult the product literature and other references to determine when it is safe to administer medications without the use of a rate controlling device.

Mechanical or electronic syringe pumps are used when the rate must be safely controlled or when a medication is given over long intervals for therapeutic reasons. Special consideration should be given to the method of packing drug-filled syringes to ensure that they do not leak,

Table 4. Manufacturer Storage of Commercial IV Solutions after Removal from Protective Overwrap[d]

Brand Name (Manufacturer)	Volume	Maximum Storage Time (room temperature only)
LifeCare™[a] and ADD-Vantage®[a] PVC Containers (HSP)	25 mL >25 mL	21 d 30 d
Viaflex™[b] PVC and AVIVA™ Containers (BA)	≤50 mL ≥100 mL	15 d 30 d
Mini-Bag Plus™[c] (BA)	50 mL 100 mL	15 d 30 d

[a]Manufacturer letter. Hospira, Inc., Medical Communications Department. April 2008.
[b]Manufacturer letter. Baxter Healthcare Corporation IV Systems Delivery. June 2012.
[c]Manufacturer letter. Baxter Healthcare Corporation, Medication Delivery. August 2006.
[d]Intact overwrap retards water loss across container wall.

NOTE: Consult product labeling for all commercial premixed and frozen medications for recommended storage times and conditions after removal of protective overwrap.

that the plungers are not accidentally pushed in, and that the plungers and other clean parts of the syringe do not come in contact with potential contaminants. Further, clinical staff and patients/caregivers must be made aware that only the interior contents of a syringe (barrel, capped hub) should be considered sterile once a syringe is filled and capped during aseptic filling processes.

Commercially prepared solutions. Always consult the most current package labeling for stability dating of commercially available premixed solutions. Labeled frozen and post-thaw stability data for each premixed drug apply only to that specific commercial product. Practitioners must not extrapolate stability data from premixed commercial preparations of drugs in solution to extemporaneously compounded preparations.

Elastomeric reservoirs. Elastomeric reservoirs are nonelectric, single-use medical devices that deliver their contents at a controlled rate. They consist of a balloon-like central container that exhibits pressure when filled, and the rate of flow is controlled by the size of a restrictor on the tubing. Each brand of elastomeric device is made of unique and proprietary materials. This precludes the extrapolation of drug stability from one brand of these device containers to another.

The manufacturers of most elastomeric reservoirs publish guidelines on the stability of drugs in these devices. Some device manufacturer guidelines cite data for selected agents extrapolated from other container studies or resources. In addition, not all of the references specify original stability studies in a given device. Practitioners should consult the most current guide for the specific brand of elastomeric device when determining the stability dating for a given agent. The contributors to this publication reviewed the manufacturers' guidelines and incorporated their data, but the contributors did not review the unpublished stability studies cited in guidelines and resources provided by the device manufacturers.

Factors affecting the accuracy of elastomeric flow rate are reviewed in detail elsewhere. They include temperature during administration, viscosity of the solution, atmospheric pressure, back pressure (affected by position relative to infusion site), partial filling, and temperature during storage.[30] Elastomeric devices have applications for many ambulatory and home infusion therapies, including intermittent dosing of anti-infective agents, continuous chemotherapy, and patient-controlled pain management. Each type of application requires a different type of elastomeric device; these are available with different specific flow rates, total volume, and bolus abilities. Practitioners should pay particular attention to the model and type of device to ensure the correct dose and rate of infusion is administered.

Other specialty devices. The medication delivery device market has responded to compatibility, stability, and beyond-use dating challenges with several innovative devices:

- **Multi-chambered bags.** One relatively new type of container system is the multi-chambered device. The AutoDose™ drug delivery system consists of a multi-chambered EVA bag with a preattached administration set and flow restrictors integral to the tubing; this allows drugs to be delivered at specific rates. The chambered bag contains the drug in saline, two chambers of saline flush, and one chamber with heparin flush, if applicable. The bag is inserted into a specific nonelectric device that is powered by the latent energy contained in a spring. This latest development is focused on minimizing patient and caregiver manipulation of the line, as well as simplifying the time and education regarding the catheter flush process.[19]
- **Dual-chambered bags.** Dual-chambered bags are designed for total parenteral nutrition (TPN) solutions. The provider prepares the amino acid, dextrose, and electrolyte solution in one chamber and places the fat emulsion in the second chamber. These chambers are separated by a removable divider. The bag is designed for separate storage of the lipid emulsion and amino acid/dextrose solution until just before the start of administration. A complete three-in-one admixture results from removing a rod that keeps the chambers separated until this point. Several brands of PVC and EVA dual-chambered bags are available.
- **Drug-bag delivery systems.** The Duplex® system is another type of dual-chambered bag. The system is stable at room temperature until the ready-to-mix drug is reconstituted with the diluent in the second chamber. This type of system is increasingly used in hospitals with automated dispensing systems (ADS), since it can be stored in the ADS cabinet until time of administration. The closed system drug activation bypasses all compounding processes.
- **Vial-bag connectors.** Several types of specialized devices and bags allow for the connection of a vial of medication to a small volume infusion container. Generally, the connection of the vial to the bag is made under aseptic conditions. The actual mixing of the medication with the IV fluid takes place immediately prior to administration. Patients and caregivers are trained to ensure that complete reconstitution, when applicable, and mixing takes place before administration. The most common application of these systems is with very short stability medications. The pharmacy must consider the specific device manufacturer's guidelines when setting policy on the storage of connected, but not activated, devices. Most recommendations are for 30 days or less. The update to USP Chapter <797> states that "storage and beyond-use times for attached and activated (where activated is defined as allowing contact of the previously separate diluent and drug contents) container pairs of drug products...shall be applied as indicated by the manufacturer."[7]
- **Ambulatory infusion systems.** The technology of ambulatory infusion devices continues to evolve. A number of electronic and mechanical devices are available on the market today.[20–22,31] Some providers standardize selection to one brand of device, which then allows for standardized training staff, patients, and caregivers.[32] When this selection includes multi-functional devices that have several programs (e.g., PCA, intermittent, continuous, and TPN ramping), then the programming and patient/caregiver education must ensure that the proper program is used for the therapy in question.
- **Implanted infusion devices.** These specialized devices are limited volume reservoirs that are implanted intradermally. They are filled with special needles similar to the process for accessing implanted ports, and their use is primarily for intraspinal pain management, spas-

ticity management, and other neurological conditions. The microinfusions must be prepared without preservatives due to their potential neurological toxicity. Since these medications will be stored at body temperature for extended periods in these reservoirs, practitioners should be especially mindful of the stability, sterility, and potential for endotoxin or other adulteration of these preparations when developing procedures for their preparation, quality assurance, dispensing, and administration.

External Factors Affecting Stability

Circumstances beyond the direct control of the pharmacy that may affect the medication's potency and stability include the following[6]:

- Available method of delivery (e.g., common carrier, courier, or a pharmacy-controlled delivery process)
- Availability of a functioning, clean refrigerator in the home or alternate care site
- Ambient temperature in the care setting, especially non–air-conditioned residences in hot weather
- The need for patients/caregivers to manipulate sterile products, sets, and other devices
- Patient and caregiver adherence to labeled storage instructions of compounded preparations

Drug Delivery Process and Control

The drug delivery and storage conditions are generally not easily controlled by the pharmacy. However, pharmacists can take a number of constructive steps to ensure that proper temperature and light protection conditions are met. The delivery process (including containers, insulating and packing materials, courier, and environmental conditions) should be validated to ensure that the contents of the shipment are maintained at a temperature within established stability parameters.[23] The pharmacy should be aware of storage and shipping limitations and should take extra precautions for extreme temperatures (summer heat, winter freezing temperatures) to ensure that preparation stability is not affected during shipping.

Patient/Caregiver Storage and Administration

The variation and fluctuation of temperatures in noncommercial home refrigerators can be a major uncontrolled factor in drug stability. Many providers have established the practice of providing reliable refrigerator thermometers and teaching the patients or caregivers to monitor these temperatures. This is particularly important when there is only one in-home refrigerator for a number of residents. Some medications and parenteral solutions are particularly sensitive to temperature fluctuations. Pharmacists should be aware of the in-home situation, should ensure that the patient or caregiver education addresses proper drug storage and handling, and should closely monitor the status of temperature control when critical stability issues are identified.

Practitioners should carefully consider specific patient circumstances and needs prior to dispensing frozen preparations. Considerations should include an assessment of freezer capabilities at the pharmacy and the patient's home or care facility. Freezer temperatures should be monitored to ensure that conditions match those reflected in the stability study or reference.

When preparation stability data are based on light-protected conditions, then the drug storage and administration conditions should incorporate light protection. Some ambulatory infusion device reservoirs and elastomeric devices are made of light-protective plastics. In the absence of these devices, several methods of light protection can be employed, including UV-blocking overwrap plastic coverings or aluminum foil wraps. The pharmacist should ensure that the overwrap and the medication container are properly labeled, just in case the overwrap is accidentally removed. A double-label system (labeling both the container and the overwrap) can help ensure that the drug will be both stored and used properly.

Patient/Caregiver Education

Pharmacists should always ensure that patients and caregivers know what to do with their medications, equipment, and supplies. The written instructions and labeling, coupled with oral reinforcement, should address proper drug storage, handling, administration, disposal, and any relevant precautions or issues to watch for and report to the pharmacist. This written and oral patient education provided by the pharmacist should be consistent with in-home instruction provided by home care nurses. Interdisciplinary (and often interorganizational) collaboration is essential to effective and accurate patient and caregiver education.

Ethanol and Antibiotic Locks

Ethanol lock therapy (ELT) and antibiotic locks (ABL) are increasingly used to prevent or manage catheter related blood stream infections.[33,34] Practitioners must consider the available stability data[35] as well as catheter compatibility information when determining a concentration and dwell time for these specialized forms of access device care. Additional research on ABL and ET stability and therapeutic efficacy continues.[36,37]

Summary

Practitioners involved in parenteral therapy (including nurses, pharmacists, and physicians) must be aware of the factors affecting the application of stability data to patient care. In addition to published stability data, practitioners must consider the type of container, intravascular infusion method, medication delivery and storage conditions, patient or caregiver abilities, as well as the quality assurance, methods, and environment for sterile compounding before establishing an appropriate beyond-use date to the CSP.

References

1. Kastango ES. The cost of quality in pharmacy. *Int J Pharm Compound.* 2002; 6(6):404–7.

2. Trissel LA. ASHP's Interactive Handbook on Injectable Drugs, 16th ed. Bethesda, MD: American Society of Health-System Pharmacists; 2011. Accessed 5/18/12.

3. Bing CM. Chapter 10: Storage and beyond-use dating. In: Buchanan EC, Schneider PJ. *Compounding Sterile Preparations.* 3rd edition. Bethesda, MD: American Society of Health-System Pharmacists; 2009.

4. Lima HA. Drug stability and compatibility: special considerations for home care. *Infusion.* 1996; 2(Aug):11–6.

5. United States Pharmacopeia (USP). Chapter <1206> *Sterile Drug Products for Home Use. USP 24– NF 19.* Rockville, MD: USP Convention Inc; 1999:2130–43.

6. United States Pharmacopeia (USP). *U.S. Pharmacopeia 28.* Chapter <797> *Pharmaceutical Compounding—Sterile Preparations.* Rockville, MD: U.S. Pharmacopeial Convention Inc; 2004:2461– 77.

7. United States Pharmacopeial Convention. Revised General Chapter <797> *Pharmaceutical compounding–Sterile Preparations.* Available at: http://www.usp.org/pdf/EN/USPNF/ generalChapter797.pdf. Accessed December 31, 2007.

8. American Society of Health-System Pharmacists (ASHP). ASHP guidelines on minimum standards for home care pharmacies. *Am J Health-Syst Pharm.* 1999; 56:629–38.

9. American Society of Health-System Pharmacists (ASHP). ASHP guidelines on quality assurance for pharmacy-prepared sterile products. *Am J Health-Syst Pharm.* 2000; 57:1150–69.

10. U.S. Food and Drug Administration. Food and drug administration modernization act of 1997, §127. Application of federal law to practice of pharmacy compounding. Pub L No. 105–115, 111 Stat. 2296. Available at: http://www.fda.gov/Drugs/GuidanceComplianceRegulatoryInformation/PharmacyCompounding/. Accessed 5/18/12.

11. U.S. Food and Drug Administration. Compliance policy guidance for FDA staff and industry. Chapter 4, Subchapter 460, Section 460.200 Pharmacy Compounding. Reissued 5/29/02. Available at: http://www.fda.gov/ICECI/ComplianceManuals/CompliancePolicyGuidanceManual/ucm074398.htm. Accessed 5/18/12.

12. Phelps J, Hak EB, Crill CM, eds. *Pediatric Injectable Drugs.* 9th edition. Bethesda, MD: American Society of Health-System Pharmacists; 2010.

13. Buchanan EC. Sterile preparation formulation. In: Buchanan EC, Schneider PJ. *Compounding Sterile Preparations.* 3rd edition. Bethesda, MD: American Society of Health-System Pharmacists; 2009:19–32.

14. Siegel F. Tonicity, osmoticity, osmolality, and osmolarity. In: *Remington's Pharmaceutical Sciences.* 18th ed. Easton, PA: Mack Publishing; 1990:1484.

15. Kuban PK. Labeling sterile preparations. In: Buchanan EC, Schneider PJ. *Compounding Sterile Preparations.* 3rd edition. Bethesda, MD: American Society of Health-System Pharmacists; 2009:129–42.

16. Poole SM, Nowobilski-Vasilios A. To push or not to push. *Infusion.* 1999; 5(9):52–5.

17. U.S. Food and Drug Administration. Safety assessment of Di(2-ethylhexyl) phthalate (DEHP) released from PVC medical devices. Available at: www.fda.gov/downloads/MedicalDevices/DeviceRegulationandGuidance/GuidanceDocuments/UCM080457.pdf. Accessed 12/16/12.

18. Barrell Counce J. DEHP in medical devices: sleeping tiger or paper tiger? *Infusion.* 2002(Sept–Oct); 8(5):18–25.

19. Closson T, Holmes H, McCoy L. Using new technology to reduce antibiotic therapy costs: a case study. *Infusion.* 2002; 8(1):18–25.

20. Saladow J. History in the making: healthcare delivery and pump technology continue to evolve. *Infusion.* 1999; 5(9):15–51.

21. Saladow J. Infusion device technologies: consolidation and change. *Infusion.* 2000; 6(8):9–39.

22. Saladow J. Delivery device update. *Infusion.* 2002; 8(5):32–5.

23. Chamallas SN, Fishwick JJ, Riesenberg M. Special delivery: keeping the product stable during shipping. *Infusion.* 1997(Dec); 4(3):30–2.

24. FDA Public Health Notification: PVC Devices Containing the Plasticizer DEHP. July 12, 2002

25. Center for the Evaluation of Risks to Human Reproduction (National Toxicology Program, US Department of Health and Human Services). NTP-CERHR Monograph on the Potential Human Reproductive and Developmental Effects of Di(2-Ethylhexyl) Phthalate (DEHP). NIH Publication No. 06-4476, November 2006.

26. Kastango ES. *The ASHP Discussion Guide for Compounding Sterile Preparations. Summary and Implementation of USP Chapter <797>.* Bethesda, MD: American Society of Health-System Pharmacists. http://www.ashp.org/s_ashp/docs/files/HACC_797guide.pdf. Accessed 5/18/12.

27. Alexander M. ed. Infusion Nursing Society standards of practice. *J Inf Nursing.* 2011:34(1S), S1–S110.

28. Task Force for the Revision of Safe Practices for Parenteral Nutrition. Safe practices for parenteral nutrition. *J Parenter Enteral Nutr.* 2004; 28(6):S39–S70.

29. Trissel LA, Xu QA, Baker M. Drug compatibility with new polyolefin infusion solution containers. *Am J Health-Syst Pharm.* 2006; 63:2379–82.

30. Skryabina EA, Dunn TA. Disposable infusion pumps. *Am J Health-Syst Pharm.* 2006; 63:1260–8.

31. Saladow J. Ambulatory infusion technologies: new developments and how they might affect alternate site care. *Infusion.* 2007; 13(4):17–22.

32. Saladow J, Prosser B. Improving the continuity of care: New infusion pump technologies. *Home infusion continuum.* 2007; 1(1):1, 8–11.

33. Bing CM, Ross KL. Antibiotic and ethanol lock therapy. *Home infusion continuum.* 2008; 1(2):1, 10–11.

34. Bestul MB, VandenBussche HL. Antibiotic lock technique: Review of the literature. *Pharmacotherapy.* 2005; 25(2):211–27.

35. Cober MP, Johnson CE. Stability of 70% alcohol solutions in polypropylene syringes for use in ethanol-lock therapy. *Am J Health-Syst Pharm.* 2007; 64:2480–2.

36. Patel D, Bing C, Goebel M, et al. Evaluating the outcomes of antibiotic lock therapy: results from a national home infusion provider. Poster presentation. National Home Infusion Association. Orlando; April 2011.

37. Ustaszewski L, Bing C, Kunzendorf C, et al. Ethanol lock therapy: patient outcomes in home infusion. Poster presentation. National Home Infusion Association. Orlando, FL; April 2011. Encore poster at Infectious Diseases Society of America. Boston, MA; October 2011.

38. *NHIA CVAD Guidelines for the Adult Home-Based Patient,* rev 6-25-2011. http://www.nhia.org/CVADGuidelines/NHIAAdultVADGuidelinesV6.pdf. Accessed 12/10/11.

Beyond-Use Dating of Parenteral Nutrition Formulations

Diane Nitzki-George, Barbara Limburg-Mancini

Parenteral nutrition (PN) is one of the most complex admixtures prepared by a pharmacy. Safety, stability, and compatibility issues should always be evaluated prior to mixing. When mixed incorrectly, calcium may form an insoluble precipitate with phosphate that can be fatal; and a cracked lipid emulsion with its free oil should never be administered to a patient. Although caregivers are instructed to inspect the bag for signs of precipitation or creamed/cracked lipids, the pharmacist is ultimately responsible for determining the stability of additives and assigning a beyond-use date. Often those decisions are based more on experience than on published stability.

Published stability on PN admixtures applies only to the test formula and conditions reported. Pharmacists are expected to extrapolate the results and apply them to different product brands and different additive concentrations. Decision-making about PN stability is based on known causes of instability, in conjunction with the upper and lower limits of tested stability, instead of knowing that a specific formulation is stable. The pharmacist should be aware that a similar formula is stable and that there are no known factors that will cause instability. This approach is associated with a degree of risk, but has been used for years.

The American Society for Parenteral and Enteral Nutrition (ASPEN) has recognized that not all products used in the preparation of PN are equivalent, and brand substitution of the amino acids, lipid emulsion, vitamins, and trace elements should not be done. Either the product formulation will affect admixture stability or the product composition will affect clinical outcome. As such, these PN additives should always be labeled by brand name. Furthermore, assumptions regarding stability should be made relative to the product differences. For example, the major stability related difference between amino acids is the pH, so stability and beyond-use dating relative to additives affected by pH (i.e., calcium phosphate solubility, lipid emulsion stability) should be brand specific.

Before making a decision about the stability or beyond-use date of PN, each pharmacist should evaluate the degree of risk they are willing to assume. Below are several questions to think about when evaluating stability risk:

- Will the nutrient lose potency through degradation?
- What are the possible degradation mechanisms?
- Will a toxic degradation product or precipitate be formed?
- Will the nutrient bind or complex with another additive or the container, and is it reversible?
- Will the nutrient cause erosion or extraction of the container or set?
- What are the professional, regulatory, and practice requirements?

The discussion and tables in this chapter are intended to assist the pharmacist with his or her evaluation of the answers to these and other questions for appropriate decision making.

Non-Formulation Factors Affecting PN Stability

There are several factors, besides the PN formulation that will affect stability. These factors are managed through product selection as well as techniques in handling and storage **(Table 1)**. Different PN formulas have different stability concerns requiring that pharmacists have knowledge about product characteristics and handling techniques.

NOTE: The beyond-use date used by another pharmacy is specific to their products, techniques, and policies that may not apply to all practices.

Table 1. Factors Affecting PN Stability

Handling

Light

- Light is a catalyst to the oxidation of several PN additives, especially vitamins[1]
- Light can affect the stability of most parenteral vitamins within 24 h, resulting in peroxide generation[2]
- Significant loss of vitamins A, C, and riboflavin (B2) occur over 48 h when PN and Total Nutrient Admixtures (TNAs) are exposed to phototherapy light[3]
- Many pharmacy refrigerators have glass doors that permit PN exposure to light during storage and can affect stability

Oxygen

- Most of the amino acids and vitamins added to PN will degrade in the presence of oxygen[4]
- During the amino acids manufacturing process, oxygen is replaced by nitrogen to ensure stability of a product through the expiration date[5]
- Not only is oxygen introduced during the compounding process, but it can also migrate through most plastic containers
- Light, heat, and trace elements can catalyze oxygen degradation[6]
- Oxygen can also affect the triglycerides in a lipid emulsion, forming peroxides that have been reported to cause harm in neonates[7]
- The process of transferring lipid emulsions to a plastic syringe or making a TNA is enough to introduce oxygen and begin the cascade of changes that lead to peroxide formation[8]

Temperature

- Dextrose degrades when autoclaved[9]
- Calcium phosphate is more likely to precipitate when the temperature is high[10]
- The integrity of a lipid emulsion is maintained longer when stored at lower temperatures, but not below freezing[11]

Products

Container

- None of the plastic containers available for compounding PN in the United States is considered an oxygen barrier and all are subject to oxygen migration through the plastic[12]
- Extraction of plasticizer from polyvinyl chloride (PVC) containers is a concern with lipid emulsions[13]
- Adsorption of drug to the container surface is a concern with vitamin A[14]
- Vitamin A stability appears to vary by the type of plastic container[15]
- Vitamin A in PVC for 21 d showed no loss of potency[16]

pH

- Vitamin C stability is improved with lower pH (i.e., pH 5.5 compared to pH 6.5), while thiamine stability is maintained best at pH 6.5[3]
- Calcium phosphate is more soluble at lower pH when equilibrium favors the monobasic form[10]
- Lipid emulsions display less evidence of instability when the admixture pH is greater than 5.5[17]
- The pH of the amino acid product is used to estimate the overall admixture pH since amino acids are strong buffers[18]

Table 1. Factors Affecting PN Stability *(continued)*

Sulfites

- Concentrations of sodium bisulfite greater than 2 mEq/L have been shown to negatively impact the stability of vitamin A and thiamine[3]
- Tryptophan, used in powder form by some pharmacies to make an amino acid solution, loses 20% potency over 4 h if mixed with sodium bisulfite. If protected from light, then only 4% is lost when stored at room temperature for 6 months[19]

Amino Acids

- The rate of amino acid conversion to Maillard products (non-enzymatic browning) is significantly increased after admixture when stored for 30 d at 4°C; the presence of electrolytes and storage at higher temperatures facilitates the formation of these degradants[20]
- Amino acid solutions can form highly colored degradants that are not reliable indicators of the solution potency or the degree of decomposition[21]

Lipids

- Lipid emulsions display less evidence of instability when the admixture pH is greater than 5.5[17]

Vitamin C (ascorbic acid)

- Ascorbic acid, when oxidized, can degrade to oxalic acid, which can form a precipitate when mixed with calcium[22]; ascorbic acid oxidation is catalyzed by the presence of trace elements[23]

Handling Tips

Several techniques that have been reported to minimize the impact of handling on PN stability are as follows:

- Add multivitamins immediately prior to infusion.
- Store PN under refrigeration to prolong stability.
- Remove air from the PN bag after mixing.
- Limit the lipid emulsion hang time on a compounder to 4 hours.
- Protect PN bags from light, especially if refrigerator has glass doors.[104]
- Vacuum-seal PN in a foil overpouch for prolonged storage.

Product Tips

Keep in mind the product features and information that may impact PN stability as follows:

- Know the pH of the amino acids product.
- Use amino acid-specific calcium phosphate solubility curves that correspond to the final PN concentration.
- Lipid emulsion stability in total nutrient admixture (TNA) should be based on the specific amino acid product used in testing and the final concentration of macro- and micronutrients.
- Ensure that the types of plastic containers used for compounding are appropriate for the PN formulation.
- In addition to the PN formulation, assign beyond-use dates relative to the container type, amino acids pH, light/oxygen exposure, and presence of sulfites.

Formulation Factors Affecting PN Stability

The basic components of a PN formula, including amino acids, dextrose, and electrolytes, appear to be stable for 2 weeks or longer. **Table 2** includes a summary of published studies. These studies set an upper limit for beyond-use dating that should not be exceeded without additional testing. However, the upper limit should not be assumed for all formulas. Exceptions related to product formulation factors are explained below.

Table 2. Summary of Published Studies on Basic PN Stability

Formulation	Conc.	Storage Time	Storage Temp.[a]	Container	Comments/Reference
Amino acids Dextrose Sodium/Potassium Magnesium Calcium phosphate Multiple vitamins Trace elements	Unspec.	Stable 28 d	Ref	PVC	No significant change in the concentration of amino acids, dextrose, sodium, potassium, calcium, phosphate, magnesium, and trace elements (European products) was seen (data not shown)[24]
Amino acids (FreAmine®) Dextrose Sodium chloride Sodium bisulfite	4.25% 25% 10 mEq/L <0.1%	Stable 12 w	Ref (4°C)	Glass	Samples stored at room temperature and 37°C showed more rapid deterioration of amino acids[21]
Amino acids (FreAmine®) Dextrose	4.25% 25%	Stable 14 d	Ref or RT	Glass	No additives. Tryptophan was the least stable amino acid[25]

[a]RT—room temperature, Ref—refrigeration.

Lipid Emulsions

TNAs combine lipid emulsion with amino acids, dextrose, and micronutrients in a single bag. The concept of TNA, first reported in the literature in the mid-1980s, has become a standard of practice in home care and in many hospital and long-term care settings.[26] Home care patients or caregivers are instructed to inject limited stability additives, such as multivitamins, immediately prior to administration. They are then able to infuse the TNA in the same manner they would other intravenous admixtures.

Parenteral lipid emulsions are small droplets of oil encapsulated by a phospholipid bilayer that is suspended in the aqueous emulsion phase. These droplets, also called globules or particles, are considered a liquid precipitate. Clinical concerns arise when either free oil is liberated, due to a cracked emulsion, or when the droplets become clumped, flocculated, or enlarged as evidenced by creaming. Since lipid emulsions, by definition, are thermodynamically unstable, all emulsions are expected to demonstrate some degree of instability over time.[27] It may take as long as 3 days for an unstable emulsion to become visually evident.[28] Lipid emulsions with more than 0.4% of droplets greater than 5 microns in diameter are considered unstable.[29] Knowing this, the pharmacist's approach to lipid emulsion stability in TNA is based primarily on known factors that will destabilize the emulsion.

The literature contains TNA studies that report stability of lipid emulsion ranging from 24 hours to 6 weeks.[17,30–38] The key to interpreting the literature is to understand the factors in the following discussion that are known to affect lipid emulsions stability.

pH

Lipid emulsions are formulated at a pH of 6–8.[39,40] Evidence of emulsion instability occurs when admixture pH is less than 5.5.[17] Since amino acid pH is used to estimate that for the overall PN, the amino acid product and concentration is critical to emulsion stability following admixture.[18] Amino acid products with pH of 5.5 or lower should not be used to compound TNA.

Dextrose Concentration

Dextrose concentrations higher than 10% are needed to prevent phase separation and creaming of lipids.[41] Dextrose concentrations of 15% (with Aminosyn II®, Liposyn II®) resulted in greater change in the lipid emulsion droplet size compared to TNA with 30% dextrose final concentrations.[38]

Divalent/Trivalent Cations

Concentrations of divalent cations (calcium or magnesium) higher than 20 mEq/liter can destabilize lipid emulsions.[42] Sodium chloride produces very little change in the surface charge (i.e., zeta potential) of a lipid emulsion (Intralipid®).[42] Trivalent cations are more disruptive to lipid emulsions than divalent cations, which are more disruptive than monovalent cations. In the late 1980s, the following formula was developed to estimate the instability of lipid emulsion based on the total cation load: (1 mono-) + (64 di-) + (729 tri-) = total load expressed as monovalent. This means that 64 mEq sodium, a monovalent cation, is as disruptive to a lipid emulsion as 1 mEq magnesium, a divalent cation.[43] The ratio of monovalent, divalent, and trivalent cations is a practical approach for use by a compounding pharmacy.[41] When applying this concept in practice, it would be difficult to destabilize a lipid emulsion using clinically appropriate doses of monovalent cations. However, trivalent cations, such as iron, can destabilize lipid emulsion even at low doses.[29] Standard doses of trace elements, many of which are divalent or trivalent cations, are low enough not to destabilize a lipid emulsion.

Temperature

Refrigerated storage maintains the integrity of lipid emulsions better than storage at room temperature.[17] Either autoclaving or freezing lipid emulsions will cause premature destabilization.[44]

Heparin

Lipid emulsion in the presence of calcium (~14.4 mEq/L) and heparin appears to undergo a phase shift toward unstable. Theoretically, calcium binds with both the lipid emulsion and heparin, forming a bridge (calcium-heparin bridging) that causes lipid emulsions to appear creamed.[45,46]

Calcium Phosphate Solubility

Pharmacists routinely screen PN formulas for calcium phosphate solubility using curves and tables found in other references.[47] Although the curves were generated based on limited data, they have been validated in clinical practice.[108] The data are typically generated over 24 or 48 hours and do not represent extended storage. The concentrations of calcium, phosphate, and amino acid as well as the calcium salt form and amino acid pH are the primary determinants of solubility,[10] although amino acids are the critical component.[105] High temperatures decrease calcium phosphate solubility while the presence of lipid emulsion does not appear to affect the solubility.

Fansel et al. studied calcium phosphate solubility over 14 days and found a significant decrease in the calcium concentration, presumably due to precipitation, and a decrease in pH suggesting that it takes several days for equilibrium to be reached in the admixture.[48] This information and the lack of long-term calcium phosphate solubility studies invalidates the typical screening done by pharmacists when beyond-use dates are assigned. The change in calcium phosphate solubility over time highlights the need for in-line filters when assigning beyond-use dates. The lower total volume of PN in neonates, infants, and pediatric patients presents additional stability challenges; the separate administration of lipids or use of a dual chamber bag helps the practitioner and/or caregiver to visualize calcium phosphate gross precipitation that would be masked in a TNA. However, visual inspection of PN, even without lipids, is not a reliable method to detect precipitation. The human eye is able to see particles as small as 50 microns, while particles as small as 5 microns may be associated with harm.[109]

Outside of the United States, organic phosphates are used to minimize the risk of phosphate precipitate with calcium. PN formulations containing 1.1 mEq/100 mL of sodium glycerophosphate, an organic phosphate, do not precipitate when mixed with concentrations of calcium gluconate as high as 1000 mg/100 mL (4.64 mEq/100 mL) when stored for 7 days.[110] While organic phosphate and organic calcium products are not currently available in the United States, pharmacists should be careful not to establish beyond-use dates based on the wrong form of phosphate.

Vitamins

Temperature, light, container type, and the presence of lipid emulsion all affect the stability of vitamins. Individual vitamin stability ranges from a few hours to several days depending on the conditions. There is no single set of conditions in which all thirteen vitamins are stable. Unfortunately, many parenteral vitamins can only be found in combination products, and should be added to PN/TNA immediately prior to administration. A summary of stability studies on individual vitamins that may be supplemented to PN/TNA follows. The individual vitamin product stability tables are listed in alphabetical order.

Trace Elements and Other Minerals

There are several contradictions in the published literature related to the stability of trace elements and other minerals, primarily due to study design and uncontrolled variables. Amino acid products with cysteine, a sulfur containing amino acid, have been reported to form complexes with several minerals including selenium, copper, and iron. In some cases, the complexes have been reported to precipitate.[49] These events appear to be a function of the mineral concentration, admixture pH, and amino acid concentrations. It is unclear if complexed minerals are bioavailable after administration.

Lipid emulsions are easily destabilized by divalent and trivalent cations. The standard doses of trace elements are low enough to avoid instability. Iron dextran has been reported to destabilize lipid emulsion and should not be added to TNA.[50] A recent study found particulate matter in iron sucrose-containing PN when stored beyond 4 hours, despite the fact that iron sucrose remained chemically stable.[107] The published studies on trace elements and other minerals in PN/TNA are summarized at the end of this chapter.

Drugs and Other Additives

Albumin is not recommended for addition to PN admixtures for several reasons as follows[106]:

- Lack of test data
- Reports of color change when mixed with trace elements

- Risk of precipitation with amino acids
- Formulated with a pH in the range of 6.6–7.4, which may increase the pH of a PN resulting in calcium phosphate instability
- Potential glycosylation with dextrose
- May clog a 1.2 micron filter
- Large aluminum contamination

Published studies on the stability of other common additives to PN/TNA are summarized alphabetically at the end of this chapter.

Commercial Products and Extemporaneous Compounding

The effect of compounding methods on lipid emulsion stability in TNA (Aminosyn®, Liposyn®, dextrose, electrolytes, trace metals, vitamins in nonphalate PVC containers) was evaluated based on sequential or simultaneous mixing (using Nutrimix® compounder). After 3 days' storage, no difference was noted based on compounding method.[51] However, a separate study reported that TNA prepared using simultaneous pumping had a higher percentage of lipid particles larger than 5 microns compared to TNA prepared by sequential pumping.[38] This suggests that the order of mixing may affect lipid emulsion stability. Manufacturer recommendations should always be followed.

Ready-to-use PN products are commercially available but still require addition of multivitamins, trace elements, and possibly electrolytes. Although these products are formulated to remain stable through the product expiration date, assigning beyond-use dating should continue to follow the general PN information presented here unless instructed otherwise by the manufacturer.

Professional, Regulatory, and Accreditation Expectations and Guidance

ASPEN has developed several guidance documents related to PN. The most important for an IV admixture pharmacist is entitled *Safe Practices for Parenteral Nutrition*.[50] This guidance document highlights the type of medication error and adverse events that have occurred from PN. The guidance also recommends techniques the pharmacy can implement to reduce the risk of subsequent errors. The guidelines are separated into five different topics and identify specific practice recommendations for the following:

1. Labeling
2. Nutrient Requirements
3. Sterile Compounding
4. Stability and Compatibility
5. Administration

The ASPEN sterile compounding recommendations include 10 practice guidelines to ensure that the compounding process does not introduce incompatibility or instability, that in-process and end-product inspection and testing are used to confirm compounding accuracy, and that pharmacies adhere to the USP Chapter <797>, *Pharmaceutical Compounding—Sterile Preparations*. Additionally, there are seven practice guidelines to assist pharmacists with their approach to making decisions about PN stability and compatibility.

The complexity of PN preparation processes includes multiple manipulations, multiple sterile source component additives, and/or the use of automated compounding equipment. The *risk* for preparation error and/or contamination increases with this complexity. For most pharmacists, compounding PN is treated as a medium risk activity following USP Chapter <797> requirements, with maximum beyond-use dating not to exceed 9 days refrigerated.[52]

The Centers for Disease Control and Prevention (CDC), in their *Guidelines for the Prevention of Intravascular Catheter-Related Infections,* recommends that lipid emulsions should be infused for no longer than 12 hours when infused alone and no longer than 24 hours as a component of a TNA. Administration sets for lipids should be changed every 24 hours.[54]

USP Chapter <729> *Globule Size Distribution in Lipid Injectable Emulsions* contains methodology for manufacturers to determine the mean particle size in lipid emulsions. Since lipid globules larger than 5 microns can be trapped in the lung, USP Chapter <729> has set a limit for mean lipid globule at no greater than 5 microns. Additionally, the percent of globules larger than 5 microns, expressed as PFAT5, should not exceed 0.05%. Although most pharmacies will not be equipped to perform particle sizing of the lipids in their TNAs, an understanding of how the test procedures are performed will enable the pharmacist to better interpret the published literature.[52]

Accrediting bodies such as The Joint Commission (TJC) and the Accreditation Commission for Health Care (ACHC) do not have specific compounding standards for PN, although compliance with USP Chapter <797>, state law, OSHA regulations, and CDC guidelines is required.

Summary

PN and TNA formulas often combine over 20 different drug and nutrient products into a single container. Calcium phosphate solubility and lipid emulsion stability are the two most important concerns when evaluating PN formulations, but certainly not the only components with potential stability and compatibility issues. Amino acid products alone are formulated to contain about 15 different nutrients, and most multiple vitamin products contain 12 or 13 vitamins plus excipients. The possible permutations and commutations of different PN or TNA formulas are too numerous to test for stability and compatibility. Pharmacists must rely on a "matrix approach" to evaluate the stability and compatibility literature—ensuring that the specific formulations of PN or TNA fall within tested parameters for all of the components.

Carnitine *in Parenteral Nutrition*

Container	Stability	Concentration	Temperature			Light		Lipids		Reference
			Refrigerator	Room	Body	Exposed	Protected	With	Without	
Unknown[a]	Stable	130 mg/L 200 mg/L	30 d	24 h		X	X	X	X	53
Unknown[b]	Stable	60 to 420 mg/L		24 h					X	99

Notes

[a]30 d refrigerated followed by 24 h at room temperature; samples exposed to light when moved to room temperature; six different formulations; neither cysteine nor ranitidine influenced carnitine stability.

[b]PN included electrolytes, multivitamins, cysteine, heparin, and trace elements; individualized dose of 10 mg/kg/d.

Chromium *in Parenteral Nutrition*

Container	Stability	Temperature			Light		Lipids		Reference
		Refrigerator	Room	Body	Exposed	Protected	With	Without	
Glass[a]	Stable		48 h		X			X	73

Note

[a]Formulas included amino acids (Travasol®) alone or in TPN (no formula provided).

Parenteral Nutrition

EXTENDED STABILITY FOR PARENTERAL DRUGS

Cimetidine *in Parenteral Nutrition*

Container	Stability	Concentration	Temperature			Light		Lipids		Reference
			Refrigerator	Room	Body	Exposed	Protected	With	Without	
EVAa	Stable	80 mg/L	28 d						X	87
EVAb	Stable	400, 800 & 1200 mg/L		24 h		X		X		88
EVAc	Stable	450 mg/L		48 h		X		X	X	89
PVCd	Stable	579 mg/L		48 h			X		X	78
PVCe	Stable	300 mg/L	24 h	24 h					X	90

EVA—ethylene vinyl acetate; PVC—polyvinyl chloride.

Notes

aFormula: amino acids (FreAmine III®, Vamin 14®, Aminoplex 12®), dextrose, electrolytes, and trace elements (European products).

bFormula: amino acids (Travasol®), dextrose, lipid emulsion (Travamulsion®), electrolytes, vitamins, and trace elements; no destabilizing effect on lipid emulsion.

cFormula: amino acids (Travasol®), dextrose, lipid emulsion (+/−) (Liposyn II®, Intralipid®), electrolytes, vitamins, and trace elements; no affect on emulsion stability.

dFormula: amino acids (Travasol 8.5%®), dextrose, electrolytes, trace elements, and cimetidine.

eFormula: amino acids (Travasol®), dextrose, electrolytes, vitamins (+/−), trace elements (+/−) (Canadian products).

(+/−) indicates that sample was mixed both with and without the nutrient.

32

Parenteral Nutrition

Copper *in Parenteral Nutrition*

Container	Stability	Temperature			Light		Lipids		Reference
		Refrigerator	Room	Body	Exposed	Protected	With	Without	
Unspecified[a]	Unstable		2 h					X	74
Unspecified[b]	Stable		24 h					X	75
EVA[c]	Stable	28 d				X		X	49
Glass[d]	Stable		48 h		X			X	73
PP[e]	Unstable	30 d						X	76
PVC[f]	Stable	2 d				X		X	77
PVC[g]	Stable	48 h				X		X	78

EVA—ethylene vinyl acetate; PP—polypropylene; PVC—polyvinyl chloride.

Notes

[a]Formulas included cysteine containing amino acids (Novamine®), glucose, electrolytes, trace elements.

[b]Formulas included cysteine containing amino acids (TrophAmine®), dextrose, and electrolytes.

[c]Formulas: amino acids, glucose, calcium, vitamins, and trace elements (European products).

[d]Formulas included amino acids (Travasol®) alone or in TPN (no formula provided).

[e]Formulas: amino acids (Travasol®), dextrose, electrolytes, vitamins, trace elements (Canadian products).

[f]Formulas: amino acids, dextrose, electrolytes, and trace elements (+/−) (European products).

[g]Studied as copper sulfate. Formulas: amino acids (Travasol 8.5%®), dextrose, electrolytes, trace elements, and cimetidine.

(+/−) indicates that sample was mixed both with and without the nutrient.

Parenteral Nutrition

Famotidine *in Parenteral Nutrition*

Container	Stability	Concentration	Temperature			Light		Lipids		Reference
			Refrigerator	Room	Body	Exposed	Protected	With	Without	
Unspecified[a]	Stable	83, 166, & 250 mg/L		48 h		X			X	91
Unspecified[b]	Stable	20 mg/L		48 h		X	X	X		92
EVA[c]	Stable	20 & 50 mg/L	24 h	24 h				X		93
EVA[d]	Stable	20 mg/L		24 h		X		X		94
EVA[e]	Stable	20 & 40 mg/L	7 d	48 h		X			X	95
EVA[f]	Stable	20 mg/L		48 h		X		X	X	89
EVA[g]	Stable	20 & 40 mg/L		72 h		X		X		96
PVC[h]	Stable	20 mg/L	35 d				X		X	97

EVA—ethylene vinyl acetate; PVC—polyvinyl chloride.

Notes

[a]Formulas included amino acids (FreAmine III®), glucose, electrolytes, heparin, iron, and trace elements (Canadian products).[91]

[b]Tested in individual solutions of either amino acids, D5W, lipid emulsion (Intralipid®), or NS (European products).[92]

[c]Stability was 48 h total (24 h refrigerated followed by 24 h at room temp). Formula: amino acids (FreAmine III®), dextrose, lipid emulsion (Intralipid 20%®), electrolytes, and trace elements; no impact on emulsion stability.[93]

[d]Formula: amino acids (Novamine®), dextrose, lipid emulsion, electrolytes, vitamins, and trace elements.[94]

[e]Formula: amino acids (FreAmine III®), dextrose, electrolytes, vitamins, heparin, trace elements.[95]

[f]Formula: amino acids (Travasol®), dextrose, lipid emulsion (+/−) (Liposyn II®, Intralipid®), electrolytes, vitamins, and trace elements; no affect on emulsion stability.[89]

[g]Formula: amino acids, glucose, lipid emulsions, electrolytes, vitamins, and trace elements.[96]

[h]Formula: amino acids (Travasol®), dextrose, electrolytes, trace elements.[97]

(+/−) indicates that sample was mixed both with and without the nutrient.

Folic acid *in Parenteral Nutrition*

Container	Stability	Temperature			Light		Lipids		Reference
		Refrigerator	Room	Body	Exposed	Protected	With	Without	
PVCᵃ	Stable	48 h	48 h		X		X	X	56
EVAᵇ	Stable		24 h		X			X	57
Glassᵃ	Stable	48 h	48 h		X		X	X	56
Glassᶜ	Stable	48 h	48 h		X	X		X	58
Glassᵈ	Stable		24 h		X	X	X		59
PVCᵉ	Stable	2 w	2 w			X		X	60
PVCᶠ	Stable		24 h			X		X	23
Unspecifiedᵍ	Stable		8 h		X			X	55
Unspecifiedᵍ	Stable	7 w				X		X	55

EVA—ethylene vinyl acetate; PVC—polyvinyl chloride.

Notes

ᵃ*Formulas included amino acids (four different brands), sulfites (+/−), dextrose, lipid emulsion (+/−), electrolytes, vitamins, and trace elements.*

ᵇ*Formula included amino acids, glucose, electrolytes, vitamins, trace elements (European products).*

ᶜ*Formula included Aminosyn® and dextrose only.*

ᵈ*Admixture of only Intralipid® and multivitamins; stability defined as greater than 80% of initial concentration.*

ᵉ*The pH must remain above 5.0 to avoid precipitation of folic acid; formula: amino acids, dextrose, electrolyte, zinc sulfate, vitamins (European products).*

ᶠ*Formula: amino acids, dextrose, electrolytes, trace elements, MVI-12® (European products).*

ᵍ*Formula included amino acids, dextrose, electrolytes, vitamins (Multivitamin Concentrate®), trace elements.*

(+/−) indicates that sample was mixed both with and without the nutrient.

Parenteral Nutrition

Heparin *in Parenteral Nutrition*

Container	Stability	Concentration	Temperature			Light		Lipids		Reference
			Refrigerator	Room	Body	Exposed	Protected	With	Without	
PVC[a]	Stable	3,000, 5,000, 10,000, & 20,000 units/L	21 d						X	98

PVC—polyvinyl chloride.

Notes

[a]Formula: amino acids (+/−) (Travasol®), dextrose, electrolytes, trace elements; longer stability with amino acids included in formula.

(+/−) indicates that sample was mixed both with and without the nutrient.

Iron *in Parenteral Nutrition*

Container	Stability	Concentration	Temperature			Light		Lipids		Reference
			Refrigerator	Room	Body	Exposed	Protected	With	Without	
EVA[a]	Unstable	2 mg/L (dextran)		30 h				X		29
Unspecified[b]	Stable	100 mg/L (dextran)		18 h					X	79
EVA[c]	Unstable	50 mg/L (dextran)		24 h		X		X		80
Glass[d]	Stable	2 mg/L (dextran)	48 h	48 h				X		81
PP[e]	Unstable	10 mg/L (dextran)		12 h			X		X	82
Unspecified[f]	Unstable	1–100 mg/L (sucrose)		8 h					X	107

EVA—ethylene vinyl acetate; PP—polypropylene.

(continued)

Parenteral Nutrition

Iron *in Parenteral Nutrition* (continued)

Notes

[a]*Formulas included amino acids (Aminosyn II®), dextrose, lipid emulsion (Liposyn III®), and electrolytes; instability defined as disruption of emulsion stability.*

[b]*Formulas included amino acids (Travasol®), dextrose, electrolytes, vitamins (+/−), trace elements (+/−).*

[c]*Formulas: amino acids (Travasol®), dextrose, lipid emulsion (Intralipid®), electrolytes, vitamins, trace elements, cimetidine; loss of iron and destabilization of emulsion noted.*

[d]*Formulas included amino acids (Travasol®), dextrose, lipid emulsions (Intralipid®, Liposyn II®), electrolytes, and heparin.*

[e]*Formulas included <2% cysteine containing amino acids (TrophAmine®), dextrose, electrolytes, heparin, vitamins (+/−), and trace elements (+/−); samples with higher concentrations of amino acid were stable for 48 h.*

[f]*Formulas included amino acids (TrophAmine® 10%), dextrose, electrolytes, trace elements, multivitamins (MVI Pediatric®), cysteine (+/−), ranitidine (Zantac®) (+/−), carnitine (+/−).*

(+/−) indicates that sample was mixed both with and without the nutrient.

Manganese *in Parenteral Nutrition*

Container	Stability	Temperature			Light		Lipids		Reference
		Refrigerator	Room	Body	Exposed	Protected	With	Without	
Glass[a]	Stable		48 h		X			X	73
PP[b]	Unstable	30 d						X	76
PVC[c]	Stable	7 d				X		X	77

PP—polypropylene; PVC—polyvinyl chloride.

Notes

[a]*Formulas included amino acids (Travasol®) alone or in TPN (no formula provided).*

[b]*Formulas: amino acids (Travasol®), dextrose, electrolytes, vitamins, trace elements (Canadian products).*

[c]*Formulas: amino acids (+/−), dextrose (+/−), electrolytes (+/−), and trace elements (European products).*

(+/−) indicates that sample was mixed both with and without the nutrient.

Ranitidine *in Parenteral Nutrition*

Container	Stability	Concentration	Temperature			Light		Lipids		Reference
			Refrigerator	Room	Body	Exposed	Protected	With	Without	
Unspecified[a]	Stable	83, 166 & 250 mg/L		72 h					X	100
EVA[b]	Stable	50 & 100 mg/L		12 h		X		X		101
EVA[c]	Stable	75 mg/L		24 h		X		X	X	89
EVA[d]	Stable	50 & 100 mg/L	48 h	48 h		X	X	X	X	102
PVC[e]	Stable	50 & 100 mg/L		24 h		X			X	103

EVA—ethylene vinyl acetate; PVC—polyvinyl chloride.

Notes

[a]*Formula: amino acids (FreAmine III®), glucose, electrolytes, vitamins, trace elements, iron, heparin (Canadian products).*

[b]*Formula: amino acids, dextrose, lipid emulsion, electrolytes, vitamins, trace elements (European products); no destabilization of emulsion.*

[c]*Formula: amino acids (Travasol®), dextrose, lipid emulsion (+/−) (Liposyn II®, Intralipid®), electrolytes, vitamins, and trace elements; no affect on emulsion stability.*

[d]*Formula: amino acids (Travasol®), dextrose, lipid emulsion (+/−) (Intralipid®); longer stability when lipid added; no affect on emulsion stability.*

[e]*Formulas included amino acids (Travasol®), dextrose, electrolytes (+/−), vitamins (including K), trace elements, and heparin.*

(+/−) indicates that sample was mixed both with and without the nutrient.

Selenium *in Parenteral Nutrition*

Container	Stability	Temperature			Light		Lipids		Reference
		Refrigerator	Room	Body	Exposed	Protected	With	Without	
Unspecified[a]	Stable							X	84
Unspecified[b]	Unstable							X	85
Unspecified[c]	Stable							X	86
PP[d]	Stable	30 d	30 d					X	76
PVC[e]	Stable	10 w						X	72

PP—polypropylene; PVC—polyvinyl chloride.

Notes

[a]*24 h. Formulas: amino acids (Travasol®), dextrose, electrolytes, vitamins, and trace elements; results only apply to solutions with pH >4.75.*

[b]*30 min storage at an unspecified temperature. Formulas included cysteine containing amino acids (+/−), dextrose (+/−), electrolytes (+/−), ascorbic acid (+/−), and trace elements (+/−) (European products).*

[c]*Formulas: amino acids, dextrose, electrolytes, ascorbic acid, and trace elements (European products).*

[d]*Formulas: amino acids (Travasol®), dextrose, electrolytes, vitamins, and trace elements (Canadian products).*

[e]*Formulas: amino acids (Aminosyn®), dextrose, electrolytes, vitamins, trace elements, and iron (Canadian products).*

(+/−) indicates that sample was mixed both with and without the nutrient.

Trace Elements *in Parenteral Nutrition*

Container	Stability	Temperature			Light		Lipids		Reference
		Refrigerator	Room	Body	Exposed	Protected	With	Without	
PVC[a]	Stable		72 h					X	83

PVC—polyvinyl chloride.

Note

[a]*Formulas included amino acids, dextrose, electrolytes, and trace elements (European products); no precipitate was identified when normal concentrations were added, but several precipitates were identified with higher concentrations including iron, manganese, and copper phosphate and insoluble selenium (due to ascorbic acid).*

Parenteral Nutrition

Vitamin A *in Parenteral Nutrition*

Container	Stability	Temperature			Light		Lipids		Reference
		Refrigerator	Room	Body	Exposed	Protected	With	Without	
EVA[b]	Stable	24 h	24 h	24 h	X		X		62
EVA[c]	Unstable		6 h		X		X	X	63
EVA[d]	Stable	6 d	24 h		X	X[d]	X		64
EVA[k]	Stable	24 h	24 h	24 h	X		X		68
EVA, Glass, PVC[e]	Stable	20 d				X	X	X	65
Glass[f]	Stable	48 h	48 h		X		X		56
Glass[g]	Stable		24 h		X	X	X		59
PVC[h]	Stable	7 d	7 d				X	X	66
PVC[i]	Stable		8 h		X				24
PVC[i]	Stable	5 d	39 h			X			24
PVC[j]	Unstable		24 h		X			X	67
Unspecified[a]	Unstable		5 h			X			61

EVA—ethylene vinyl acetate; PVC—polyvinyl chloride.

(continued)

Vitamin A *in Parenteral Nutrition* (continued)

Notes

[a]Loss of potency attributed to tubing adsorption; samples tested as vitamins alone or plus TPN (formula not identified).[61]

[b]Formula: amino acids, glucose, lipid emulsion, electrolytes, vitamins, and trace elements (European products).[62]

[c]Formula: amino acids, glucose, lipid emulsion (+/−), electrolytes, and trace elements. (European products).[63]

[d]Retinyl palmitate. Formula: amino acids, glucose, lipid emulsion (Intralipid®), electrolytes, vitamins, and trace elements (European products); refrigerated samples were protected from light; stability defined as greater than 80% of initial concentration; room temperature storage followed 6 d refrigeration.[64]

[e]Formula: amino acids, glucose, lipid emulsion (+/−), electrolytes, MVI-12®, trace elements (+/−) (European products); stability defined as greater than 80% of initial concentration.[65]

[f]Formulas included amino acids (four different brands), sulfites (+/−), dextrose, lipid emulsion, electrolytes, vitamins, and trace elements; unstable if lipid not in formula or if stored in PVC plastic.[56]

[g]Retinol admixture of only Intralipid® and multivitamins; stability defined as greater than 80% of initial concentration.[59]

[h]Formula: amino acids (+/−), glucose (+/−), lipid emulsion (+/−), vitamins, trace elements (+/−); no electrolytes (European products).[66]

[i]Formulas included amino acids, glucose, electrolytes, and trace elements (European products); also stable 8 h at room temperature when exposed to light.[24]

[j]Formula: amino acid, dextrose, electrolytes, vitamins, and trace elements (Canadian products); in-line filtration did not affect stability.[67]

[k]Retinol formulas included amino acids, glucose, lipid emulsions (Liposyn 20%®, Intralipid 20%®, ClinOleic 20%®), electrolytes, vitamins, and trace elements; no change in emulsion stability over 4 d.[68]

(+/−) indicates that sample was mixed both with and without the nutrient.

Vitamin B1 *in Parenteral Nutrition*

Container	Stability	Temperature			Light		Lipids		Reference
		Refrigerator	Room	Body	Exposed	Protected	With	Without	
PVC, Glass[f]	Stable	48 h			X		X	X	56
Glass[e]	Stable		24 h		X	X	X		59
EVA[a]	Stable	96 h				X	X		64
EVA[b]	Stable		24 h		X			X	57
PVC[h]	Stable		22 h					X	69
PVC[d]	Stable	5 d	5 d		X	X		X	24
PVC, Glass[f]	Unstable		12 h		X		X	X	56
EVA[i]	Unstable	72 h	72 h	72 h	X		X		62
PVC[g]	Unstable		5 h					X	69
Unspecified[c]	Unstable		8 h		X			X	55
ML[j]	Stable	72 h	72 h		X	X		X	111

EVA—ethylene vinyl acetate; ML—multilayer; PVC—polyvinyl chloride.

Notes

[a]Form: thiamine. Formula: amino acids, glucose, lipid emulsion (Intralipid®), electrolytes, vitamins, and trace elements (European products); stability defined as greater than 80% of initial concentration. Room temp studied followed 6 d refrigerated.

[b]Form: thiamine hydrochloride. Formula: amino acids, glucose, electrolytes, vitamins, trace elements (European products).

[c]Form: thiamine. Formula: amino acids, dextrose, electrolytes, vitamins (Multivitamin Concentrate®), trace elements.

[d]Form: thiamine. Formulas included amino acids, glucose, electrolytes, and trace elements (European products).

[e]Form: thiamine. Admixture of only Intralipid® and multivitamins; stability defined as greater than 80% of initial concentration.

[f]Form: thiamine. Formulas included amino acids (Novamine®, Neopham®, FreAmine III®, Travasol®), sulfites (+/−), dextrose, lipid emulsion (Intralipid®) (+/−), electrolytes, vitamins (MVI 12®), and trace elements; thiamine is less stable in FreAmine III® (pH=6.5) than other amino acids; thiamine stability decreased at high pH and high sulfite content.

[g]Form: thiamine. Mixed in amino acids with sulfites (<0.05%) and no other additives.

[h]Form: thiamine. Amino acids with sulfites, dextrose, vitamins.

[i]Form: thiamine. Formula: amino acids, glucose, lipid emulsion, electrolytes, vitamins, and trace elements (European products).

[j]Formula: amino acids, dextrose, electrolytes, trace elements, pediatric multivitamins, high concentration calcium and organic phosphate (Brazilian products).

(+/−) indicates that sample was mixed both with and without the nutrient.

Parenteral Nutrition

Vitamin B2 *in Parenteral Nutrition*

Container	Stability	Temperature			Light		Lipids		Reference
		Refrigerator	Room	Body	Exposed	Protected	With	Without	
EVA[a]	Stable	6 d	24 h		X	X	X		64
EVA[b]	Unstable	24 h			X			X	57
Unspecified[c]	Unstable		4 h		X			X	55
PVC, Glass[d]	Stable	48 h	48 h		X		X	X	56
Glass[e]	Stable		24 h		X	X	X		59
ML[f]	Stable	72 h	72 h		X	X		X	111

EVA—ethylene vinyl acetate; ML—multilayer; PVC—polyvinyl chloride.

Notes

[a]*Form: riboflavin. Formula: amino acids, glucose, lipid emulsion (Intralipid®), electrolytes, vitamins, and trace elements (European products); stability defined as greater than 80% of initial concentration. Room temp studied followed 6 d refrigerated.*

[b]*Form: riboflavin 5 phosphate sodium. Formula: amino acids, glucose, electrolytes, vitamins, trace elements (European products).*

[c]*Form: riboflavin. Formula: amino acids, dextrose, electrolytes, vitamins (Multivitamin Concentrate®), trace elements.*

[d]*Form: riboflavin. Formulas included amino acids (four different brands), dextrose, lipid emulsion (+/−), electrolytes, vitamins, and trace elements.*

[e]*Form: riboflavin. Admixture of only Intralipid® and multivitamins; stability defined as greater than 80% of initial concentration.*

[f]*Formula: amino acids, dextrose, electrolytes, trace elements, pediatric multivitamins, high-concentration calcium and organic phosphate (Brazilian products).*

(+/−) indicates that sample was mixed both with and without the nutrient.

Parenteral Nutrition

Vitamin B3 *in Parenteral Nutrition*

Container	Stability	Temperature			Light		Lipids		Reference
		Refrigerator	Room	Body	Exposed	Protected	With	Without	
EVAª	Stable	96 h				X	X		64
EVAᵇ	Stable	24 h			X			X	57
Unspecifiedᶜ	Stable		8 h		X			X	55

EVA—ethylene vinyl acetate.

Notes

ªForm: nicotinamide. Formula: amino acids, glucose, lipid emulsion (Intralipid®), electrolytes, vitamins, and trace elements (European products); stability defined as greater than 80% of initial concentration.

ᵇForm: nicotinamide. Formula: amino acids, glucose, electrolytes, vitamins, trace elements (European products).

ᶜForm: niacinamide. Formula: amino acids, dextrose, electrolytes, vitamins (Multivitamin Concentrate®), trace elements.

Vitamin B5 *in Parenteral Nutrition*

Container	Stability	Temperature			Light		Lipids		Reference
		Refrigerator	Room	Body	Exposed	Protected	With	Without	
EVAª	Stable	96 h				X	X		64

EVA—ethylene vinyl acetate.

Note

ªForm: pantothenate. Formula: amino acids, glucose, lipid emulsion (Intralipid®), electrolytes, vitamins, and trace elements (European products); stability defined as greater than 80% of initial concentration.

Vitamin B6 *in Parenteral Nutrition*

Container	Stability	Temperature			Light		Lipids		Reference
		Refrigerator	Room	Body	Exposed	Protected	With	Without	
EVA[a]	Stable	96 h				X	X		64
EVA[b]	Stable	24 h			X			X	57
Unspecified[c]	Unstable		8 h		X			X	55
Glass[d]	Stable		24 h		X	X	X		59
ML[e]	Stable	72 h	72 h		X	X		X	111

EVA—ethylene vinyl acetate; ML—multilayer.

Notes

[a]*Form: pyridoxine. Formula: amino acids, glucose, lipid emulsion (Intralipid®), electrolytes, vitamins, and trace elements (European products); stability defined as greater than 80% of initial concentration. Room temp studied followed 6 d refrigerated.*

[b]*Form: pyridoxine hydrochloride. Formula: amino acids, glucose, electrolytes, vitamins, trace elements (European products).*

[c]*Form: pyridoxine. Formula: amino acids, dextrose, electrolytes, vitamins (Multivitamin Concentrate®), trace elements.*

[d]*Form: pyridoxine. Admixture of only Intralipid® and multivitamins; stability defined as greater than 80% of initial concentration.*

[e]*Formula: amino acids, dextrose, electrolytes, trace elements, pediatric multivitamins, high-concentration calcium and organic phosphate (Brazilian products).*

Vitamin B12 *in Parenteral Nutrition*

Container	Stability	Temperature			Light		Lipids		Reference
		Refrigerator	Room	Body	Exposed	Protected	With	Without	
EVA[a]	Stable	96 h				X	X		64

EVA—ethylene vinyl acetate.

Note

[a]*Form: cyanocobalamin. Formula: amino acids, glucose, lipid emulsion (Intralipid®), electrolytes, vitamins, and trace elements (European products); stability defined as greater than 80% of initial concentration.*

Vitamin C *in Parenteral Nutrition*

Container	Stability	Temperature			Light		Lipids		Reference
		Refrigerator	Room	Body	Exposed	Protected	With	Without	
PVC, Glass[a]	Stable	48 h			X		X	X	56
Glass[b]	Unstable		24 h		X	X	X		59
Glass[c]	Unstable		12 h			X		X	71
Glass, PVC[d]	Unstable	3 h	3 h			X		X	70
EVA[e]	Unstable		24 h		X			X	57
EVA[f]	Unstable	6 h	6 h	X	X		X		62
EVA[g]	Unstable	24 h				X	X		64
ML[h]	Unstable	24 h	24 h				X		62
PVC[i]	Stable	39 h				X		X	24
PVC[j]	Unstable	24 h	24 h		X	X		X	23
ML[k]	Stable	72 h	24 h		X	X		X	111

EVA—ethylene vinyl acetate; ML—multilayer (oxygen barrier); PVC—polyvinyl chloride.

(continued)

Vitamin C *in Parenteral Nutrition* (continued)

Notes

[a]*Formulas included amino acids (four different brands), sulfites (+/−), dextrose, lipid emulsion (+/−), electrolytes, vitamins, and trace elements.*

[b]*Ascorbate; Admixture of only Intralipid® and multivitamins; stability defined as greater than 80% of initial concentration.*

[c]*Ascorbic acid; Formula: amino acids, glucose, electrolytes, and trace elements (+/−) (European products).*

[d]*Ascorbic acid; Tested in the presence of copper; formula: amino acids, glucose, electrolytes, vitamins, and trace elements (European products).*

[e]*Ascorbic acid; Formula: amino acids, glucose, electrolytes, vitamins, trace elements (European products).*

[f]*Formula: amino acids, glucose, lipid emulsion, electrolytes, vitamins, and trace elements (European products).*

[g]*Formula: amino acids, glucose, lipid emulsion (Intralipid®), electrolytes, vitamins, and trace elements (European products); stability defined as greater than 80% of initial concentration.*

[h]*Formula: amino acids, glucose, lipid emulsions (MCT/LCT), electrolytes (European products); three different ML bags evaluated; minimum of 11.8% ascorbic acid loss in 24 h.*

[i]*Formulas included amino acids, glucose, electrolytes, and trace elements (European products).*

[j]*Ascorbic acid; Formula: amino acids, glucose, electrolytes, MVI-12®, trace elements (European products).*

[k]*Formula: amino acids, dextrose, electrolytes, trace elements, pediatric multivitamins, high-concentration calcium and organic phosphate (Brazilian products).*

(+/−) indicates that sample was mixed both with and without the nutrient.

Vitamin D *in Parenteral Nutrition*								
Container	**Stability**	**Temperature**			**Light**		**Lipids**		**Reference**
		Refrigerator	Room	Body	Exposed	Protected	With	Without	
Glass[a]	Stable		24 h		X	X	X		59
PVC[b]	Unstable		24 h		X			X	67

PVC—polyvinyl chloride.

Notes

[a]*Ergocalciferol; Admixture of only Intralipid® and multivitamins; stability defined as greater than 80% of initial concentration.*

[b]*Formula: amino acid, dextrose, electrolytes, vitamins, and trace elements (Canadian products); in-line filtration did not affect stability.*

Vitamin E *in Parenteral Nutrition*

Container	Stability	Temperature			Light		Lipids		Reference
		Refrigerator	Room	Body	Exposed	Protected	With	Without	
PVC, Glass[a]	Stable	48 h	48 h		X		X	X	56
EVA[b]	Stable	6 d	24 h		X	X	X		64
EVA[c]	Stable	72 h	72 h	72 h	X		X		62
EVA[d]	Stable	24 h	24 h	24 h	X		X		68
EVA, Glass, PVC[e]	Stable	20 d				X	X	X	65
EVA[f]	Unstable		1 h		X		X	X	63
Glass[g]	Stable		24 h		X	X	X		59
PVC[h]	Stable		24 h		X			X	72
PVC[i]	Unstable		24 h		X			X	67

EVA—ethylene vinyl acetate; PVC—polyvinyl chloride.

Notes

[a]*Formulas included amino acids (four different brands), sulfites (+/−), dextrose, lipid emulsion (+/−), electrolytes, vitamins, and trace elements.*

[b]*Formula: amino acids, glucose, lipid emulsion (Intralipid®), electrolytes, vitamins, and trace elements (European products); refrigerated samples were protected from light; stability defined as greater than 80% of initial concentration.*

[c]*Formula: amino acids, glucose, lipid emulsion, electrolytes, vitamins, and trace elements (European products).*

[d]*Tocopherol; Formulas included amino acids, glucose, lipid emulsions (Liposyn 20%®, Intralipid 20%®, ClinOleic 20%®), electrolytes, vitamins, and trace elements; no change in emulsion stability over 4 d.*

[e]*Formula: amino acids, glucose, lipid emulsion (+/−), electrolytes, MVI-12®, trace elements (+/−) (European products); stability defined as greater than 80% of initial concentration.*

[f]*Formula: amino acids, glucose, lipid emulsion (+/−), electrolytes, and trace elements. (European products).*

[g]*Tocopherol; Admixture of only Intralipid® and multivitamins; stability defined as greater than 80% of initial concentration.*

[h]*Formula: amino acids (Aminosyn®), dextrose, electrolytes, vitamins, trace elements, and iron (Canadian products).*

[i]*Formula: amino acid, dextrose, electrolytes, vitamins, and trace elements (Canadian products); in-line filtration did not affect stability.*

(+/−) indicates that sample was mixed both with and without the nutrient.

Vitamin K *in Parenteral Nutrition*

Container	Stability	Temperature			Light		Lipids		Reference
		Refrigerator	Room	Body	Exposed	Protected	With	Without	
Glass[a]	Stable		24 h		X	X	X		59
EVA, Glass, PVC[b]	Stable	20 d				X	X	X	65

EVA—ethylene vinyl acetate; PVC—polyvinyl chloride.

Notes

[a]*Phylloquinone; Admixture of only Intralipid® and multivitamins; stability defined as greater than 80% of initial concentration.*

[b]*Vitamin K1; Formula: amino acids, glucose, lipid emulsion (+/−), electrolytes, MVI-12®, trace elements (+/−) (European products); stability defined as greater than 80% of initial concentration.*

(+/−) indicates that sample was mixed both with and without the nutrient.

Zinc *in Parenteral Nutrition*

Container	Stability	Temperature			Light		Lipids		Reference
		Refrigerator	Room	Body	Exposed	Protected	With	Without	
Glass[a]	Stable		48 h		X			X	73
PVC[b]	Stable	7 d				X		X	77
PP[c]	Unstable	30 d						X	76

PP—polypropylene; PVC—polyvinyl chloride.

Notes

[a]*Formulas included amino acids (Travasol)® alone or in TPN (no formula provided).*

[b]*Formulas: amino acids, dextrose, electrolytes, and trace elements (+/−) (European products).*

[c]*Formulas: amino acids (Travasol®), dextrose, electrolytes, vitamins, trace elements (Canadian products).*

(+/−) indicates that sample was mixed both with and without the nutrient.

References

1. Brawley V, Bhatia J, Karp WB. Hydrogen peroxide generation in a model paediatric parenteral amino acid solution. *Clin Sci.* 1993; 85(6):709–12.

2. Laborie S, Lavoie JC, Pineault M, et al. Contribution of multivitamins, air, and light in the generation of peroxides in adult and neonatal parenteral nutrition solutions. *Ann Pharmacother.* 2000; 34(Apr):440–5.

3. Smith JL, Canham JE, Wells PA. Effect of phototherapy light, sodium bisulfite, and pH on vitamin stability in total parenteral nutrition admixtures. *J Parent Enteral Nutr.* 1988; 12(4):394–402.

4. Li S, Schoneich C, Borchardt RT. Chemical pathways of peptide degradation. Part 8. Oxidation of methionine in small model peptides by prooxidant/transition metal ion systems: influence of selective scavengers for reactive oxygen intermediates. *Pharm Res.* 1995; 12(Mar):348–55.

5. Guerret J, Murano RA. The unique challenges of manufacturing parenteral nutrition products. *Eur J Parent Sci.* 2002; 7(4):127–30.

6. Allwood MC, Hardy G, Sizer T, et al. Effects of air and oxygen on parenteral nutrition admixtures—an underrated risk? *Nutrition.* 1996; 12(3):222–3.

7. Weinberger B, Watorek K, Strauss R, et al. Association of lipid peroxidation with hepatocellular injury in preterm infants. *Crit Care Med.* 2002; 6(6):521–5.

8. Pironi L, Guidetti M, Zolezzi C, et al. Peroxidation potential of lipid emulsions after compounding in all-in-one solutions. *Nutrition.* 2003; 19(9):784–8.

9. Postaire E, Pradier F, Postaire M, et al. Various techniques for the routine evaluation of the degradation of glucose in parenteral solutions—a critical study. *J Pharmaceut Biomed Anal.* 1987; 5(4):309–18.

10. Driscoll DF, Newton DW, Bistrian BR. Precipitation of calcium phosphate from parenteral nutrient fluids. *Am J Hosp Pharm.* 1994; 51(Nov 15):2834–6.

11. Lee MD, Yoon JE, Kim SI, et al. Stability of total nutrient admixtures in reference to ambient temperatures. *Nutrition.* 2003; 19(10):886–90.

12. Cutter CN. Microbial control by packaging: a review. *Crit Rev Food Sci Nutr.* 2002; 42(2):151–61.

13. Mazur HI, Stennett DJ, Egging, PK. Extraction of diethylhexylphthalate from total nutrient solution-containing polyvinyl chloride bags. *J Parent Enteral Nutr.* 1989; 13(Jan–Feb):59–62.

14. Gutcher GR, Lax AA, Farrell PM. Vitamin A losses to plastic intravenous infusion devices and an improved method of delivery. *Am J Clin Nutr.* 1984; 40(1):8–13.

15. Henton DH, Merritt RJ. Vitamin A sorption to polyvinyl and polyolefin intravenous tubing. *J Parent Enteral Nutr.* 1990; 14(Jan–Feb):79–81.

16. Bluhm DP, Summers RS, Lowes MM, et al. Influence of container on vitamin A stability in TPN admixtures. *Int J Pharmaceut.* 1991; 68(Feb 1):281–3.

17. Bettner FS, Stennett DJ. Effects of pH, temperature, concentration and time on particle counts in lipid containing total parenteral nutrition admixtures. *J Parent Enteral Nutr.* 1986; 10(Jul–Aug):375–80.

18. Lundgren P, Landersjo L. Studies on the stability and compatibility of drugs in infusion fluids. I. pH and buffer capacity of infusion fluids. *Acta Pharmaceutica Suecica.* 1970; 7(4):407–22.

19. Kleinman LM, Tangrea JA, Gallelli JF, et al. Stability of solutions of essential amino acids. *Am J Hosp Pharm.* 1973; 30(Nov):1054–7.

20. Fry LK, Stegink LD. Formation of Maillard reaction products in parenteral alimentation solutions. *J Nutr.* 1982; 112(8):1631–7.

21. Laegeler WL, Tio JM, Blake MI. Stability of certain amino acids in a parenteral nutrition solution. *Am J Hosp Pharm.* 1984; 31(8):776–9.

22. Das Gupta V. Stability of vitamins in total parenteral nutrient solutions. *Am J Hosp Pharm.* 1986; 43(9):2132, 38, 43.

23. Nordfjeld K, Pedersen JL, Rasmussen M, et al. Storage of mixtures of total parenteral nutrition III. Stability of vitamins in TPN mixtures. *J Clin Hosp Pharm.* 1984; 9(4):293–301.

24. Shine B, Farwell JA. Stability and compatibility in parenteral nutrition solutions. *Br J Parenter Ther.* 1984; 5(Mar):42–6.

25. Jurgens RW Jr, Henry RS, Welco A. Amino acids stability in a mixed parenteral nutrition solution. *Am J Hosp Pharm.* 1981; 38(9):1358–9.

26. Daly JM, Masser E, Hanse L, et al. Peripheral vein infusion of dextrose/amino acid solutions +/− 20% fat emulsion. *J Parent Enteral Nutr.* 1985; 9(3):296–99.

27. Washington C. Stability of intravenous fat emulsions in total parenteral nutrition mixtures. *Int J Pharmaceut.* 1990; 66(Dec 1):1–21.

28. Black CD, Popovich NG. A study of intravenous emulsion compatibility: effects of dextrose, amino acids, and selected electrolytes. *Drug Intel Clin Pharm.* 1981; 15(3):184–93.

29. Driscoll DF, Bhargava HN, Li L, et al. Physicochemical stability of total nutrient admixtures. *Am J Health-Syst Pharm.* 1995; 52(Mar 15):623–34.

30. Lea PJ, Calvieri B. Electron microscopy of all-in-one admixture liposomes. *Nutr Support Serv.* 1987; 7(Oct):26.

31. Thomas SM. Stability of Intralipid in a parenteral nutrition solution. *Aust J Hosp Pharm.* 1987; 17(Jun):115–7.

32. Turner SA. Stability and clinical use of intravenous admixtures containing lipid emulsions. *Pharmaceut J.* 1985; 234(Jun 22):799–800.

33. Ang SD, Canham JE, Daly JM. Parenteral infusion with an admixture of amino acids, dextrose and fat emulsion solution: compatibility and clinical safety. *J Parent Enteral Nutr.* 1987; 11(Jan–Feb):23–7.

34. Barat AC, Harrie K, Jacob M, et al. Effect of amino acid solutions on total nutrient admixture stability. *J Parent Enteral Nutr.* 1987; 11(Jul–Aug):384–8.

35. Bullock L, Fitzgerald JF, Walter WV. Emulsion stability in total nutrient admixtures containing a pediatric amino acid formulation. *J Parent Enteral Nutr.* 1992; 16(Jan–Feb):64–8.

36. Driscoll DF, Bacon MN, Bistrian BR. Effects of in-line filtration on lipid particle size distribution in total nutrient admixtures. *J Parent Enteral Nutr.* 1996; 20(Jul–Aug):296–301.

37. Tripp MG, Menon SK, Mikrut BA. Stability of total nutrient admixtures in a dual chamber flexible container. *Am J Hosp Pharm.* 1990; 47(Nov):2496–503.

38. Li LC, Sampogna TP. Factorial design study on the physical stability of 3-in-1 admixtures. *J Pharm Pharmacol.* 1993; 45(Nov):985–7.

39. Intralipid package insert. Deerfield, IL: Baxter Healthcare Corporation; April 2000.

40. Liposyn III package insert. North Chicago, IL: Abbott Laboratories; May 2000.

41. Washington C, Ferguson JA, Irwin SE. Computational prediction of the stability of lipid emulsions in total nutrient admixtures. *J Pharmaceut Sci.* 1993; 82(Aug):808–12.

42. Washington C. Electrokinetic properties of phospholipid stabilized fat emulsions. Part 6. Zeta potentials of Intralipid 20% in TPN mixtures. *Int J Pharmaceut.* 1992; 87(Nov 10):167–74.

43. Davis SS, Galloway M. Studies on fat emulsion in combined nutrition solutions. *J Clin Hosp Pharm.* 1986; 11(1):33–45.

44. Washington C, Koosha F, Davis SS. Physicochemical properties of parenteral fat emulsions containing 20% triglyceride: Intralipid and Ivelip. *J Clin Pharm Therapeut.* 1993; 18(2):123–31.

45. Raupp P, Von Kries R, Schmidt E, et al. Incompatibility between fat emulsion and calcium plus heparin in parenteral nutrition of premature babies. *Lancet.* 1988; 1(Mar 26):700.

46. Johnson OL, Washington C, Davis SS, et al. The destabilization of parenteral feeding emulsions by heparin. *Int J Pharmaceut.* 1989; 53(Aug 1):237–40.

47. Trissel LA. *Calcium and Phosphate Compatibility in Parenteral Nutrition.* Houston, TX: TriPharma Communications; 2001.

48. Fansel CA, Newton DW, Driscoll DF, et al. Effect of fat emulsion and supersaturation on calcium phosphate solubility in parenteral nutrient admixtures. *Int J Pharmaceut Comp.* 1997; 1(1):54–9.

49. Allwood MC, Martin H, Greenwood M, et al. Precipitation of trace elements in parenteral nutrition mixtures. *Clin Nutr.* 1998; 17(5):223–6.

50. Mirtallo J, Canada T, Johnson D, et al. Safe practices for parenteral nutrition. *J Parent Enteral Nutr.* 2004; 28(6):S39–S70.

51. Tripp, MG. Automated 3-in-1 admixture compounding: comparative study of simultaneous versus sequential pumping of core substrates on admixture stability. *Hosp Pharm.* 1990; 25(Dec):1090–3, 1096.

52. The United States Pharmacopeial Convention. *USP 35/NF 30. Chapter <797>*. Rockville, MD: The United States Pharmacopeial Convention; 2012.

53. Storm C, Wang B, Helms RA. Stability of carnitine in pediatric TPN and TNA formulations. *J Parenter Enteral Nutr.* 1998; 22:S18. Abstract 71.

54. O'Grady NP, Alexander M, Dellinger EP, et al. Guidelines for the prevention of intravascular catheter-related infections. Appendix B. Centers for Disease Control and Prevention. *MMWR Recomm Rep.* 2002; 51(RR-10):1–29.

55. Chen MF, Boyce HW Jr, Triplett L. Stability of the B vitamins in mixed parenteral nutrition solutions. *J Parent Enteral Nutr.* 1983; 7(5):462–4.

56. Smith JL, Canham JE, Kirkland WD, et al. Effect of Intralipid, amino acids, container, temperature, and duration of storage on vitamin stability in total parenteral nutrition admixtures. *J Parent Enteral Nutr.* 1988; 12(5):478–83.

57. Van Der Horst A, Martens HJ, De Goede PN. Analysis of water-soluble vitamins in total parenteral nutrition solution by high pressure liquid chromatography. *Pharm Weekly Sci.* 1989; 11(Oct 20):169–74.

58. Louie N, Stennet DJ. Stability of folic acid in 25% dextrose, 3.5 amino acids, and multivitamin solution. *J Parent Enteral Nutr.* 1984; 8(4):421–6.

59. Dahl GB, Svensson L, Kinnander NJ, et al. Stability of vitamins in soybean oil fat emulsion under conditions simulating intravenous feeding of neonates and children. *J Parent Enteral Nutr.* 1994; 18(3):234–9.

60. Barker A, Hebron BS, Beck PR, et al. Folic acid and total parenteral nutrition. *J Parent Enteral Nutr.* 1984; 8(Jan–Feb):3–8.

61. Riggle MA, Brandt RB. Decrease of available vitamin A in parenteral nutrition solutions. *J Parent Enteral Nutr.* 1986; 10(Jul–Aug):388–92.

62. Dupertuis YM, Morch A, Fathi M, et al. Physical characteristics of total parenteral nutrition bags significantly affect the stability of vitamins C and B1: a controlled prospective study. *J Parent Enteral Nutr.* 2002; 26(5):310–6.

63. Allwood MC, Martin HJ. The photodegradation of vitamins A and E in parenteral nutrition mixtures during infusion. *Clin Nutr.* 2000; 19(5):339–42.

64. Dahl GB, Jeppsson RI, Tengborn HJ. Vitamin stability in a TPN mixture stored in an EVA plastic bag. *J Clin Hosp Pharm.* 1986; 11(4):271–9.

65. Billion-Rey F, Guillaumont M, Frederich A, et al. Stability of fat-soluble vitamins A (retinol palmitate), E (tocopherol acetate), and K1 (phylloquinone) in total parenteral nutrition at home. *J Parent Enteral Nutr.* 1993; 17(Jan–Feb):56–60.

66. Bluhm DP, Summers RS, Lowes MM, et al. Lipid emulsion content and vitamin A stability in TPN admixtures. *Int J Pharmaceut.*1991; 68(Feb 1):277–80.

67. Gillis J, Jones G, Pencharz P. Delivery of vitamins A, D and E in total parenteral nutrition solutions. *J Parent Enteral Nutr.* 1983; 7(Jan–Feb):11–4.

68. Sforzini A, Bersani G, Stancari A, et al. Analysis of all-in-one parenteral nutrition admixtures by liquid chromatography and laser diffraction: study of stability. *J Pharmaceut Biomed Anal.* 2001; 24(5–6):1099–109.

69. Bowman BB, Nguyen P. Stability of thiamin in parenteral nutrition solutions. *J Parent Enteral Nutr.* 1983; 7(6):567–8.

70. Allwood MC. Factors influencing the stability of ascorbic acid in total parenteral nutrition infusions. *J Clin Hosp Pharm.* 1984; 9(2):75–85.

71. Gibbons E, Allwood MC, Neal T, et al. Degradation of dehydroascorbic acid in parenteral nutrition mixtures. *J Pharm Biomed Anal.* 2001; 25:605–11.

72. McGee CD, Mascarenhas MG, Ostro MJ, et al. Selenium and vitamin E stability in parenteral solutions. *J Parent Enteral Nutr.* 1985; 9(Sep–Oct):568–70.

73. Boddapati S, Yang K, Murty R. Intravenous solution compatibility and filter retention characteristics of trace element preparations. *Am J Hosp Pharm.* 1981; 38(Nov):1731–6.

74. Bates CG, Greiner G, Gegenheimer A. Precipitate in admixtures of new amino acid injection. *Am J Hosp Pharm.* 1984; 41(Jul):1312.

75. Cochran EB, Boehm KA. Prefilter and postfilter cysteine/cystine and copper concentrations in pediatric parenteral nutrition solutions. *J Parent Enteral Nutr.* 1992; 16(Sep–Oct):460–3.

76. Pluhator-Murton MM, Fedorak RN, Audette RJ, et al. Trace element contamination of total parenteral nutrition. Part 2. Effect of storage duration and temperature. *J Parent Enteral Nutr.* 1999; 23(Jul–Aug):228–32.

77. Allwood MC. Compatibility of four trace elements in total parenteral nutrition infusions. *Int J Pharmaceut.* 1983; 16(Aug):57–63.

78. Mitrano FP, Baptista RJ. Stability of cimetidine HCl and copper sulfate in a TPN solution. *DICP Ann Pharmacother.* 1989; 23(May):429–30.

79. Kee Wan K, Tsallas G. Dilute iron dextran formulation for addition to parenteral nutrient solutions. *Am J Hosp Pharm.* 1980; 37(2):206–10.

80. Vaughan LM, Small C, Plunkett V. Incompatibility of iron dextran and a total nutrient admixture. *Am J Hosp Pharm.* 1990; 47(Aug):1745–6.

81. Tu YH, Knox NL, Biringer JM, et al. Compatibility of iron dextran with total nutrient admixtures. *Am J Hosp Pharm.* 1992; 49(Sep):2233–5.

82. Mayhew SL, Quick MW. Compatibility of iron dextran with neonatal parenteral nutrient solutions. *Am J Health-Syst Pharm.* 1997; 54(5):570–1.

83. Allwood MC, Greenwood M. Assessment of trace element compatibility in total parenteral nutrition infusions. *Pharm Weekly Sci.* 1992; 14(Oct 16):321–4.

84. Ganther HE, Kraus RJ. Chemical stability of selenious acid in total parenteral nutrition solutions containing ascorbic acid. *J Parent Enteral Nutr.* 1989; 13(2):185–8.

85. Postaire E, Le Hoang MD, Anglade P, et al. Stability and behavior of selenium in total parenteral nutrition solutions. *Int J Pharmaceut.* 1989; 55(Oct 15):99–103.

86. Postaire E, Anglade P. Selenium stability in total parenteral nutrition solutions. *J Parent Enteral Nutr.* 1990; 14(2):223–4.

87. Allwood MC, Martin HJ. Long-term stability of cimetidine in total parenteral nutrition. *J Clin Pharm Ther.* 1996; 21(1):19–21.

88. Baptista RJ, Palombo JD, Tahan SR, et al. Stability of cimetidine hydrochloride in a total nutrient admixture. *Am J Hosp Pharm.* 1985; 42(Oct):2208–10.

89. Hatton J, Luer M, Hirsch J, et al. Histamine receptor antagonists and lipid stability in total nutrient admixtures. *J Parent Enteral Nutr.* 1994; 18(4):308–12.

90. Tsallas G, Allen LC. Stability of cimetidine hydrochloride in parenteral nutrition solutions. *Am J Hosp Pharm.* 1982; 39(Mar):484–5.

91. Walker SE, Iazzetta J, Lau DW, et al. Famotidine stability in total parenteral nutrient solutions. *Can J Hosp Pharm.* 1989; 42(3):97–103.

92. Underberg WJ, Koomen JM, Beijnen JH. Stability of famotidine in commonly used nutritional infusion fluids. *J Parent Sci Tech.* 1998; 42(3):94–7.

93. Bullock L, Fitzgerald JF, Glick MR. Stability of famotidine 20 and 50 mg/L in total nutrient admixtures. *Am J Hosp Pharm.* 1989; 46(Nov):2326–9.

94. Shea BF, Souney PF. Stability of famotidine in a 3-in-1 total nutrient admixture. *DICP Ann Pharmacother.* 1990; 24(Mar):232–5.

95. Bullock L, Fitzgerald JF, Glick MR, et al. Stability of famotidine 20 and 40 mg/L and amino acids in total parenteral nutrient solutions. *Am J Hosp Pharm.* 1989; 46(Nov):2321–5.

96. Montoro JB, Pou L, Salvador P, et al. Stability of famotidine 20 and 40 mg/L in total nutrient admixtures. *Am J Hosp Pharm.* 1989; 46(Nov):2329–32.

97. DiStefano JE, Mitrano FP, Baptista RJ, et al. Long-term stability of famotidine 20 mg/L in a total parenteral nutrient solution. *Am J Hosp Pharm.* 1989; 46(Nov):2333–5.

98. Hensrud DD, Burritt MF, Hall LG. Stability of heparin anticoagulant activity over time in parenteral nutrition solutions. *J Parent Enteral Nutr.* 1996; 20(May–Jun):219–21.

99. Borum PR. Is L-carnitine stable in parenteral nutrition solutions prepared for preterm neonates? *Neonatal Intensive Care.* 1993; Sept/Oct:30–2.

100. Walker SE, Bayliff CD. Stability of ranitidine hydrochloride in total parenteral nutrient solution. *Am J Hosp Pharm.* 1985; 42(Mar):590–2.

101. Cano SM, Montoro JB, Pastor C, et al. Stability of ranitidine hydrochloride in total nutrient admixtures. *Am J Hosp Pharm.* 1988; 45(May):1100–2.

102. Williams MF, Hak LJ, Dukes G. In vitro evaluation of the stability of ranitidine hydrochloride in total parenteral nutrient mixtures. *Am J Hosp Pharm.* 1990; 47(Jul):1574–9.

103. Bullock L, Parks RB, Lampasona V, et al. Stability of ranitidine hydrochloride and amino acids in parenteral nutrient solutions. *Am J Hosp Pharm.* 1985; 42(12):2683–7.

104. Allwood MC. Light protection during parenteral nutrition infusion: is it really necessary? *Nutrition.* 2000; 16:234–5.

105. Klang MG, Lewars K, Nguyen H. Calcium-phosphate precipitation in amino acid-dextrose solutions as measured by nephelometric analysis. *Clinical Nutrition Week.* 2008. Poster 50–524.

106. Lester LR, Crill CM, Hak EB. Should adding albumin to parenteral nutrient solutions be considered an unsafe practice? *Am J Health-Syst Pharm.* 2006; 63:1656–61.

107. MacKay M, Rusho W, Jackson D, et al. Physical and chemical stability of iron sucrose in parenteral nutrition. *Nutr Clin Pract.* 2009; Dec 24(6):733–7.

108. MacKay M, Jackson D, Eggert L, et al. Practice-based validation of calcium and phosphorous solubility limits for pediatric parenteral nutrition solutions. *Nutr Clin Pract.* 2011; Dec 26(6):708–13.

109. Matsusue S. White milky color veils dirt. *J Parenter Enteral Nutr.* 1996; Nov–Dec 20(6):435.

110. Ribeiro DO, Lobo BW, Volpato NM, et al. Influence of the calcium concentration in the presence of organic phosphorous on the physicochemical compatibility and stability of all-in-one admixtures for neonatal use. *Nutr J.* 2009; Oct 26(8):51.

111. Ribeiro DO, Pinto DC, Lima LM, et al. Chemical stability study of vitamins thiamine, riboflavin, pyridoxine and ascorbic acid in parenteral nutrition for neonatal use. *Nutr J.* 2011; May 14(10):47.

Part II

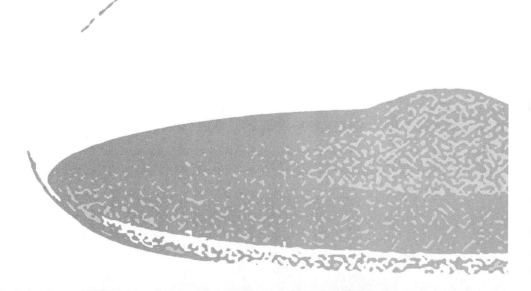

Acetaminophen[a]

Storage Conditions

	Drug Manufacturer	Concentration	Diluents	Osmolality (mOsm/kg)	pH	Temperature			Post-thaw Temp			Refer.
						Room	Refrig	Frozen	Room	Refrig	Body Temp	
CONTAINER												
Bags, Plastic	CAD	10 mg/mL	undiluted	c	b	6 h	n/a	n/a	n/a	n/a	n/a	1
Polyolefin	CAD	10 mg/mL	undiluted	c	b	6 h	n/a	n/a	n/a	n/a	n/a	2
Polyvinyl Chloride (PVC)	CAD	10 mg/mL	undiluted	c	b	6 h	n/a	n/a	n/a	n/a	n/a	2
Syringes, Plastic (BD)	CAD	10 mg/mL	undiluted	c	b	6 h	n/a	n/a	n/a	n/a	n/a	1, 2
Syringes, Polypropylene	CAD	10 mg/mL	undiluted	c	b	84 h	n/a	n/a	n/a	n/a	n/a	4, 5
OTHER INFUSION CONTAINERS												
Glass	CAD	10 mg/mL	undiluted[d]	c	b	6 h	n/a	n/a	n/a	n/a	n/a	1
	BMS	10 mg/mL	undiluted[d,e]	n/a	3.7–6.6	48 h	n/a	n/a	n/a	n/a	n/a	3
	CAD	10 mg/mL	undiluted[d]	c	b	84 h	n/a	n/a	n/a	n/a	n/a	4, 5

Flush Compatibility: Heparin sodium and normal saline.[2]
Special Considerations: Store at room temperature; do not refrigerate or freeze.[1]

Notes

[a]Acetaminophen is known internationally as paracetamol.[1]
[b]pH of undiluted solution is approximately 5.5.[1]
[c]Osmolality of undiluted solution is approximately 290 mOsm/kg.[1]
[d]Undiluted, after opening and within original glass vial.
[e]With ketoprofen (Profenid, SAV) 100 mg added to paracetamol[a] (Perfalgan, BMS) 10 mg/mL in original glass vial.

References

1. Ofirmev™ [package insert]. San Diego, CA: Cadence Pharmaceuticals, Inc.; November 2010.
2. Navarrete T, Medical Information Services [personal communication]. San Diego CA: Cadence Pharmaceuticals; September 27, 2012.
3. Kambia NK, Lyuckx M, Dine T, et al. Stability and compatibility of paracetamol injection admixed with ketoprofen. Eur J Hosp Pharm. 2006; 12:81–4.
4. Kwiatkowski JL. Extended stability of intravenous acetaminophen in syringes and opened glass bottles. ICHP Annual Meeting, September 2012.
5. Kwiatkowski JL, Johnson CE, Wagner DS. Extended stability of intravenous acetaminophen in syringes and opened vials. Am J Health-Syst Pharm. 2012; 69:1999–2001.

Acyclovir Sodium

continued on next page

Acyclovir Sodium[a]

CONTAINER	Drug Manufacturer	Concentration	Diluents	Osmolality (mOsm/kg)	pH[h]	Temperature Room	Temperature Refrig	Temperature Frozen	Post-thaw Temp Room	Post-thaw Temp Refrig	Body Temp	Refer.
Ethyvinyl Acetate (EVA)	WEL	2.5, 5 mg/mL	NS	n/a	h	28 d[g]	n/a	n/a	n/a	n/a	n/a	1
Polyvinyl Chloride (PVC)	BW	1 mg/mL	D5W	c	h	35 d[d]	35 d[b,e]	n/a	n/a	n/a	n/a	1
	BW	1, 7 & 10 mg/mL	NS	c	h	7 d[d]	35 d[b,e]	n/a	n/a	n/a	n/a	1
	BW	5 mg/mL	NS	316	h	37 d	37 d[b]	n/a	n/a	n/a	n/a	1
	BW	5 mg/mL	D5W	289	h	37 d	37 d[b]	n/a	n/a	n/a	n/a	1
	BW	7 mg/mL	D5W	c	h	28 d[d]	35 d[b,e]	n/a	n/a	n/a	n/a	1
	BW	10 mg/mL	D5W	c	h	21 d[d]	35 d[b,e]	n/a	n/a	n/a	n/a	1
Syringes, Plastic	unspec.	8.3 mg/mL	NS	n/a	h	24 h	7 d	n/a	n/a	n/a	n/a	5
	unspec.	8.3 mg/mL	D5W	n/a	h	24 h	n/a	n/a	n/a	n/a	n/a	5
Syringes, Polypropylene	APP	10 mg/mL	NS	n/a	10.4–10.7	30 d	i	n/a	n/a	n/a	n/a	1
OTHER INFUSION CONTAINERS												
AccuFlo™/ AccuFlux™/ AccuRX® (B. Braun)	unspec.	10 mg/mL	NS	n/a	n/a	10 d[f]	30 d[f]	n/a	n/a	n/a	n/a	4
Homepump®/ Homepump Eclipse® (I-Flow Corp)	unspec.	10 mg/mL	NS	c	h	10 d	30 d[b]	n/a	n/a	n/a	n/a	3
INTERMATE (Baxter)	WEL	1–10 mg/mL	D5W, NS	c	h	4 d	n/a	n/a	n/a	n/a	n/a	2
	WEL	10 mg/mL	NS, D5W	c	h	29 d	n/a	n/a	n/a	n/a	n/a	2

Acyclovir Sodium (cont'd)

Flush Compatibility: Heparin lock flush and normal saline.[1]

Special Considerations: n/a

Notes

[a]Do not use bacteriostatic water for injection containing parabens or benzyl alcohol for reconstitution. Special attention must be paid to the drug's potential for precipitation. Precipitation depends on preparation, storage conditions, concentration, pH, and diluent.

[b]Refrigeration may cause precipitation; product will resolubilize at room temperature but should be used immediately due to reformation of microprecipitates. Physical instability is the principal limitation to long-term storage due to persistent subvisual microprecipitates and frank persistent precipitates after as few as 7 d.[1]

[c]Acyclovir 10 mg/mL has an osmolality of 342 and 316 mOsm/kg in NS and D5W respectively; at 7 mg/mL osmolality is 299 and 278 mOsm/kg in NS and D5W respectively.[1]

[d]Solutions were maintained at room temperature only, protected from light.

[e]Authors recommend using refrigerated admixtures immediately after warming to room temperature.

[f]Manufacturer(s) extrapolated data from other sources.

[g]No significant increases in subvisual particulates in EVA container after 28 d.[1]

[h]pH of reconstituted solution is 10.5–11.6.[1]

[i]Precipitate formed within 5 d stored at 5°C.[1]

References

1. Trissel LA. ASHP's Interactive Handbook on Injectable Drugs. Bethesda, MD: American Society of Health-System Pharmacists. Accessed 2012 Jan.
2. Intermate/Infusor Drug Stability Information. Deerfield, IL: Baxter Healthcare Corporation; 2008.
3. Stability Data for Drugs Using Homepump Disposable Elastomeric Infusion Systems. Lake Forest, CA: I-Flow Corporation; October 2009.
4. Drug Stability Data Using Elastomeric Infusion Systems. B. Braun Medical Production Ltd. (Thailand); August 2011.
5. Rapp RP, Hatton J, Record K. Drug Stability in Plastic Syringes. HealthTek™ and University of KY Lexington; Repro-Med Systems Inc.; 1998.

Aldesleukin[a,b]

Storage Conditions

Drug Manufacturer	Concentration	Diluents	Osmolality (mOsm/kg)	pH[e]	Temperature			Post-thaw Temp		Body Temp	Refer.
					Room	Refrig	Frozen	Room	Refrig		
CONTAINER											
Polyvinyl Chloride (PVC)	CHI	0.005–0.06 mg/mL[d]	D5W	n/a	e	6 d[c]	n/a	n/a	n/a	n/a	n/a	1
	CHI	0.1–0.5 mg/mL	D5W	n/a	e	6 d[c]	n/a	n/a	n/a	n/a	n/a	1, 2
Syringes, Plastic	CHI	0.22 mg/mL	D5W	n/a	e	n/a	14 d	n/a	n/a	n/a	n/a	1, 2
	CHI	18 million I.U./mL	W	n/a	e	48 h	5 d	n/a	n/a	n/a	n/a	2
OTHER INFUSION CONTAINERS											
CADD° Cassette (SIMS Deltec)	CHI	0.1–0.5 mg/mL	D5W	n/a	e	6 d[c]	n/a	n/a	n/a	n/a	n/a	1, 2
	CHI	5, 40 mcg/mL[d]	D5W	n/a	e	6 d[c]	n/a	n/a	n/a	n/a	n/a	1, 2

Flush Compatibility: Heparin lock flush.[1,2]
Special Considerations: Do not mix with normal saline.[1]

Notes

[a]Various measurement units have been used and reported for this agent. The International Unit (I.U.) is now the standard measure of activity. Consult current manufacturer's literature for conversion factors.
[b]Do not use in-line filters. Reconstitution or dilution with NS or BWFI may cause aggregation (deactivation).[1,2]
[c]Solutions stored at 32°C.
[d]Solutions also contained human serum albumin (HSA) for a final albumin concentration of 0.1%. Addition of HSA to aldesleukin 5–60 mcg/mL prevents sorption to the container, as well as microaggregation.
[e]pH of reconstituted product is 7.2–7.8.[2]

References

1. Professional Services [personal communication]. Emeryville, CA: Chiron Therapeutics; August 31, 1994.
2. Trissel LA. ASHP's Interactive Handbook on Injectable Drugs. Bethesda, MD: American Society of Health-System Pharmacists. Accessed 2012 May.

Amikacin Sulfate

Container	Drug Manufacturer	Concentration	Diluents	Osmolality (mOsm/kg)	pH[e]	Temperature Room	Temperature Refrig	Temperature Frozen	Post-thaw Temp Room	Post-thaw Temp Refrig	Body Temp	Refer.
CONTAINER												
Ethyvinyl Acetate (EVA)	n/a	0.25, 5 mg/mL	NS	n/a	e	7 d[d]	30 d[d]	n/a	n/a	n/a	n/a	1
Glass	BR	50 mg/mL	NS	n/a	e	n/a	n/a	6 m	n/a	n/a	n/a	2
Polyvinyl Chloride (PVC)	BR	0.25, 5 mg/mL	NS	a	e	24 h	60 d	30 d	24 h	24 h	n/a	1
	BR	0.25, 5 mg/mL	D5W	b	e	24 h	60 d	30 d	24 h	24 h	n/a	1
	BR	20 mg/mL	D5W	n/a	e	n/a	n/a	30 d	24 h	n/a	n/a	1
Syringes, Plastic	BR	187.5 mg/mL	NS	n/a	e	48 h	n/a	n/a	n/a	n/a	n/a	1
OTHER INFUSION CONTAINERS												
AccuFlo™/ AccuFlux™/ AccuRX® (B. Braun)	unspec.	10 mg/mL	NS	n/a	e	24 h	14 d	n/a	n/a	n/a	n/a	6
	unspec.	10 mg/mL	NS	n/a	e	24 h[c]	10 d[c]	30 d[c]	n/a	n/a	n/a	6
	unspec.	10–20 mg/mL	NS	n/a	e	24 h[c]	28 d[c]	n/a	n/a	n/a	n/a	6
AutoDose (Tandem Medical)	n/a	0.25, 5 mg/mL	NS	n/a	e	7 d	30 d	n/a	n/a	n/a	n/a	5
Homepump Eclipse®/ Homepump® C-Series (I-Flow Corp.)	unspec.	10 mg/mL	NS	n/a	e	24 h	10 d	30 d	n/a	n/a	n/a	4
	unspec.	10–20 mg/mL	NS	n/a		24 h	28 d	n/a	n/a	n/a	n/a	4
INTERMATE/ INFUSOR (Baxter)	BMS	0.25–20 mg/mL	D5W, NS	n/a	e	48 h[f]	28 d	n/a	n/a	n/a	n/a	3
	BMS	20 mg/mL	D5W, NS	n/a	e	24 h	n/a	30 d	24 h	n/a	n/a	3

(Storage Conditions spans the Temperature, Post-thaw Temp, and Body Temp columns.)

Flush Compatibility: Normal saline. Incompatible with heparin; immediate precipitation occurs.[1]
Special Considerations: n/a

continued on next page

Amikacin Sulfate (cont'd)

Notes

[a]Amikacin sulfate 5 mg/mL in NS has an osmolality of 349 mOsm/kg.[1]

[b]Amikacin sulfate 5 mg/mL in D5W has an osmolality of 319 mOsm/kg.[1]

[c]Manufacturer(s) extrapolated data from other sources.

[d]Protected from light.

[e]pH of undiluted solution is 3.5–5.5.[1]

[f]After 28 d at 2–8°C.[3]

References

1. Trissel LA. ASHP's Interactive Handbook on Injectable Drugs. Bethesda, MD: American Society of Health-System Pharmacists. Accessed 2012 May.
2. Chedru-Legros V, Fines-Guyon M, Cherel A, et al. In vitro stability of fortified ophthalmic antibiotics stored at −20 deg C for 6 months. Cornea 2010; 29:807–11.
3. Intermate/Infusor Drug Stability Information. Deerfield, IL: Baxter Healthcare Corporation; 2008.
4. Stability Data for Drugs Using Homepump Disposable Elastomeric Infusion Systems. Lake Forest, CA: I-Flow Corporation; October 2009.
5. AutoDose Stability Reference. San Diego, CA: Tandem Medical Inc.; 2002.
6. Drug Stability Data Using Elastomeric Infusion Systems. B. Braun Medical Production Ltd. (Thailand); August 2011.

Amiodarone Hydrochloride

	Drug Manufacturer	Concentration	Diluents	Osmolality (mOsm/kg)	pH[e]	Storage Conditions						
						Temperature			Post-thaw Temp		Body Temp	Refer.
						Room	Refrig	Frozen	Room	Refrig		
CONTAINER												
Polyolefin	BED	2 mg/mL	D5W	n/a	e	21 d[a]	38 d[a]	n/a	n/a	n/a	n/a	1
Polyolefin VISIV (Hospira)	BED	1 mg/mL	D5W	n/a	e	24 h	n/a	n/a	n/a	n/a	n/a	3, 4
OTHER INFUSION CONTAINERS												
Glass	LZ	0.6 mg/mL	D5W	n/a	n/a	5 d	n/a	n/a	n/a	n/a	n/a	3
Glass	BED	2 mg/mL	D5W	n/a	e	32 d	32 d	n/a	n/a	n/a	n/a	3
Glass	WY	2 mg/mL	D5W	n/a	n/a	32 d[c]	32 d[c]	n/a	n/a	n/a	18 d[c,d]	3
Glass Vial	BED	50 mg/mL	undiluted	n/a	4.08	14 d[b]	14 d[b]	n/a	n/a	n/a	n/a	1

Flush Compatibility: D5W.[2]

Special Considerations: Use only glass or polyolefin bags to administer infusions exceeding 2 h due to adsorption to PVC as well as leaching of plasticizers. The use of evacuated glass containers is not recommended since the buffer in these containers may cause precipitation of amiodarone. The manufacturer recommends the use of an in-line filter.[2] Dilute only with D5W due to conflicting stability data in other solutions.[3]

Notes

[a]*Braun Excel bags (polyolefin).*
[b]*Multidose vials (preserved) were punctured three times at initiation of study, day 7, and at day 14.*
[c]*In amber glass container.*
[d]*Stored at 40°C.*
[e]*pH of undiluted solution is 4.08.[3]*

References

1. Van Dine M [internal memo to sales force]. Bedford, OH: Bedford Laboratories; January 15, 2003.
2. Amiodarone Hydrochloride Injection [prescribing information]. Bedford, OH: Bedford Laboratories; March 2006.
3. Trissel LA. ASHP's Interactive Handbook on Injectable Drugs. Bethesda, MD: American Society of Health-System Pharmacists. Accessed 2012 Jun.
4. Aloumanis V, Ben M, Kupiec TC, et al. Drug compatibility with a new generation of VISIV polyolefin infusion solution containers. *International Journal of Pharmaceutical Compounding* 2009; 13(2):162–5.

Amphotericin B

| | Drug Manufacturer | Concentration | Diluents | Osmolality (mOsm/kg) | pH[c] | Storage Conditions | | | | | | |
| | | | | | | Temperature | | | Post-thaw Temp | | Body Temp | Refer. |
						Room	Refrig	Frozen	Room	Refrig		
CONTAINER												
Polyvinyl Chloride (PVC)	SQ	0.05 mg/mL, 0.1 mg/mL, 0.5 mg/mL	D5W	n/a	c	24 h	n/a	n/a	n/a	n/a	n/a	1
	SQ	0.1, 0.25 mg/mL	D5W	256[a], n/a	5.7[1]	n/a	35 d[b]	n/a	n/a	n/a	n/a	1, 3
	SQ	0.2 mg/mL, 0.5 mg/mL, 1 mg/mL	D5W	n/a	c	5 d	5 d	n/a	n/a	n/a	n/a	1
OTHER INFUSION CONTAINERS												
AccuFlo™/ AccuFlux™/ AccuRX® (Medpro)	unspec.	0.2 mg/mL	D5W	n/a	n/a	24 h[f]	10 d[e,f]	n/a	n/a	n/a	n/a	5
Homepump Eclipse®/ Homepump® C-Series (I-Flow Corp.)	unspec.	0.2 mg/mL[d]	D5W	r/a	c	24 h	10 d	n/a	n/a	n/a	n/a	4
INTERMATE (Baxter)	SQ	0.2–0.5 mg/mL	D5W	n/a	c	n/a	10 d	n/a	n/a	n/a	n/a	2

Flush Compatibility: Incompatible with normal saline and heparin lock flush. Flush all sodium-chloride-containing solutions from lines with D5W before and after amphotericin B administration.[1]

Special Considerations: In situations where filtration is necessary, the filter pore size must be 1 micron or larger.[1] Protect from light.

Notes

[a] A 0.1-mg/mL solution in D5W is 256 mOsm/kg.[1]

[b] 4% amphotericin loss. Stored protected from light.

[c] pH of 0.1 mg/mL in D5W is 5.7.[1]

[d] Special attention must be paid to the drug's potential for precipitation, which may occur depending on preparation, storage conditions, concentration, pH, and diluents.

[e] Susceptible to crystallization when refrigerated.

[f] Manufacturer(s) extrapolated data from other sources.

continued on next page

Amphotericin B (cont'd)

References

1. Trissel LA. ASHP's Handbook on Injectable Drugs. Bethesda, MD: American Society of Health-System Pharmacists. Accessed 2012 Jan.
2. Intermate/Infusor Drug Stability Information. Deerfield, IL: Baxter Healthcare Corporation; October 2008.
3. Mitrano FP, Outman WR, Baptista RJ, et al. Chemical and visual stability of amphotericin B in 5% dextrose injection stored at 4°C for 35 days. Am J Health-Syst Pharm. 1991; 48:2635–7.
4. Stability Data for Drugs Using Homepump Disposable Elastomeric Infusion Systems. Lake Forest, CA: I-Flow Corporation; October 2009:2.
5. Drug Stability Data Using Elastomeric Infusion Systems. B. Braun Medical Production Ltd. (Thailand); August 2011:1.

Amphotericin B Cholesteryl Sulfate Complex

Drug Manufacturer	Concentration	Diluents	Osmolality (mOsm/kg)	pH	Storage Conditions						Refer.
					Temperature			Post-thaw Temp		Body Temp	
					Room	Refrig	Frozen	Room	Refrig		
CONTAINER											
Polyvinyl Chloride (PVC) SEQ[a]	0.1, 2.0 mg/mL	D5W	n/a	n/a	7 d[b]	7 d[b]	c	n/a	n/a	n/a	1, 2
OTHER INFUSION CONTAINERS											
Glass Vial SEQ[a]	5 mg/mL	W	n/a	n/a	7 d	7 d	c	n/a	n/a	n/a	1

Flush Compatibility: Flush sodium chloride containing solutions from lines with D5W before and after amphotericin B administration. Amphotericin B is incompatible with saline and heparin.[2]

Special Considerations: Be certain to resuspend these emulsions by gently shaking the admixtures before infusion. Amphotericin B Cholesteryl Sulfate Complex is a colloidal dispersion. DO NOT FILTER.

Notes

[a]Amphotericin B Cholesteryl Complex (Amphotec®) stability limitations include an increase in particle size above 10 microns over time.
[b]Protected from light.
[c]Do not freeze.[3]

References

1. Xu QA, Trissel LA. Stability of amphotericin B cholesteryl sulfate complex after reconstitution and admixture. Hosp Pharm. 1998; 33(10):1203–7.
2. Trissel LA. ASHP's Interactive Handbook on Injectable Drugs. Bethesda, MD: American Society of Health-System Pharmacists; 2011. Accessed 2012 Jun.
3. Amphotec® [package insert]. Bedford, OH: Ben Venue Laboratories, Inc.; July 2005.

Amphotericin B Lipid Complex

CONTAINER	Drug Manufacturer	Concentration	Diluents	Osmolality (mOsm/kg)	pH[b]	Storage Conditions						Refer.
						Temperature			Post-thaw Temp		Body Temp	
						Room	Refrig	Frozen	Room	Refrig		
Polyolefin Bag	ZNS	0.4 mg/mL[c], 0.8 mg/mL[c], 2 mg/mL[c]	D5W	n/a	b	7 d	7 d[d]	n/a	n/a	n/a	n/a	3
Unspecified	SIT[a]	1 mg/mL	D5W	n/a	b	6 h	10 d	n/a	n/a	n/a	n/a	1

Flush Compatibility: Flush line with D5W before and after administration; incompatible with saline and heparin.[2]

Special Considerations: Be certain to resuspend these emulsions by gently shaking the admixtures before infusion, and every 2 h during longer infusions. Do not administer with an in line filter.[1]

Notes

[a]Amphotericin B Lipid Complex Injection (Abelcet®).
[b]pH of undiluted product is 5–7.[2]
[c]Protect from light.
[d]Stored at 4°C.

References

1. Abelcet® stability letter [personal communication]. Gaithersburg, MD: Sigma-Tau Pharmaceuticals, Inc.; January 10, 2012.
2. Trissel LA. ASHP's Interactive Handbook on Injectable Drugs. Bethesda, MD: American Society of Health-System Pharmacists. Accessed 2012 Jun.
3. Vanneaux V, Proust B, Cheron M, et al. A physical and chemical stability study of amphotericin B lipid complexes (Abelcet®) after dilution in dextrose 5%. *Europ J Hosp Pharm Science* 2007; 13:10–3.

Amphotericin B Liposome[a]

CONTAINER	Drug Manufacturer	Concentration	Diluents	Osmolality (mOsm/kg)	pH[b]	Temperature			Post-thaw Temp			Refer.
						Room	Refrig	Frozen	Room	Refrig	Body Temp	
Polyolefin	ASL	0.2 mg/mL	D5W	n/a	b	24 h[c]	11 d[d]	n/a	n/a	n/a	n/a	2
	ASL	0.2 mg/mL	D10W	n/a	b	n/a	48 h[d]	n/a	n/a	n/a	n/a	2
	ASL	2 mg/mL	D5W	n/a	b	24 h[c]	14 d[d]	n/a	n/a	n/a	n/a	2
	ASL	2 mg/mL	D10W, D20W, D25W	n/a	b	n/a	48 h[d]	n/a	n/a	n/a	n/a	2
Polyvinyl Chloride (PVC)	ASL	0.5 mg/mL	D5W	n/a	b	n/a	14 d[d]	n/a	n/a	n/a	n/a	2
	ASL	2 mg/mL	D5W	n/a	b	n/a	14 d[d]	n/a	n/a	n/a	n/a	2
Syringes, Plastic	ASL	4 mg/mL	W	n/a	b	n/a	14 d[d]	n/a	n/a	n/a	n/a	2
OTHER INFUSION CONTAINERS												
Glass Vial	ASL	4 mg/mL	W	n/a	b	n/a	14 d[d]	n/a	n/a	n/a	n/a	2
Homepump Eclipse® (B. Braun)	ASL	0.2 mg/mL	D5W	n/a	b	n/a	7 d[d]	n/a	n/a	n/a	n/a	2
	ASL	2 mg/mL	D5W	n/a	b	n/a	14 d[d]	n/a	n/a	n/a	n/a	2

Storage Conditions

Flush Compatibility: Flush administration line with D5W before and after administration or use a separate administration line. Incompatible with saline containing solutions.[1]

Special Considerations: Increased concentrations of dextrose (>D5W) reduce the stability.[2] After dilution (suspension) of product in W, shake the vial vigorously to form a completely dispersed suspension. Withdraw the suspension required into a sterile syringe; attach the manufacturer-provided, 5-micron filter to the syringe and add the contents into the diluent/container. Use only one filter per vial of product. May administer through an in-line membrane filter with a mean pore diameter not less than 1.0 micron.[1]

Notes

[a]Amphotericin B liposome for injection (Am**B**isome®).
[b]pH of suspension following reconstitution with W to 4 mg/mL is 5–6.[1]
[c]Exposed to fluorescent light.
[d]Protected from light.

References

1. Am**B**isome® [package insert]. Deerfield, IL: Astellas Pharma US Inc.; March 2012.
2. Medical Information Department [personal communication]. Deerfield, IL: Astellas Pharma US Inc.; January 10, 2012.

Ampicillin Sodium

Container	Drug Manufacturer	Concentration	Diluents	Osmolality (mOsm/kg)	pH[a]	Temperature Room	Temperature Refrig	Temperature Frozen	Post-thaw Temp Room	Post-thaw Temp Refrig	Body Temp	Refer.
CONTAINER												
Ethyvinyl Acetate (EVA)	APO	10 mg/mL	NS	n/a	a	24 h	3 d	n/a	n/a	n/a	n/a	1
Polyvinyl Chloride (PVC)	BE	10 mg/mL	NS	n/a	a	n/a	48 h	n/a	n/a	n/a	n/a	1
	BR	20 mg/mL	D5W	n/a	a	2 h[d]	n/a	n/a	n/a	n/a	n/a	1
	AY	20 mg/mL	NS	n/a	a	24 h	24 h	n/a	n/a	n/a	n/a	1
	WY	20 mg/mL	NS	n/a	a	24 h	4 d	n/a	n/a	n/a	n/a	1
Syringes, Plastic	WY	2.1–33.33 mg/mL	NS	288–439	a	8 h	48 h	n/a	n/a	n/a	n/a	5
	WY	2.1–33.33 mg/mL	D5W	264–416	a	2 h	4 h	n/a	n/a	n/a	n/a	5
Unspecified	APO[c]	Up to 20 mg/mL	D5W	n/a	a	2 h	4 h	n/a	n/a	n/a	n/a	1
		Up to 2 mg/mL	D5W	n/a	a	4 h	n/a	n/a	n/a	n/a	n/a	1
	APO[c]	Up to 20 mg/mL	NS	n/a	a	n/a	48 h	n/a	n/a	n/a	n/a	1
		Up to 30 mg/mL	NS	n/a	a	8 h	n/a	n/a	n/a	n/a	n/a	1
		30 mg/mL	NS	n/a	a	n/a	24 h	n/a	n/a	n/a	n/a	1
	APO[c]	Up to 20 mg/mL	W	n/a	a	n/a	72 h	n/a	n/a	n/a	n/a	1
		Up to 30 mg/mL	W	n/a	a	8 h	n/a	n/a	n/a	n/a	n/a	1
		30 mg/mL	W	n/a	a	n/a	48 h	n/a	n/a	n/a	n/a	1
OTHER INFUSION CONTAINERS												
AccuFlo™/AccuFlux™/AccuRX® (B. Braun)	unspec.	20 mg/mL	NS	372[1]	8.7[1]	8 h[b]	3 d[b]	n/a	n/a	n/a	n/a	2
AutoDose (Tandem Medical)	APO	10 mg/mL	NS	328[1]	a	24 h	3 d	n/a	n/a	n/a	n/a	1

Storage Conditions

continued on next page

Drug Manufacturer	Concentration	Diluents	Osmolality (mOsm/kg)	pH[a]	Storage Conditions							Refer.
					Temperature			Post-thaw Temp			Body Temp	
					Room	Refrig	Frozen	Room	Refrig			
Homepump Eclipse®/ Homepump® C-Series (I-Flow Corp.)	20 mg/mL	NS	372[1]	8.7[1]	8 h	3 d	n/a	n/a	n/a	n/a	n/a	4
INTERMATE (Baxter)	20 mg/mL	NS	372[1]	8.7[1]	8 h	72 h	n/a	n/a	n/a	n/a	n/a	3
INTERMATE/ INFUSOR (Baxter)	20–30 mg/mL	NS	n/a	[a]	8 h	48 h	n/a	n/a	n/a	n/a	n/a	3

Flush Compatibility: Heparin lock flush and normal saline.[1]

Special Considerations: Ampicillin stability decreases as concentration increases. Stability is greatly decreased in D5W. Storage temperature and pH of the solution affect stability. Do not freeze.[1]

Notes

[a]pH range of 10 mg/mL in recommended diluents and concentrations is 8–10. pH range of 20–100 mg/mL in W, NS or D5W is 8.7–9.3.[1]

[b]Manufacturer extrapolated data from other source(s).

[c]This data is applicable to other brands of ampicillin sodium injection, as this is part of the Abbreviated New Drug Application (ANDA) FDA-approved labeling. Refer to manufacturer-specific package inserts.

[d]Followed by 1 h simulated infusion.

References

1. Trissel LA. ASHP's Interactive Handbook on Injectable Drugs. Bethesda, MD: American Society of Health-System Pharmacists. Accessed 2012 Jun.
2. Drug Stability Data Using Elastomeric Infusion Systems. B. Braun Medical Production Ltd. (Thailand); August 2011.
3. Intermate/Infusor Drug Stability Information. Deerfield, IL: Baxter Healthcare Corporation; 2008.
4. Stability Data for Drugs Using Homepump Disposable Elastomeric Infusion Systems. Lake Forest, CA: I-Flow Corporation; October 2009.
5. Rapp RP, Hatton J, Record K. Drug Stability in Plastic Syringes. HealthTek™ and University of KY Lexington. Chester, NY: Repro-Med Systems Inc.; 1998–9.

Ampicillin Sodium–Sulbactam Sodium

CONTAINER	Drug Manufacturer	Concentration	Diluents	Osmolality (mOsm/kg)	pH[e]	Temperature Room	Temperature Refrig	Temperature Frozen	Post-thaw Temp Room	Post-thaw Temp Refrig	Body Temp	Refer.
Polyvinyl Chloride (PVC)	RR	20 mg/mL[a]	NS	n/a	e	32 h	68 h	n/a	n/a	n/a	n/a	1
Syringes, Plastic	WY	8.3, 16.7, 33.33 mg/mL[b]	NS	345, 413, n/a	e	8 h	48 h	n/a	n/a	n/a	n/a	4
	WY	8.3, 16.7, 33.33 mg/mL[b]	D5W	322, 390, n/a	e	2 h	4 h	n/a	n/a	n/a	n/a	4
Unspecified	PF	20 mg/mL[b]	NS, W	n/a	e	n/a	72 h	n/a	n/a	n/a	n/a	1
	PF	30 mg/mL[b]	NS, W	n/a	e	8 h	48 h	n/a	n/a	n/a	n/a	1
OTHER INFUSION CONTAINERS												
AccuFlo™/ AccuFlux™/ AccuRX® (B. Braun)	unspec.	30 mg/mL[b]	NS	n/a	e	n/a	3 d[g]	n/a	n/a	n/a	n/a	5
ADD-Vantage® (Abbott)	RR	20 mg/mL[b]	NS	n/a	e	8 h[f]	n/a	n/a	n/a	n/a	n/a	3
Glass	PF	20 mg/mL[a,d]	NS	n/a	e	n/a	72 h	n/a	n/a	n/a	n/a	3
	PF	20 mg/mL[a,d]	D5W	n/a	e	2 h	4 h	n/a	n/a	n/a	n/a	3
	PF	30 mg/mL[c,d]	NS	n/a	e	8 h	48 h	n/a	n/a	n/a	n/a	3
Homepump Eclipse®/ Homepump® C-Series (I-Flow Corp.)	unspec.	30 mg/mL[b]	NS	n/a	e	n/a	3 d	n/a	n/a	n/a	n/a	2

continued on next page

Ampicillin Sodium–Sulbactam Sodium (cont'd)

Flush Compatibility: Heparin lock flush and normal saline.[1]
Special Considerations: n/a

Notes

[a]Concentration studied was 20 mg/mL ampicillin plus 10 mg/mL sulbactam.
[b]Ampicillin concentration.
[c]Concentration studied was 30 mg/mL ampicillin plus 15 mg/mL sulbactam.
[d]Concentration of final dilutions is unspecified. See manufacturer's instructions for preparation.
[e]pH of solutions is 8–10.[1]
[f]After activation.
[g]Manufacturer extrapolated from other source(s).

References

1. Trissel LA. ASHP's Interactive Handbook on Injectable Drugs. Bethesda, MD: American Society of Health-System Pharmacists. Accessed 2011 Dec.
2. Stability Data for Drugs Using Homepump Elastomeric Infusion Systems. Lake Forest, CA: I-Flow Corporation; October 2009.
3. Unasyn® [product information]. New York, NY: Pfizer; April 2007.
4. Rapp RP, Hatton J, Record K. Drug Stability in Plastic Syringes. HealthTek™ and University of KY Lexington. Chester, NY: Repro-Med Systems Inc.; 1998.
5. Drug Stability Data Using Elastomeric Infusion Systems. B. Braun Medical Production Ltd. (Thailand); August 2011.

Azithromycin

Drug Manufacturer	Concentration	Diluents	Osmolality (mOsm/kg)	pH	Temperature Room	Temperature Refrig	Temperature Frozen	Post-thaw Temp Room	Post-thaw Temp Refrig	Body Temp	Refer.
CONTAINER											
Unspecified											
PF	1–2 mg/mL	D5W, NS[a]	n/a	6.4–6.6	24 h	7 d	n/a	n/a	n/a	n/a	1
OTHER INFUSION CONTAINERS											
AccuFlo™/ AccuFlux™/ AccuRX® (B. Braun)	1–2 mg/mL	NS, D5W	n/a	n/a	24 h[b]	7 d[b]	n/a	n/a	n/a	n/a	2
unspec.											

Flush Compatibility: Saline.
Special Considerations: Do not administer via IV bolus or IM. Infuse over no less than 60 min.

Notes

[a]Equivalent stability in $^1/_2$S, LR, D5$^1/_2$S, D5LR, D5$^1/_3$S, D5$^1/_2$S with KCl 20 mEq, NM in D5W, NR in D5W.
[b]Manufacturer extrapolated data from other sources.

References

1. Trissel LA. ASHP's Interactive Handbook on Injectable Drugs. Bethesda, MD: American Society of Health-System Pharmacists. Accessed 2012 May.
2. *Drug Stability Data Using Elastomeric Infusion Systems.* B. Braun Medical Production Ltd. (Thailand); August 2011.

Aztreonam

Container	Drug Manufacturer	Concentration	Diluents	Osmolality (mOsm/kg)	pH[a]	Temperature Room	Temperature Refrig	Temperature Frozen	Post-thaw Temp Room	Post-thaw Temp Refrig	Body Temp	Refer.
CONTAINER												
Polyvinyl Chloride (PVC)	SQ	10 mg/mL	NS	n/a	a	96 h	96 h	n/a	n/a	n/a	n/a	1
	SQ	10 & 20 mg/mL	NS, D5W	n/a	a	48 h	7 d	n/a	n/a	n/a	n/a	1
Syringes, Plastic	SQ	0.83, 16.7, 33.3 mg/mL	NS	312, 347, 415	a	48 h	7 d	90 d	n/a	n/a	n/a	5
Unspecified	SQ	10, 20 mg/mL	NS, D5W	n/a	a	n/a	n/a	3 m	24 h	72 h	n/a	1
	SQ	20 mg/mL	NS	n/a	a	37 d	120 d	120 d	n/a	n/a	n/a	1
OTHER INFUSION CONTAINERS												
AccuFlo™/ AccuFlux™/ AccuRX® (B. Braun)	unspec.	5–20 mg/mL	NS	n/a	a	n/a	28 d[c]	n/a	n/a	n/a	n/a	6
	unspec.	13.3–26.7 mg/mL	NS	n/a	a	7 d[c]	7 d[c]	n/a	n/a	n/a	n/a	6
	unspec.	20–30 mg/mL	NS	n/a	a	n/a	14 d[c]	n/a	n/a	n/a	n/a	6
	unspec.	60 mg/mL	NS	n/a	a	24 h[c]	28 d[c]	n/a	n/a	n/a	n/a	6
Homepump Eclipse®/ Homepump® C-Series (I-Flow Corp.)	unspec.	5–20 mg/mL	NS	n/a	a	n/a	28 d	n/a	n/a	n/a	n/a	4
	unspec.	20–30 mg/mL	NS	n/a	a	n/a	14 d	n/a	n/a	n/a	n/a	4
	unspec.	26.7 mg/mL	NS	n/a	a	7 d	7 d	n/a	n/a	n/a	n/a	4
	unspec.	60 mg/mL	NS	n/a	a	24 h	28 d	n/a	n/a	n/a	n/a	4
INTERMATE (Baxter)	BMS	5 mg/mL	NS, D5W	n/a	a	48 h[d]	28 d	n/a	n/a	n/a	n/a	3
	SQ	5–20 mg/mL	NS, D5W	n/a	a	24 h	14 d	30 d	24 h	n/a	n/a	3
	BMS	5–60 mg/mL	NS, D5W	n/a	a	24 h[d]	28 d	n/a	n/a	n/a	n/a	3
	BMS	10 mg/mL	W	n/a	a	n/a	10 d	n/a	n/a	n/a	n/a	3
COMMERCIAL PREPARATIONS (RTU)												
Galaxy Plastic Container (Baxter)	BMS	20, 40 mg/mL	D	iso	4.5–7.5	n/a	n/a	b	48 h[b]	14 d[b]	n/a	2

continued on next page

Aztreonam (cont'd)

Flush Compatibility: Heparin lock flush and normal saline.[1]
Special Considerations: n/a

Notes

[a]pH of aqueous solutions is 4.5–7.5.[1]
[b]Frozen expiration date per manufacturer's label. Do not extrapolate commercial premix stability data to extemporaneously compounded solutions.
[c]Manufacturer extrapolated data from other source(s).
[d]Following 28 d refrigerated.

References

1. Trissel LA. ASHP's Interactive Handbook on Injectable Drugs. Bethesda, MD: American Society of Health-System Pharmacists. Accessed 2012 Jun.
2. Azactam® in Galaxy Plastic Container [prescribing information]. Princeton, NJ: Bristol-Myers Squibb Company; January 2010.
3. Intermate/Infusor Drug Stability Information. Deerfield, IL: Baxter Healthcare Corporation; 2008.
4. Stability Data for Drugs Using Homepump Disposable Elastomeric Infusion Systems. Lake Forest, CA: I-Flow Corporation; October 2009.
5. Rapp RP, Hatton J, Record K. Drug Stability in Plastic Syringes. HealthTek™ and University of KY Lexington. Chester, NY: Repro-Med Systems Inc.; 1998.
6. Drug Stability Data Using Elastomeric Infusion Systems. B. Braun Medical Production Ltd. (Thailand); August 2011.

Baclofen

Drug Manufacturer	Concentration	Diluents	Osmolality (mOsm/kg)	pH[g]	Storage Conditions					Body Temp	Refer.
					Temperature			Post-thaw Temp			
					Room	Refrig	Frozen	Room	Refrig		
OTHER INFUSION CONTAINERS											
Fresenius Implantable Pump unspec.	0.5 mg/mL	undiluted	l	g	n/a	n/a	n/a	n/a	n/a	56 d	1
Glass CI	0.2 mg/mL[j]	NS	n/a	g	n/a	n/a	n/a	n/a	n/a	30 d	1
SH	1 mg/mL[e]	NS	n/a	g	n/a	n/a	n/a	n/a	n/a	70 d	1, 4
CI	1.5 mg/mL[i]	NS	r/a	g	n/a	n/a	n/a	n/a	n/a	30 d	1
Implantable Pump (Infusaid) CI	0.2 mg/mL[a]	NS	r/a	g	n/a	n/a	n/a	n/a	n/a	30 d	1
CI	0.8 mg/mL[b]	NS	r/a	g	n/a	n/a	n/a	n/a	n/a	29 d	1
CI	0.8 mg/mL[c]	NS	r/a	g	n/a	n/a	n/a	n/a	n/a	30 d	1
CI	1 mg/mL[d]	NS	154.6	g	n/a	n/a	n/a	n/a	n/a	30 d	1, 3
Synchromed® Implantable Pump (Medtronic) NVS	0.25, 0.5, 1 mg/mL	NS	n/a	g	n/a	n/a	n/a	n/a	n/a	14 w[f]	5
CI	0.5, 2 mg/mL	undiluted	l	g	n/a	n/a	n/a	n/a	n/a	90 d	2
NVS	1.5 mg/mL[h]	undiluted[h]	n/a	5.8	n/a	n/a	n/a	n/a	n/a	12 d	6
BB	2 mg/mL[k]	k	n/a	6.0	n/a	n/a	n/a	n/a	n/a	20 d	6

Flush Compatibility: Normal saline.[1]
Special Considerations: n/a

Notes

[a]*With morphine sulfate 1 mg/mL and 1.5 mg/mL.*
[b]*With morphine sulfate 1 mg/mL.*
[c]*With morphine sulfate 1.5 mg/mL.*
[d]*With morphine sulfate 15 mg/mL.*
[e]*Also stable when mixed with clonidine hydrochloride 0.2 mg/mL (both from powder).*
[f]*Combined with clonidine 0.25, 0.5 and 1 mg/mL.*
[g]*pH of undiluted solution is 5–7.[1]*
[h]*With ziconotide 25 mcg/mL.*
[i]*With morphine sulfate 7.5 mg/mL.*
[j]*With morphine sulfate 21 mg/mL.*

continued on next page

Baclofen (cont'd)

[k]Baclofen powder dissolved in ziconotide (ELN) 25 mcg/mL.
[l]Undiluted baclofen injection is an isotonic solution.[1]

References

1. Trissel LA. ASHP's Interactive Handbook on Injectable Drugs. Bethesda, MD: American Society of Health-System Pharmacists. Accessed 2012 Jun.
2. *Intrathecal Baclofen Therapy Clinical Reference Guide for Spasticity Management.* Minneapolis, MN: Medtronic Inc.; 1997:7–2.
3. Sitaram BR, Tsui M, Rawicki HB, et al. Stability and compatibility of intrathecal admixtures containing baclofen and high concentrations of morphine. *Int J Pharm (AMST).* 1997; 153:13–24.
4. Godwin DA, Kim NH, Zuniga R. Stability of a baclofen and clonidine hydrochloride admixture for intrathecal administration. *Hosp Pharm.* 2001; 36:950–4.
5. Alvarez JC, Mazancourt P, Chartier-Kastler E, et al. Drug stability testing to support clinical feasibility investigations for intrathecal baclofen-clonidine admixture. *J Pain Symptom Manage.* 2004; 28:268–72.
6. Shields D, Montenegro R, Aclan A. Chemical stability of admixtures combining ziconotide with baclofen during simulated intrathecal administration. *Neuromodulation* 2007; 10:S12–7.

Bevacizumab

CONTAINER	Drug Manufacturer	Concentration	Diluents	Osmolality (mOsm/kg)	pH[a]	Temperature Room	Temperature Refrig	Temperature Frozen	Post-thaw Temp Room	Post-thaw Temp Refrig	Body Temp	Refer.
Glass Vial	GEN	25 mg/mL[c]	undiluted[d]	n/a	6.2	n/a	3 m	n/a	n/a	n/a	n/a	2
Polyolefin Bag	GEN	unspec.[b]	NS	n/a	a	n/a	8 h	n/a	n/a	n/a	n/a	1
Polyvinyl Chloride (PVC)	GEN	unspec.[b]	NS	n/a	a	n/a	8 h	n/a	n/a	n/a	n/a	1
Syringes, Plastic	GEN	25 mg/mL[c]	undiluted	n/a	6.2	n/a	3 m	n/a	n/a	n/a	n/a	2

Flush Compatibility: Normal saline.
Special Considerations: Do not freeze. Do not administer or mix with dextrose solutions. Do not shake. Dilute desired dose in a total volume of 100 mL NS.[1] Not compatible with dextrose.[1]

Notes

[a] pH of undiluted solution is 6.2.[1]
[b] Concentrations may vary; calculated dosage should be diluted to a total volume of 100 mL NS.
[c] Do not administer as IV push or bolus. Must be diluted prior to administration.[1]
[d] Pierced vial.

References

1. Avastin® [prescribing information]. South San Francisco, CA: Genentech Inc.; May 2012.
2. Bakri SJ, Snyder MR, Pulido JS, et al. Six-month stability of Bevacizumab (Avastin) binding to vascular endothelial growth factor after withdrawal into a syringe and refrigeration or freezing. Retina 2006; 26:519–22.

Bleomycin Sulfate

Container	Drug Manufacturer	Concentration	Diluents	Osmolality (mOsm/kg)	pH[b]	Storage Conditions						Refer.
						Temperature			Post-thaw Temp		Body Temp	
						Room	Refrig	Frozen	Room	Refrig		
CONTAINER												
Polyvinyl Chloride (PVC)	unspec.	0.15 units/mL	NS	n/a	b	28 d[a]	n/a	n/a	n/a	n/a	n/a	1
OTHER INFUSION CONTAINERS												
INTERMATE (Baxter)	LUN	0.109 units/mL	NS	n/a	b	2 d[a]	n/a	n/a	n/a	n/a	n/a	2

Flush Compatibility: Heparin lock flush and normal saline.[1]

Special Considerations: Because of the risk of microbial contamination in products without preservatives, it is recommended that solutions be used within 24 hours of reconstitution.[1]

Notes

[a]*Protected from light.*
[b]*pH of reconstituted solutions is 4.0–6.*[1]

References

1. Trissel LA. ASHP's Interactive Handbook on Injectable Drugs. Bethesda, MD: American Society of Health-System Pharmacists. Accessed 2012 Jun.
2. *Intermate/Infusor Drug Stability Information.* Deerfield, IL: Baxter Healthcare Corporation; October 2008.

Bortezomib

Container / Drug Manufacturer	Concentration	Diluents	Osmolality (mOsm/kg)	pH[c]	Storage Conditions						Refer.
					Temperature			Post-thaw Temp		Body Temp	
					Room	Refrig	Frozen	Room	Refrig		
CONTAINER											
Syringes, Polypropylene	JC	1 mg/mL	NS	n/a	c	4 d[d]	7 d[a]	n/a	n/a	n/a	n/a	1, 4
OTHER INFUSION CONTAINERS											
Glass	JC	1 mg/mL	NS	n/a	c	n/a	5 d[b]	n/a	n/a	n/a	n/a	1, 4
Glass	JC	1 mg/mL[f]	NS	n/a	c	42 d	42 d	n/a	n/a	n/a	n/a	4, 5
Vial[f]	OB	1 mg/mL	NS	n/a	4–7	8 h	28 d[e]	n/a	n/a	n/a	n/a	2

Flush Compatibility: Normal saline.

Special Considerations: Handle according to guidelines for cytotoxic drugs. Storage time of reconstituted solution must not exceed 8 h if exposed to normal indoor lighting.[3]

Notes

[a] Protected from light, with air bubbles removed.
[b] In original container at 5°C and protected from light.
[c] pH of reconstituted preparation in NS is approximately 6.0.[1]
[d] Not protected from light.
[e] Protected from light.
[f] Stored in the original container.

References

1. Andre P, Cisternino S, Chiadmi F, et al. Stability of bortezomib solution in plastic syringe and glass vial. *Ann Pharmacother*. 2005; 39:1462–6.
2. Friess D, Nguyen HC, Lipp HP. HPLC stability data with reconstituted solutions containing bortezomib [translated from German]. *Deutscher Apotheker Verlag*. 2005; 6:206–10.
3. Velcade® for injection [prescribing information]. Cambridge, MA: Millennium Pharmaceuticals Inc.; January 2012.
4. Trissel LA. ASHP's Interactive Handbook on Injectable Drugs. Bethesda, MD: American Society of Health-System Pharmacists. Accessed 2012 Jun.
5. Walker SE, Milliken D, Law S. Stability of bortezomib reconstituted with 0.9% sodium chloride at 4°C and room temperature (23°C). *Can J Hosp Pharm*. 2008; 61:14–20.

Bumetanide

Container	Drug Manufacturer	Concentration	Diluents	Osmolality (mOsm/kg)	pH[a]	Storage Conditions							Refer.
						Temperature			Post-thaw Temp		Body Temp		
						Room	Refrig	Frozen	Room	Refrig			
Polyvinyl Chloride (PVC)	RC	0.02 mg/mL	D5W	n/a	n/a	72 h	n/a	n/a	n/a	n/a	n/a		1
	RC	0.2 mg/mL	D5W	n/a	n/a	72 h	n/a	n/a	n/a	n/a	n/a		1
	RC	0.25 mg/mL	undiluted	n/a	a	72 h	n/a	n/a	n/a	n/a	n/a		1, 2

Flush Compatibility: Normal saline.[1]
Special Considerations: n/a

Note
[a]pH of undiluted solution is ~7.[1]

References

1. Trissel LA. Interactive Handbook on Injectable Drugs. Bethesda, MD: American Society of Health-System Pharmacists. Accessed 2012 Jan.
2. Cornish LA, Montgomery PA, Johson PE. Stability of bumetanide in 5% dextrose injection. Am J Health-Syst Pharm. 1997; 54:422–3.

Bupivacaine Hydrochloride

Bupivacaine Hydrochloride[a,b]

continued on next page

Container	Drug Manufacturer	Concentration	Diluents	Osmolality (mOsm/kg)	pH[c]	Temperature Room	Temperature Refrig	Temperature Frozen	Post-thaw Temp Room	Post-thaw Temp Refrig	Body Temp	Refer.
CONTAINER												
Non-DEHP Bags (INTRAVIA, Baxter)	HSP	0.01 mg/mL[l]	NS	n/a	3.3–5.9	n/a	28 d[l,x,y]	n/a	n/a	n/a	n/a	7
	HSP	20 mg/mL[m]	NS	n/a	3.4–4.9	n/a	28 d[m,x,y]	n/a	n/a	n/a	n/a	7
	HSP	37.5 mg/mL[w]	NS	n/a	4.0–4.9	n/a	28 d[w,x,y]	n/a	n/a	n/a	n/a	7
Polyvinyl Chloride (PVC)	unspec.	0.6 mg/mL[p]	NS	n/a	n/a	30 d[p]	30 d[p]	n/a	n/a	n/a	n/a	1
	AB	0.625 mg/mL, 1.25 mg/mL	NS	r/a	[c]	72 h	n/a	n/a	n/a	n/a	n/a	1
	unspec.	0.85 mg/mL	NS	n/a	[c]	28 d	28 d	n/a	n/a	n/a	n/a	1
	unspec.	1.25 mg/mL[d]	NS	n/a	n/a	30 d[d]	30 d[d]	n/a	n/a	n/a	n/a	1
	AST	4 mg/mL[e]	NS	n/a	n/a	28 d[e,f]	n/a	n/a	n/a	n/a	n/a	4
Syringes, Polypropylene	HSP	0.01 mg/mL[l]	NS	n/a	3.3–6.0	n/a	28 d[l,x,y]	n/a	n/a	n/a	n/a	7
	AST	1 mg/mL	NS	n/a	[c]	30 d[y]	30 d[y]	n/a	n/a	n/a	30 d[y]	1, 5
	AST	1 mg/mL[g]	NS	n/a	n/a	30 d[g,y]	30 d[g,y]	n/a	n/a	n/a	30 d[g,y]	5
	AST	1.25 mg/mL	NS	n/a	[c]	32 d	32 d[x]	n/a	n/a	n/a	n/a	1
	AST	2.5 mg/mL[h]	NS[h]	n/a	n/a	91 d[h]	91 d[h]	n/a	n/a	n/a	n/a	6
	HSP	20 mg/mL[m]	NS	n/a	3.4–5.3	n/a	28 d[m,x,y]	n/a	n/a	n/a	n/a	7
	HSP	37.5 mg/mL[w]	NS	n/a	4.6–5.0	n/a	28 d[w,x,y]	n/a	n/a	n/a	n/a	7
OTHER INFUSION CONTAINERS												
AccuFlo™/ AccuFlux™/ AccuRX® (B. Braun)	unspec.	0.125%	NS	n/a	[c]	30 d	30 d	n/a	n/a	n/a	n/a	8
	unspec.	0.5%	NS	n/a	[c]	30 d	30 d	n/a	n/a	n/a	n/a	8
CADD® Cassette (SIMS Deltec)	WI	0.44 mg/mL[n]	[n]	n/a	n/a	20 d[o]	20 d[o]	n/a	n/a	n/a	n/a	1
	AST	1.25 mg/mL	NS	n/a	[c]	4 d	7 d	n/a	n/a	n/a	n/a	2
	AST	2 mg/mL[z]	NS	n/a	n/a	n/a	30 d[z]	n/a	n/a	n/a	30 d[z]	1
	unspec.	3 mg/mL[za]	NS	n/a	n/a	10 d[za]	10 d[za]	n/a	n/a	n/a	10 d[za]	1
	AST	5 mg/mL	NS	n/a	[c]	7 d	7 d	n/a	n/a	n/a	n/a	2

Bupivacaine Hydrochloride (cont'd)

Drug Manufacturer	Concentration	Diluents	Osmolality (mOsm/kg)	pH[c]	Storage Conditions					Refer.
					Temperature			Post-thaw Temp		Body Temp	
					Room	Refrig	Frozen	Room	Refrig		

Drug Manufacturer	Concentration	Diluents	Osmolality (mOsm/kg)	pH[c]	Room	Refrig	Frozen	Room	Refrig	Body Temp	Refer.
INFUSOR (Baxter)											
AST	0.5–7.5 mg/mL[u]	NS, D5W	n/a	n/a	n/a	30 d[u,v]	n/a	n/a	n/a	n/a	3
AST	0.6–7.5 mg/mL	NS, D5W, W	n/a	c	30 d	180 d[q]	n/a	n/a	n/a	n/a	3
AST	6.75 mg/mL[s]	NS	n/a	n/a	28 d[r,s]	93 d[s,t]	n/a	n/a	n/a	n/a	3
AST	6.75 mg/mL[s]	NS	n/a	n/a	14 d[s,t]	n/a	n/a	n/a	n/a	n/a	3
Synchromed® Implanted Pump (Medtronic)											
unspec.	7.5 mg/mL[j]	j	n/a	c	n/a	n/a	n/a	n/a	n/a	12 w[k]	1
unspec.	25 mg/mL[l]	W[i]	n/a	n/a	n/a	n/a	n/a	n/a	n/a	90 d[k]	1

Flush Compatibility: n/a: not used intravenously.
Special Considerations: n/a

Notes

[a]Do not use products or diluents containing preservatives for intraspinal or epidural administration.
[b]Avoid freezing.
[c]pH range of undiluted product is 4–6.5.[1]
[d]Admixed with fentanyl citrate 0.002 mg/mL and 0.02 mg/mL.
[e]Combined with morphine tartrate 1 mg/mL and midazolam hydrochloride 0.5 mg/mL.
[f]Protected from light at 22°C ± 2°C.
[g]Combined with fentanyl citrate 35 mcg/mL and clonidine hydrochloride 9 mcg/mL at 4°C, 21°C, 25°C.
[h]Stored at 22°C, exposed to light, at 6°C protected from light; also contained hydromorphone 0.02 or 0.04 mg/mL.
[i]With clonidine HCl 2 mg/mL and morphine sulfate 50 mg/mL.
[j]In Dextrose 8.25% (Marcaine™ spinal).
[k]Stored at 37°C.
[l]With hydromorphone (SZ) 0.01 mg/mL or 43 mg/mL; or morphine (SZ) 0.01 mg/mL or 43 mg/mL; or fentanyl (SZ) 0.15 mcg/mL or 43 mcg/mL.
[m]With hydromorphone (SZ) 0.01 mg/mL or 25 mg/mL; or morphine (SZ) 0.01 mg/mL or 25 mg/mL; or fentanyl (SZ) 0.15 mcg/mL or 25 mcg/mL.
[n]With fentanyl citrate (IN) 1.25 mcg/mL and epinephrine hydrochloride (AB) 0.69 mcg/mL.
[o]Followed by a 48 h infusion at near body temperature (30°C).
[p]With fentanyl 0.002 mg/mL.
[q]Followed by 14 d at room temperature.
[r]Followed by 2 d at 33°C.
[s]With sufentanil citrate (IN) 5 mcg/mL.
[t]Followed by 7 d at 33°C.

continued on next page

Bupivacaine Hydrochloride (cont'd)

uWith fentanyl citrate (JN) 1–5 mcg/mL.
vFollowed by 3 d at room temperature, followed by 5 d at 33°C.
wWith hydromorphone (SZ) 0.01 mg/mL; or morphine (SZ) 0.01 mg/mL; or fentanyl (SZ) 0.15 mcg/mL.
xProtected from light.
yAlthough pH remained within stability range for the drug, this does not definitively demonstrate stability.l
zWith sufentanil 5 mcg/mL at 4°C and at 32°C.
zaWith sufentanil 0.2 mg/mL.

References

1. Trissel LA. ASHP's Interactive Handbook on Injectable Drugs. Bethesda, MD: American Society of Health-System Pharmacists. Accessed 2012 Jul.
2. Astra Pain Control AB. CADD Ambulatory Infusion Pump System Stability Data. St. Paul, MN: SIMS Deltec Inc.; 1995.
3. Intermate/Infusor Drug Stability Information. Deerfield, IL: Baxter Healthcare Corporation; October 2008.
4. La Forgia SP, Sharley NA, Burgess NG, et al. Stability and compatibility of morphine, midazolam, and bupivacaine combinations for intravenous infusion. J Pharm Practice Res. 2002; 32:65–8.
5. Jappinen A, Kokki H, Naaranlahti T. pH stability of injectable fentanyl, bupivacaine, or clonidine solution or a ternary mixture in 0.9% sodium chloride in two types of polypropylene syringes. Int J Pharm Compound. 2002; 6:471–4.
6. Donnelly RF. Physical compatibility and chemical stability of bupivacaine and hydromorphone in polypropylene syringes. Can J Hosp Pharm. 2004; 57:230–5.
7. Donnelly RF, Wong K, Spencer J. Physical compatibility of high-concentration bupivacaine with hydromorphone, morphine, and fentanyl. Can J Hosp Pharm. 2010; 63:154–5.
8. Drug Stability Data Using Elastomeric Infusion Systems. B. Braun Medical Production Ltd. (Thailand); August 2011.

Calcitriol

CONTAINER	Drug Manufacturer	Concentration	Diluents	Osmolality (mOsm/kg)	pH	Storage Conditions Temperature Room	Refrig	Frozen	Post-thaw Temp Room	Refrig	Body Temp	Refer.
Polyvinyl Chloride (PVC)[a]	n/a	n/a	n/a	n/a	n/a	n/a	n/a	n/a	n/a	n/a	n/a	1
Syringes, Plastic	n/a	0.8, 1, 2 mcg/mL[b]	undiluted	iso	d,e	n/a	7 d	n/a	n/a	n/a	n/a	2
	AB	1, 2 mcg/mL[b]	undiluted	iso	d,e	20 d[c]	n/a	n/a	n/a	n/a	n/a	1

Flush Compatibility: Normal saline.[1]
Special Considerations: n/a

Notes

[a]Adsorbs rapidly to PVC (50% in 2 h).
[b]In polypropylene syringes.
[c]4% loss within 20 d due to sorption.
[d]The pH of undiluted Calcijex (AB) is 5.9 to 7.0.[1]
[e]The pH of undiluted calcitriol injection (AMR) is 6.7 to to 7.7.[1]

References

1. Trissel LA. ASHP's Interactive Handbook on Injectable Drugs. Bethesda, MD: American Society of Health-System Pharmacists. Accessed 2012 May.
2. Vargas-Ruiz M, Bushman LR, Hillegas MS, et al. Stability of parenteral calcitriol in a tuberculin syringe. Paper presented at: ASHP Midyear Clinical Meeting; Miami, FL. 1994; 29:P-243. Abstract.

Calcitriol

Carboplatin

continued on next page

CONTAINER	Drug Manufacturer	Concentration	Diluents	Osmolality (mOsm/kg)	pH[a,f]	Temperature			Post-thaw Temp		Body Temp	Refer.
						Room	Refrig	Frozen	Room	Refrig		
Ethyvinyl Acetate (EVA)	BMS	1 mg/mL	D5W	n/a	f	28 d[b]	28 d[b]	n/a	n/a	n/a	28 d[b,e]	1, 6
Polyvinyl Chloride (PVC)	BMS	0.5, 4 mg/mL	D5W	n/a	f	21 d	21 d	n/a	n/a	n/a	n/a	2
	TE	0.7, 2.15 mg/mL	D5W	n/a	a	24 h	84 d[b,d]	n/a	n/a	n/a	n/a	6, 7
	BMS	1 mg/mL	D5W	n/a	f	28 d[b]	28 d[b]	n/a	n/a	n/a	28 d[b,e]	1, 6
	BMS	1 mg/mL	W	n/a	f	n/a	14 d	n/a	n/a	n/a	14 d	6
	BR	2.4 mg/mL	D5W	n/a	f	9 d[b]	n/a	n/a	n/a	n/a	n/a	1, 6
Syringes, Plastic	BMS	10 mg/mL	W	n/a	f	n/a	5 d	n/a	n/a	n/a	24 h	3, 6
Syringes, Polypropylene	BMS	10 mg/mL	W	n/a	f	8 d[b]	n/a	n/a	n/a	n/a		4, 6
OTHER INFUSION CONTAINERS												
CADD® Cassette (Pharmacia Deltec)	BR	6 mg/mL	D5W	n/a	f	n/a	n/a	n/a	n/a	n/a	14 d[b]	6
	BR	10 mg/mL	W	n/a	f	n/a	n/a	n/a	n/a	n/a	14 d[b]	6
Glass	BMS	0.5, 4 mg/mL	D5W	n/a	f	21 d[b]	21 d[b]	n/a	n/a	n/a	n/a	6
	BMS	0.75, 2 mg/mL	D5W	n/a	f	7 d[b]	7 d[b]	n/a	n/a	n/a	n/a	6
	BM	1 mg/mL	D5W	n/a	f	28 d[b]	28 d[b]	n/a	n/a	n/a	28 d[b,e]	1, 6
	unspec.	1 mg/mL	W	n/a	f	14 d	n/a	n/a	n/a	n/a	n/a	6
INFUSOR (Baxter)	BMS	0.5–10 mg/mL	D5W	n/a	f	n/a	91 d[c]	n/a	n/a	n/a	7 d[c]	5
	BMS	1 mg/mL	D5W	n/a	f	28 d	28 d	n/a	n/a	n/a	n/a	6
Polyolefin (Fresenius Kabi UK)	TE	0.7, 2.15 mg/mL	D5W	n/a	a	24 h	84 d[b,d]	n/a	n/a	n/a	n/a	6, 7

Storage Conditions

Flush Compatibility: Normal saline.[6]
Special Considerations: n/a

86

Carboplatin (cont'd)

Notes

[a] pH range for the concentrations and diluent in this study was 4.16–4.67 at various time points and storage conditions.[7]

[b] Protected from light.

[c] Stored 91 d refrigerated followed by 7 d at body temperature.

[d] Infusions were stored refrigerated for 84 d, then stored at 25°C for 24 h, then again refrigerated for another 7 d.

[e] Stored at 35°C.

[f] pH of a 1% solution is 5–7.[1]

References

1. Rochard E, Barthes D, Courtois P. Stability and compatibility study of carboplatin with three portable infusion pump reservoirs. *Int J Pharm.* 1994; 101:257–62.
2. Amador FD, Azzati ES, Lopez-Coterilla A. Stability of carboplatin in polyvinyl chloride bags. *Am J Health-Syst Pharm.* 1998; 55:602, 604.
3. Sewell GJ, Riley CM, Rowland CG. The stability of carboplatin in ambulatory continuous infusion regimens. *J Clin Pharm Ther.* 1987; 12:427–32.
4. Valiere C, Arnaud P, Caroff E, et al. Stability and compatibility study of a carboplatin solution in syringes for continuous ambulatory infusion. *Int J Pharm.* 1996; 138:125–8.
5. Intermate/Infusor Drug Stability Information. Deerfield, IL: Baxter Healthcare Corporation; October 2008.
6. Trissel LA. ASHP's Interactive Handbook on Injectable Drugs. Bethesda, MD: American Society of Health-System Pharmacists. Accessed 2012 Jul.
7. Kaestner S, Sewell G. A sequential temperature cycling study for the investigation of carboplatin infusion stability to facilitate "dose banding." *J Oncol Pharm Practice* 2007; 13:119–26.

Caspofungin Acetate

Drug Manufacturer	Concentration	Diluents	Osmolality (mOsm/kg)	pH[a]	Temperature			Post-thaw Temp			Refer.
					Room	Refrig	Frozen	Room	Refrig	Body Temp	
CONTAINER											
Unspecified[b]	ME	0.2 mg–≤0.5 mg/mL	NS, LR 1/2S, 1/4S	266–303[c]	a	24 h	48 h	n/a	n/a	n/a	n/a	2
OTHER INFUSION CONTAINERS											
Homepump®/ Homepump Eclipse® (I-Flow Corp.)	ME	0.2, 0.28, 0.5 mg/mL	NS	n/a	a	60 h	14 d	n/a	n/a	n/a	n/a	1
INTERMATE (Baxter)	ME	0.2, 0.28, 0.5 mg/mL	NS	n/a	a	60 h	14 d	n/a	n/a	n/a	n/a	1

Flush Compatibility: Normal saline.

Special Considerations: Do not mix with dextrose-containing solutions. Final concentration should not exceed 0.5 mg/mL. The reconstituted solution (vial) may be stored for up to 1 h at controlled room temperature.[2]

Notes

[a]pH of saturated aqueous solution is approximately 6.0.[2]

[b]IV bag or bottle.[2]

[c]At these concentrations in NS or LR, osmolality was 266–303 mOsm/kg.[1]

References

1. Merck Global Medical Information [personal communication]. North Wales, PA: Merck & Co., Inc.; January 2012.

2. Cancidas® [package insert]. Whitehouse Station, NJ: Merck & Co Inc.; June 2010.

Cefazolin Sodium

Storage Conditions

Container	Drug Manufacturer	Concentration	Diluents	Osmolality (mOsm/kg)	pH[e]	Temperature Room	Temperature Refrig	Temperature Frozen	Post-thaw Temp Room	Post-thaw Temp Refrig	Body Temp	Refer.
CONTAINER												
Ethyvinyl Acetate (EVA)	unspec.	10 mg/mL	NS	n/a	e	7 d	30 d	n/a	n/a	n/a	n/a	7
Glass	LI	20 mg/mL	D5W, NS	n/a	e	24 h	7 d	n/a	n/a	n/a	n/a	1
	SCN	20 mg/mL	D5W, NS	n/a	e	n/a	n/a	12 w	24 h	n/a	n/a	1
	SKF	73.2 mg/mL	W	n/a	e	n/a	n/a	30 d	n/a	4 d	24 h	1
Polyvinyl Chloride (PVC)	unspec.	5 mg/mL	D5W	n/a	e	4 d	14 d	n/a	n/a	n/a	n/a	1
	LI	10 mg/mL	D5W	n/a	e	24 h	n/a	30 d	24 h	n/a	n/a	1
	BR	10 mg/mL	D5W	n/a	e	n/a	30 d	n/a	n/a	n/a	n/a	1
	LI, SKF	10 mg/mL	D5W, NS	n/a	e	n/a	n/a	48 h	4 h	n/a	n/a	1
	LI	20 mg/mL	NS	n/a	e	7 d	15 d	n/a	n/a	n/a	n/a	1
	LI	20 mg/mL	D5W	n/a	e	5 d	24 d	n/a	n/a	n/a	n/a	1
	SKF	20 mg/mL	NS, D5W	n/a	e	5 d	15 d	n/a	n/a	n/a	n/a	4
	SKF	20 mg/mL	D5W, NS	n/a	e	24 h	24 h	30 d	n/a	n/a	n/a	1
	SKF	73.2 mg/mL	W	n/a	e	n/a	n/a	30 d	n/a	4 d	24 h	1
Syringes, Plastic	unspec.	8.33, 16.7, 33.3 mg/mL	NS	309, 341, 404	n/a	24 h	96 h	26 w	n/a	n/a	n/a	8
	unspec.	8.33, 16.7, 33.3 mg/mL	D5W	285, 317, 380	n/a	24 h	96 h	26 w	n/a	n/a	n/a	8
	SKF	100, 200 mg/mL	W	340, 680	e	13 d[a]	28 d[a]	3 m	n/a	n/a	n/a	1, 2
Syringes, Polypropylene	APO	50 mg/mL	NS	n/a	e	12 d	22 d	n/a	n/a	n/a	n/a	1
OTHER INFUSION CONTAINERS												
AccuFlo™/ AccuFlux™/ AccuRX® (B. Braun)	unspec.	20 mg/mL	NS	n/a	e	24 h[i]	7 d[i]	n/a	n/a	n/a	n/a	11

continued on next page

Cefazolin Sodium (cont'd)

Cefazolin Sodium (cont'd)

Drug Manufacturer	Concentration	Diluents	Osmolality (mOsm/kg)	pH[e]	Temperature Room	Temperature Refrig	Temperature Frozen	Post-thaw Temp Room	Post-thaw Temp Refrig	Body Temp	Refer.
AutoDose (Tandem Medical) unspec.	10 mg/mL	NS	n/a	e	7 d	30 d	n/a	n/a	n/a	n/a	6
Homepump®/ Homepump Eclipse® (I-Flow Corp.) unspec.	20 mg/mL	NS	n/a	e	24 h	7 d	n/a	n/a	n/a	n/a	5
INTERMATE/ INFUSOR (Baxter) LI	5–40 mg/mL	NS, D5W	n/a	e	24 h	10 d	30 d	24 h	n/a	n/a	3
SKF	10–40 mg/mL	D5W	n/a	e	4 d[i]	17 d[i]	n/a	n/a	n/a	n/a	3
LI	20 mg/mL	W	n/a	e	n/a	10 d	n/a	n/a	n/a	n/a	3
Unspecified LI	3.33 mg/mL	NS	n/a	n/a	3 d	7 d	n/a	n/a	n/a	3 d[d]	1, 9
LI	5 mg/mL	NS	n/a	e	4 d	7 d	n/a	n/a	n/a	n/a	1
unspec.	5, 222.2, 400 mg/mL	W, D5W, NS	n/a	e	n/a	n/a	26 w[c]	n/a	n/a	n/a	1
unspec.	250 mg/mL	W	n/a	e	4 d	14 d	n/a	n/a	n/a	n/a	1
COMMERCIAL PREPARATIONS											
Duplex® Flexible Dual-Chambered Container (B. Braun) BRN	20 mg/mL	f	iso	n/a	24 h[g]	7 d[g]	n/a	n/a	n/a	n/a	1, 10
Galaxy Bag (Baxter)[b] unspec.	20 mg/mL	D5W	iso	4.5–7[1]	n/a	n/a	b, h	48 h	30 d	n/a	7

Storage Conditions

Flush Compatibility: Heparin lock flush and normal saline.[1]
Special Considerations: n/a

continued on next page

Cefazolin Sodium (cont'd)

Notes

[a]Manufacturer recommends discarding solutions after 24 h at room temperature and 10 d refrigeration to reduce potential for microbial growth, color change, and pH change.

[b]Frozen expiration date per manufacturer's label. Do not extrapolate commercial premix stability data to extemporaneously compounded solutions.

[c]When frozen within 1 h of reconstitution.

[d]Tested at 35°C.

[e]pH of reconstituted solutions 225 to 300 mg/mL in W is 4.5–6.[10]

[f]Diluent in the Duplex® dual-chamber system is iso-osmotic hydrous dextrose USP.[10]

[g]Prior to activation, expiration date is per manufacturer's label. To avoid inadvertent activation, DUPLEX container should remain folded until intended activation time. Protect from light after removal of foil strip. Once light-protecting foil strip is removed, product must be activated and used within 7 d.

[h]Thaw at room temperature or under refrigeration. Do not force thaw. Do not refreeze.

[i]17 d refrigerated may be followed by 4 d at room temperature.

[j]Manufacturer extrapolated data from other sources.

References

1. Trissel LA. ASHP's Interactive Handbook on Injectable Drugs. Bethesda, MD: American Society of Health-System Pharmacists. Accessed 2012 Jan.
2. Garrelts JC, Ast D, LaRocca J, et al. Postinfusion phlebitis after intravenous push versus intravenous piggyback administration of antimicrobial agents. Clin Pharm. 1988; 7:760–5.
3. Intermate/Infusor Drug Stability Information. Deerfield, IL: Baxter Healthcare Corporation; 2008.
4. Das Gupta V, Stewart KR. Quantitation of carbenicillin disodium, cefazolin sodium, cephalothin sodium, nafcillin sodium, and ticarcillin disodium by high pressure liquid chromatography. J Pharm Sci. 1980; 69(11):1264–7.
5. Stability Data for Drugs Using Homepump Disposable Elastomeric Infusion Systems. Lake Forest, CA: I-Flow Corporation; October 2009.
6. AutoDose Stability Reference. San Diego, CA: Tandem Medical Inc.; 2002.
7. Cefazolin Injection USP in Galaxy® Container (PL 2040 Plastic). Deerfield, IL: Baxter Healthcare Corporation; May 2006.
8. Rapp RP, Hatton J, Record K. Drug Stability in Plastic Syringes. HealthTek™ and University of KY Lexington. Chester, NY: Repro-Med Systems Inc.; 1998.
9. McEvoy GK, ed. AHFS Drug Information 2008. Bethesda, MD: American Society of Health-System Pharmacists; 2008:107.
10. Cefazolin for Injection USP and Dextrose Injection USP in Duplex® Drug Delivery System [package insert]. Irvine, CA: B. Braun Medical Inc.; April 2008.
11. Drug Stability Data Using Elastomeric Infusion Systems. B. Braun Medical Production Ltd. (Thailand); August 2011.

Cefepime Hydrochloride

Container	Drug Manufacturer	Concentration	Diluents	Osmolality (mOsm/kg)	pH[f]	Temperature Room	Temperature Refrig	Temperature Frozen	Post-thaw Temp Room	Post-thaw Temp Refrig	Body Temp	Refer.
CONTAINER												
Ethyvinyl Acetate (EVA)	BMS	10 mg/mL	NS	n/a	f	2 d	30 d	n/a	n/a	n/a	n/a	4
	BMS	40 mg/mL	NS	n/a	f	24 h	7 d	n/a	n/a	n/a	n/a	4
Polyvinyl Chloride (PVC)	BMS	1, 40 mg/mL	NS, D5W, D5S	n/a	f	24 h	7 d	n/a	n/a	n/a	n/a	1
	BMS	2.5 mg/mL	D5W	n/a	f	3 d	7 d	n/a	n/a	n/a	n/a	5
	BMS	2.5 mg/mL	NS	n/a	f	5 d	7 d	n/a	n/a	n/a	n/a	5
	BMS	5 mg/mL	D5W	n/a	f	24 h	7 d	n/a	n/a	n/a	n/a	5
	BMS	5 mg/mL	NS	n/a	f	3 d	7 d	n/a	n/a	n/a	n/a	5
	BMS	10 mg/mL	D5W	n/a	f	2 d	7 d	n/a	n/a	n/a	n/a	5
	BMS	10 mg/mL	NS	n/a	f	24 h	7 d	n/a	n/a	n/a	n/a	1
	BMS	20 mg/mL	NS, D5W	n/a	f	2 d	23 d	n/a	n/a	n/a	n/a	1
	BMS	20 mg/mL	D5W, NS	n/a	f	3 d	7 d	n/a	n/a	n/a	n/a	5
	BMS	20 mg/mL	D5W	n/a	f	n/a	n/a	30 d	n/a	11 d	n/a	1
Syringes, Plastic	BMS	100, 200 mg/mL	W, NS, D5W	n/a	f	n/a	5 d[k]	n/a	n/a	n/a	n/a	1
	BMS	100, 200 mg/mL	W, NS, D5W	n/a	n/a	1 d	14 d	90 d	n/a	n/a	n/a	1
Syringes, Polypropylene	BMS	20 mg/mL	NS	n/a	n/a	2 d	21 d	n/a	n/a	n/a	n/a	1
	BMS	100, 200 mg/mL	W, NS, D5W	n/a	n/a	n/a	n/a	90 d	n/a	7 d	n/a	1
	BMS	100, 200 mg/mL	W, NS, D5W	n/a	n/a	n/a	n/a	90 d	1 d[J]	3 d[d]	n/a	5, 6
	BMS	100, 200 mg/mL	W, NS, D5W	n/a	n/a	n/a	n/a	60 d	1 d[e]	7 d[e]	n/a	5, 6
OTHER INFUSION CONTAINERS												
AccuFlo™/ AccuFlux™/ AccuRX® (B. Braun)	unspec.	20 mg/mL	NS	n/a	f	24 h[l]	14 d[ll]		n/a	n/a	n/a	8

continued on next page

92

Cefepime Hydrochloride (cont'd)

	Drug Manufacturer	Concentration	Diluents	Osmolality (mOsm/kg)	pH^i	Storage Conditions						Refer.
						Temperature			Post-thaw Temp		Body Temp	
						Room	Refrig	Frozen	Room	Refrig		
ADD-Vantage® Container (Abbott)	BMS/ELN^g	10, 20, 40 mg/mL	NS, D5W	n/a	n/a	24 h^h	7 d^h	n/a	n/a	n/a	n/a	7
AutoDose (Tandem Medical)	BMS	10 mg/mL	NS	n/a	f	2 d	30 d	n/a	n/a	n/a	n/a	4
	BMS	40 mg/mL	NS	n/a	f	24 h	7 d	n/a	n/a	n/a	n/a	4
Homepump®/ Homepump Eclipse® (I-Flow Corp.)	unspec.	20 mg/mL	NS	n/a	f	24 h	14 d	n/a	n/a	n/a	n/a	3
INTERMATE/ INFUSOR (Baxter)	BMS	1–5 mg/mL	NS, D5W	n/a	f	2 d	14 d^a	n/a	n/a	n/a	n/a	2
	BMS	1–5 mg/mL	NS, D5W	n/a	f	2 d	7 d^b	n/a	n/a	n/a	n/a	2
	BMS	1–5 mg/mL	NS, D5W	n/a	f	n/a	n/a	63 d	48 h	7 d^c	n/a	2
	BMS	5–60 mg/mL	NS, D5W	n/a	f	24 h	n/a	63 d	24 h	n/a	n/a	2
Unspecified	BMS/ELN^g	1–40 mg/mL	NS, D5W, D5S, D5LR, D10W	n/a	n/a	24 h	7 d	n/a	n/a	n/a	n/a	7
COMMERCIAL PREPARATIONS (RTU)												
Duplex® Flexible Dual Chambered Container (B. Braun)	BRN	20, 40 mg/mL	i	iso	n/a	12 h^i	5 d^i	n/a	n/a	n/a	n/a	9

Flush Compatibility: Heparin lock flush and normal saline.[1]
Special Considerations: n/a

continued on next page

Cefepime Hydrochloride (cont'd)

Notes

[a]May be followed by 24 h at room temperature.

[b]May be followed by 48 h at room temperature.

[c]May be followed by 2 d at room temperature.

[d]90 d at −20°C followed by 3 d at 4°C followed by 1 d at 22°C to 24°C.

[e]90 d at −20°C followed by 7 d at 4°C followed by 1 d at 22°C to 24°C.

[f]pH of reconstituted preparation is 4–6.[1]

[g]Manufactured for BMS; distributed by ELN.

[h]After activation of ADD-Vantage® container, reconstitute and dilute medication per labeled instructions.

[i]Diluent in the Duplex® dual chamber system is iso-osmotic hydrous dextrose USP.[9]

[j]Prior to activation, expiration date is per manufacturer's label. Protect from light after removal of foil strip. If light-protecting foil strip is removed, product must be activated within 7 d.

[k]Followed by 24 h at room temperature.

[l]Manufacturer extrapolated data from other sources.

References

1. Trissel LA. ASHP's Interactive Handbook on Injectable Drugs. Bethesda, MD: American Society of Health-System Pharmacists. Accessed 2012 Jan.
2. Intermate/Infusor Drug Stability Information. Deerfield, IL: Baxter Healthcare Corporation; 2008.
3. Stability Data for Drugs Using Homepump Disposable Elastomeric Infusion Systems. Lake Forest, CA: I-Flow Corporation; October 2009.
4. AutoDose Stability Reference. San Diego, CA: Tandem Medical Inc.; 2002.
5. Stewart JT, Maddox FC, Warren FW. Stability of cefepime hydrochloride injection and metronidazole in polyvinyl chloride bags at 4° and 22°–24°C. Hosp Pharm. 2000; 35:1061–4.
6. Medical Information Department [personal communication]. San Diego, CA: Elan Pharmaceuticals Inc.; March 2008.
7. Maxipime™ [product information]. San Diego, CA: Elan Pharmaceuticals Inc.; March 2009.
8. Drug Stability Data Using Elastomeric Infusion Systems. B. Braun Medical Production Ltd. (Thailand); August 2011.
9. Cefepime for Injection USP and Dextrose Injection USP in Duplex® Drug Delivery System [package insert]. Irvine, CA: B. Braun Medical Inc.; June 2011.

Cefotaxime Sodium

Cefotaxime Sodium

Container	Drug Manufacturer	Concentration	Diluents	Osmolality (mOsm/kg)	pH[g]	Temperature Room	Temperature Refrig	Temperature Frozen	Post-thaw Room	Post-thaw Refrig	Body Temp	Refer.
CONTAINER												
Polyvinyl Chloride (PVC)	SAV	c	D5W, NS	n/a	n/a	24 h	5 d	13 w	n/a	n/a	n/a	1, 2
	HO	c	D5W, NS	n/a	n/a	n/a	n/a	13 w	24 h	5 d	n/a	1
	HO	10 mg/mL	NS, D5W	344, 319	n/a	24 h	22 d	63 d	n/a	n/a	n/a	1
	HO	20 mg/mL	D5W	327	n/a	24 h	24 h	n/a	n/a	n/a	n/a	1
	HO	20 mg/mL	NS	351	n/a	24 h	n/a	n/a	n/a	n/a	n/a	1
Syringes, Plastic	HO	c	D5W, NS	n/a	n/a	n/a	n/a	13 w	24 h	5 d	n/a	1
	HO	16.7, 33.3 mg/mL	NS	340, 403	n/a	24 h	5 d	13 w	n/a	n/a	n/a	7
	HO	16.7, 33.3 mg/mL	D5W	317, 380	n/a	24 h	5 d	13 w	n/a	n/a	n/a	7
	SAV	50, 95 mg/mL	W	h	g	24 h	5 d	i	n/a	n/a	n/a	2
	SAV	180, 230, 300, 330 mg/mL	W	h	g	12 h	5 d	i	n/a	n/a	n/a	2
Syringes, Polypropylene	AVE	50 mg/mL	NS	n/a	n/a	2 d	18 d	n/a	n/a	n/a	n/a	1
OTHER INFUSION CONTAINERS												
AccuFlo™/ AccuFlux™/ AccuRX® (B. Braun)	unspec.	16.66 mg/mL	NS	n/a	n/a	24 h[a]	n/a	n/a	n/a	n/a	n/a	3
	unspec.	20 mg/mL	NS	n/a	n/a	24 h	14 d	n/a	n/a	n/a	n/a	3
Glass	SAV	10–40 mg/mL[k]	D5W, NS	n/a	n/a	24 h	10 d	n/a	n/a	n/a	n/a	2
	SAV	50, 95 mg/mL[k]	W	h	g	24 h	7 d	n/a	n/a	n/a	n/a	2
	SAV	180, 230, 300, 330 mg/mL[k]	W	h	g	12 h	7 d	n/a	n/a	n/a	n/a	2
Homepump Eclipse®/ Homepump® C-Series (I-Flow Corp.)	unspec.	16.66 mg/mL	NS	n/a	n/a	24 h	n/a	n/a	n/a	n/a	n/a	6

continued on next page

95

Cefotaxime Sodium (cont'd)

Cefotaxime Sodium (cont'd)

Drug Manufacturer	Concentration	Diluents	Osmolality (mOsm/kg)	pH[g]	Temperature			Post-thaw Temp		Body Temp	Refer.
					Room	Refrig	Frozen	Room	Refrig		
INTERMATE/ INFUSOR (Baxter) HO	5–40 mg/mL	D5W, NS	n/a	n/a	24 h	n/a	30 d	24 h	n/a	n/a	5
HO	40 mg/mL	NS	n/a	n/a	24 h	10 d	n/a	n/a	n/a	n/a	5
COMMERCIAL PREPARATIONS (RTU)											
ADD-Vantage® Flexible Container (Abbott) SAV	unspec.[c]	NS, D5W	n/a	n/a	24 h[f]	j	n/a	n/a	n/a	n/a	2
Duplex® Flexible Dual-Chambered Container (B. Braun) BRN	20, 40 mg/mL	f	iso	n/a	12 h[d]	5 d[d]	n/a	n/a	n/a	n/a	4
Galaxy Bag (Baxter) HO	20, 40 mg/mL	D	iso	n/a	n/a	n/a	b, e	24 h[b]	10 d[b]	n/a	2

Flush Compatibility: Heparin lock flush and normal saline.[1]
Special Considerations: n/a

Notes

[a]Manufacturer(s) extrapolated data from other sources.
[b]Frozen expiration date per manufacturer's label. Do not extrapolate commercial premix stability data to extemporaneously compounded solutions.
[c]Concentrations of dilutions based on reconstitution and/or dilution per manufacturer's labeling. Refer to current package insert for instructions.
[d]Following reconstitution (activation) of Duplex® container.
[e]Thaw at room temperature or under refrigeration. Do not force thaw. Do not refreeze.
[f]After activation of ADD-Vantage® container (reconstituted and diluted medication) per labeled instructions.
[g]pH of injectable solutions is 5–7.5.[2]
[h]A solution of 71 mg/mL in W is isotonic.
[i]Reconstituted solutions stored in original containers remain stable for 13 w frozen.
[j]Do not freeze.[2]
[k]In original container.

continued on next page

Cefotaxime Sodium (cont'd)

References

1. Trissel LA. ASHP's Interactive Handbook on Injectable Drugs. Bethesda, MD: American Society of Health-System Pharmacists. Accessed 2012 Jun.

2. Claforan® [prescribing information]. Bridgewater, NJ: Sanofi-Aventis US LLC; September 2008.

3. Drug Stability Data Using Elastomeric Infusion Systems. B. Braun Medical Production Ltd. (Thailand); August 2011.

4. Cefotaxime for Injection USP and Dextrose Injection USP in Duplex Drug Delivery System [prescribing information]. Irvine, CA: B. Braun Medical Inc.; January 2007.

5. Intermate/Infusor Drug Stability Information. Deerfield, IL: Baxter Healthcare Corporation; 2008.

6. Stability Data for Drugs Using Homepump Disposable Elastomeric Infusion Systems. Lake Forest, CA: I-Flow Corporation; October 2009.

7. Rapp RP, Hatton J, Record K. Drug Stability in Plastic Syringes. HealthTek™ and University of KY Lexington. Chester, NY: Repro-Med Systems Inc.; 1998.

Cefotetan Disodium

Container	Drug Manufacturer	Concentration	Diluents	Osmolality (mOsm/kg)	pH[b]	Temperature			Post-thaw Temp		Body Temp	Refer.
						Room	Refrig	Frozen	Room	Refrig		
CONTAINER												
Polyvinyl Chloride (PVC)	STU	2 mg/mL	D5W	n/a	b	14 d	14 d	n/a	n/a	n/a	n/a	1
	STU	20 mg/mL	NS, D5W	n/a	b	2 d	41 d	60 d	n/a	n/a	n/a	1
	AY	20, 40 mg/mL	NS	n/a	b	3.5 d	14 d	n/a	n/a	n/a	n/a	1
	AY	20, 40 mg/mL	D5W	n/a	b	3.5 d	13 d	n/a	n/a	n/a	n/a	1
Syringes, Plastic	STU	16.7, 33.3 mg/mL	NS	346, 415	b	24 h	96 h	1 w	n/a	n/a	n/a	2
	STU	16.7, 33.3 mg/mL	D5W	323, 391	b	24 h	96 h	n/a	n/a	n/a	n/a	2
OTHER INFUSION CONTAINERS												
AccuFlo™/ AccuFlux™/ AccuRX® (B. Braun)	unspec.	10–40 mg/mL	NS, D5W	n/a	b	24 h[a]	4 d[a]	1 w[a]	r/a	n/a	n/a	3
Homepump Eclipse®/ Homepump® C-Series (I-Flow Corp.)	unspec.	10–40 mg/mL	NS, D5W	n/a	b	24 h[a]	4 d[a]	7 d[a]	n/a	n/a	n/a	5
	unspec.	20 mg/mL	NS, D5W	n/a	b	n/a	n/a	60 d	n/a	n/a	n/a	5
INTERMATE/ INFUSOR (Baxter)	STU	5–60 mg/mL	D5W	n/a	b	24 h	10 d	n/a	n/a	n/a	n/a	4
	STU	5–60 mg/mL	NS	n/a	b	n/a	10 d	n/a	n/a	n/a	n/a	4
	STU	30 mg/mL	W	n/a	b	n/a	10 d	n/a	n/a	n/a	n/a	4
	STU	60 mg/mL	NS, D5W	n/a	b	24 h	10 d	30 d	24 h	n/a	n/a	4
Unspecified	unspec.	10–40 mg/mL	D5W, NS	n/a	b	24 h	96 h	n/a	n/a	n/a	n/a	1

Storage Conditions

continued on next page

Cefotetan Disodium (cont'd)

Drug Manufacturer	Concentration	Diluents	Osmolality (mOsm/kg)	pH[b]	Storage Conditions						Refer.
					Temperature			Post-thaw Temp			
					Room	Refrig	Frozen	Room	Refrig	Body Temp	
COMMERCIAL PREPARATIONS (RTU)											
Duplex® Flexible Dual-Chambered Container (B. Braun)	20, 40 mg/mL	c	290	4–6.5	12 h[d]	5 d[d]	e	n/a	n/a	n/a	6

BRN appears in the Drug Manufacturer column for the Duplex row.

Flush Compatibility: Normal saline, heparin flush (y-site compatibility at 50 units/mL heparin with 40 mg/mL cefotetan).[1]

Special Considerations: n/a

Notes

[a] Manufacturer(s) extrapolated data from other sources.

[b] pH of reconstituted solutions is 4.5–6.5.[1]

[c] Diluent in the Duplex® dual chamber system is Hydrous Dextrose Injection at a concentration that renders the reconstituted solution iso-osmotic.

[d] Prior to activation, expiration date is per manufacturer's label. To avoid inadvertent activation, DUPLEX container should remain folded until intended activation time. Protect from light after removal of foil strip. If light-protecting foil strip is removed, product must be activated within 7 d.

[e] Do not freeze.[6]

References

1. Trissel LA. ASHP's Interactive Handbook on Injectable Drugs. Bethesda, MD: American Society of Health-System Pharmacists. Accessed 2012 Jun.

2. Rapp RP, Hatton J, Record K. Drug Stability in Plastic Syringes. HealthTek™ and University of KY Lexington. Chester, NY: Repro-Med Systems Inc.; 1998.

3. Drug Stability Data Using Elastomeric Infusion Systems. B. Braun Medical Production Ltd. (Thailand); August 2011.

4. Intermate/Infusor Drug Stability Information. Deerfield, IL: Baxter Healthcare Corporation; 2008.

5. Stability Data for Drugs Using Homepump Disposable Elastomeric Infusion Systems. Lake Forest, CA: I-Flow Corporation; October 2009.

6. Cefotetan for Injection and Dextrose Injection in Duplex® Drug Delivery System [package insert.] Irvine, CA: B. Braun Medical Inc.; February 2012.

Cefoxitin Sodium

Container	Drug Manufacturer	Concentration	Diluents	Osmolality (mOsm/kg)	pH[c]	Storage Conditions Temperature Room	Refrig	Frozen	Post-thaw Temp Room	Refrig	Body Temp	Refer.
CONTAINER												
Glass	MSD	1 mg/mL	NS	n/a	c	24 h	n/a	n/a	n/a	n/a	n/a	1
	MSD	10, 20 mg/mL	NS	n/a	c	24 h	48 h	n/a	n/a	n/a	n/a	1
	MSD	20 mg/mL	D5W, NS	n/a	c	48 h	n/a	n/a	n/a	n/a	n/a	1
	MSD	20 mg/mL	D5W	n/a	c	24 h	7 d	13 w	n/a	n/a	n/a	1
Polyvinyl Chloride (PVC)	MSD	1 mg/mL	NS	n/a	c	48 h	n/a	n/a	n/a	n/a	n/a	1
	MSD	1 mg/mL	D5W	n/a	c	24 h	n/a	n/a	n/a	n/a	n/a	1
	unspecified	10, 20 mg/mL	D5W, NS	n/a	c	n/a	n/a	72 h[f]	6 h[f]	n/a	n/a	1
	MSD	20 mg/mL	NS	352	c	24 h	13 d	n/a	n/a	n/a	n/a	1
	MSD	20 mg/mL	D5W	326	c	24 h	13 d	30 d	24 h	n/a	n/a	1
	MSD	40 mg/mL	W	n/a	c	n/a	n/a	30 d[a]	n/a	4 d[a]	24 h[a]	1
Syringes, Plastic	MSD	16.7, 33.3 mg/mL	NS	344, 411	n/a	24 h	7 d	30 w	n/a	n/a	n/a	2
	MSD	16.7, 33.3 mg/mL	D5W	321, 388	n/a	24 h	7 d	30 w	n/a	n/a	n/a	2
	MSD	100 mg/mL	W	n/a	c	48 h	23 d	3 m	n/a	n/a	n/a	1
	MSD	200 mg/mL	W	n/a	c	48 h	23 d	3 m	n/a	n/a	n/a	1
OTHER INFUSION CONTAINERS												
AccuFlo™/ AccuFlux™/ AccuRX® (B. Braun)	unspec.	10 mg/mL	D5W, NS	n/a	n/a	24 h[b]	7 d[b]	n/a	n/a	n/a	n/a	3
Homepump Eclipse®/ Homepump® C-Series (I-Flow Corp.)	unspec.	20 mg/mL	NS, D5W	n/a	c	24 h[b]	13 d[b]	n/a	n/a	n/a	n/a	5

continued on next page

Cefoxitin Sodium (cont'd)

Drug Manufacturer	Concentration	Diluents	Osmolality (mOsm/kg)	pH[c]	Temperature Room	Temperature Refrig	Temperature Frozen	Post-thaw Room	Post-thaw Refrig	Body Temp	Refer.
INTERMATE (Baxter)											
MSD	5 mg/mL	NS	n/a	c	n/a	n/a	30 d	24 h	n/a	n/a	4
MSD	5–60 mg/mL	D5W	n/a	c	n/a	10 d	30 d	24 h	n/a	n/a	4
MSD	30 mg/mL	W	n/a	c	n/a	10 d	n/a	n/a	n/a	n/a	4
MSD	60 mg/mL	NS	n/a	c	n/a	10 d	n/a	n/a	n/a	n/a	4
Unspecified											
unspec.	100 mg/mL	W	n/a	n/a	48 h	7 d	30 w	24 h	7 d	n/a	1
unspec.	250 mg/mL	W	n/a	n/a	48 h	7 d	13 w	n/a	n/a	n/a	1
unspec.	500 mg/mL	W	n/a	n/a	48 h	1 m	n/a	n/a	n/a	n/a	1
COMMERCIAL PREPARATIONS (RTU)											
Duplex® Flexible Dual-Chambered Container (B. Braun)	20, 40 mg/mL	d	290	6.5	12 h[e]	7 d[e]	g	n/a	n/a	n/a	6
Galaxy Bag (Baxter)	20, 40 mg/mL	D5W	iso	n/a	n/a	n/a	n/a	24 h	21 d	n/a	7

Flush Compatibility: Heparin lock flush and normal saline.[1]
Special Considerations: n/a

Notes

[a]Stable for 24 h at 37°C after 30 d frozen, then 4 d refrigerated temperature.
[b]Manufacturer(s) extrapolated data from other sources.
[c]pH of reconstituted solution is 4.2–7.[1]
[d]Diluent in the Duplex® dual-chamber system is Hydrous Dextrose Injection at a concentration that renders the reconstituted solution iso-osmotic.
[e]Prior to activation, expiration date is per manufacturer's label. To avoid inadvertent activation, DUPLEX container should remain folded until intended activation time. Protect from light after removal of foil strip. If light-protecting, foil strip is removed; product must be activated within 7 d.
[f]Thawed in a microwave.
[g]Do not freeze.

continued on next page

101

Cefoxitin Sodium (cont'd)

References

1. Trissel LA. ASHP's Interactive Handbook on Injectable Drugs. Bethesda, MD: American Society of Health-System Pharmacists. Accessed 2012 Jan.
2. Rapp RP, Hatton J, Record K. Drug Stability in Plastic Syringes. HealthTek™ and University of KY Lexington. Chester, NY: Repro-Med Systems Inc.; 1998.
3. Drug Stability Data Using Elastomeric Infusion Systems. B. Braun Medical Production Ltd. (Thailand); August 2011.
4. Intermate/Infusor Drug Stability Information. Deerfield, IL: Baxter Healthcare Corporation; 2008.
5. Stability Data for Drugs Using Homepump Disposable Elastomeric Infusion Systems. Lake Forest, CA: I-Flow Corporation; October 2009.
6. Cefoxitin for Injection and Dextrose Injection in Duplex® Drug Delivery System [product information]. Irvine, CA: B. Braun Medical Inc.; June 2010.
7. Cefoxitin Injection USP in Galaxy® Container (PL 2040 Plastic). Deerfield, IL: Baxter Healthcare Corporation; September 2010.

Ceftaroline Fosamil

Container	Drug Manufacturer	Concentration	Diluents	Osmolality (mOsm/kg)	pH	Temperature			Post-thaw Temp		Body Temp	Refer.
						Room	Refrig	Frozen	Room	Refrig		
Unspecified	FOR	unspec.	NS, D5W, D2.5W, 1/2S, LR	n/a	a	6 h	24 h	n/a	n/a	n/a	n/a	1

Flush Compatibility: Normal saline.[1]
Special Considerations: The compatibility of Teflaro with other drugs has not been established. Teflaro should not be mixed with or physically added to solutions containing other drugs. Reconstitute vial with 20 mL W, NS, D5W, or LR, then dilute total dose in 50–250 mL solution prior to infusion over approximately 1 h.[1]

Note
a pH of constituted solution is 4.8–6.5.[1]

Reference
1. Teflaro® [package insert]. St. Louis, MO: Forest Pharmaceuticals; Inc.; October 2012.

Ceftazidime

continued on next page

Container	Drug Manufacturer	Concentration	Diluents	Osmolality (mOsm/kg)	pH^c	Temperature Room	Temperature Refrig	Temperature Frozen	Post-thaw Temp Room	Post-thaw Temp Refrig	Body Temp	Refer.
CONTAINER												
Ethyvinyl Acetate (EVA)	GSK	20 mg/mL	NS	n/a	c	24 h	7 d	n/a	n/a	n/a	n/a	1
Glass	GL	20 mg/mL	NS, D5W	n/a	c	n/a	n/a	12 w	n/a	n/a	n/a	1
	GL	40 mg/mL	D5W	n/a	c	2 d	21 d	n/a	n/a	n/a	n/a	1
Polyvinyl Chloride (PVC)	GL^g	2, 6 mg/mL	D5W, NS	n/a	n/a	24 h	n/a	n/a	n/a	n/a	n/a	1
	GL	4 mg/mL	D5W, NS	n/a	n/a	24 h	24 h	n/a	n/a	n/a	n/a	1
	GW	10 mg/mL	D5W, NS	n/a	n/a	24 h	24 h	n/a	n/a	n/a	n/a	1
	GL^g	40 mg/mL	NS	n/a	c	24 h	14 d	n/a	n/a	n/a	n/a	1
	GL^g	40 mg/mL	D5W	n/a	c	24 h	10 d	n/a	n/a	n/a	n/a	1
Syringes, Plastic	unspec.	8.33, 16.7, 33.3 mg/mL	NS^k	304, 330, 383	n/a	24 h	7 d	12 w	n/a	n/a	n/a	7
	unspec.	8.33, 16.7, 33.3 mg/mL	D5W^k	281, 306, 360	n/a	24 h	7 d	12 w	n/a	n/a	n/a	7
Syringes, Polypropylene	GL	100, 200 mg/mL	W^k	n/a	c	8 h	96 h	91 d	8 h	4 d	n/a	1, 3
OTHER INFUSION CONTAINERS												
AccuFlo™/	unspec.	5–30 mg/mL	NS	n/a	c	n/a	28 d^e	n/a	n/a	n/a	n/a	4
AccuFlux™/	unspec.	5–40 mg/mL	NS	n/a	c	24 h^e	14 d^e	n/a	n/a	n/a	n/a	4
AccuRX® (B. Braun)	unspec.	20 mg/mL	NS	n/a	c	18 h^e	7 d^e	84 d^e	n/a	n/a	n/a	4
	unspec.	40 mg/mL	NS	n/a	c	24 h	14 d	n/a	n/a	n/a	n/a	4
	unspec.	60 mg/mL	NS	n/a	c	n/a	14 d^e	14 d^e	n/a	n/a	n/a	4
	unspec.	60 mg/mL	NS	n/a	c	n/a	14 d^e	n/a	n/a	n/a	n/a	4
AutoDose (Tandem Medical)	GSK	20 mg/mL	NS	n/a	c	24 h	7 d	n/a	n/a	n/a	n/a	1

Ceftazidime (cont'd)

Drug Manufacturer	Concentration	Diluents	Osmolality (mOsm/kg)	pH[c]	Temperature Room	Temperature Refrig	Temperature Frozen	Post-thaw Temp Room	Post-thaw Temp Refrig	Body Temp	Refer.
HomePump®/ Homepump Eclipse® (I-Flow Corp.)											
unspec.	5–30 mg/mL	NS	n/a	c	n/a	28 d	n/a	n/a	n/a	n/a	6
unspec.	5–40 mg/mL	NS	n/a	c	24 h	14 d	n/a	n/a	n/a	n/a	6
unspec.	20 mg/mL	NS	n/a	c	18 h	7 d	84 d	n/a	n/a	n/a	6
GL	60 mg/mL	NS	n/a	c	n/a	14 d[d]	14 d[d]	n/a	n/a	n/a	1
INFUSOR (Baxter)											
GL	10–40 mg/mL	D5W	n/a	c	18 h	4 d	n/a	n/a	n/a	n/a	5
INTERMATE (Baxter)											
GL	5–40 mg/mL	NS, D5W	n/a	c	24 h	7 d	n/a	n/a	n/a	n/a	5
GL	5–40 mg/mL	NS, D5W	n/a	c	24 h	10 d	30 d	24 h	n/a	n/a	5
GL	5–40 mg/mL	D5W	n/a	c	n/a	5 d	n/a	n/a	n/a	n/a	5
GL	5–60 mg/mL	NS	n/a	c	n/a	n/a	8 w	n/a	7 d	n/a	5
GL	20 mg/mL	W	n/a	c	n/a	10 d	n/a	n/a	n/a	n/a	5
Unspecified											
GSK, HSP	1–40 mg/mL	D5W, NS, D5S, D51/4S, D51/2S, D10W, LR	n/a	c	24 h	7 d	n/a	n/a	n/a	n/a	2, 8
GL	20 mg/mL	NS	n/a	c	n/a	n/a	97 d	24 h	4 d	n/a	1
GL[g]	20 mg/mL	D5W, D5S, NS	n/a	n/a	24 h	48 h	n/a	n/a	n/a	n/a	1
GL	36.6 mg/mL	W	n/a	c	n/a	n/a	30 d	n/a	4 d	24 h	1
LI	40 mg/mL	NS, D5W	n/a	c	n/a	n/a	90 d	n/a	n/a	n/a	1
unspec.	95–280 mg/mL	W	n/a	c	24 h	7 d	n/a	n/a	n/a	n/a	1
GSK	100–180 mg/mL	NS, W	n/a	c	n/a	n/a	6 m	24 h	7 d	n/a	1
HSP	100–180 mg/mL	NS, D5W	n/a	c	n/a	n/a	3 m	8 h	4 d	n/a	1
unspec.	280 mg/mL	BWFI[a]	n/a	c	24 h	7 d	n/a	n/a	n/a	n/a	1
GSK, HSP	280 mg/mL	W	n/a	c	n/a	n/a	3 m	8 h	4 d	n/a	1

Storage Conditions

continued on next page

Ceftazidime (cont'd)

Drug Manufacturer	Concentration	Diluents	Osmolality (mOsm/kg)	pH[c]	Storage Conditions					Body Temp	Refer.
					Temperature			Post-thaw Temp			
					Room	Refrig	Frozen	Room	Refrig		
COMMERCIAL PREPARTIONS (RTU)											
Duplex® Flexible Dual-Chambered Container (B. Braun)	BRN	20, 40 mg/mL	D[i]	iso	5–7.5	12 h[j]	3 d[i]	n/a	n/a	n/a	n/a	10
Galaxy Bag (Baxter)	GL	1, 2 gm/50 mL	D	iso	5–7.5	n/a	n/a	f, h	8 h[b]	3 d[b]	n/a	2, 9

Flush Compatibility: Heparin lock flush and normal saline.[1]

Special Considerations: In January 2008, GlaxoSmithKline notified wholesalers about stability changes for Fortaz® product. Room temperature stability for Fortaz formulations is labeled as 3 d.[9] The L-arginine containing formulation of ceftazidime was discontinued.[11]

Notes

[a]Also tested in lidocaine HCl 0.5% and 1% for IM injection.

[b]In January 2008, GlaxoSmithKline notified wholesalers that Fortaz® premixed in Galaxy bags post-thaw are stable for 8 h at room temperature and 3 d refrigerated.[9]

[c]pH of reconstituted solutions is 5–8.[1]

[d]Protected from light. Potentially toxic pyridine 0.53 mg/mL was found in the refrigerated solution. The authors of the study recommend freezing such solution if long-term storage is needed.[1]

[e]Manufacturer(s) extrapolated data from other sources.

[f]Frozen expiration date per manufacturer's label. Do not extrapolate commercial premix stability data to extemporaneously compounded solutions.

[g]Sodium carbonate containing formulation.

[h]Thaw at room temperature or under refrigeration. Do not force thaw. Do not refreeze.

[i]Diluent in the Duplex® dual-chamber system is iso-osmotic hydrous dextrose USP.

[j]After activation. Prior to activation, expiration date is per manufacturer's label. To avoid inadvertent activation, DUPLEX container should remain folded until intended activation time. Protect from light after removal of foil strip. If light-protecting foil strip is removed, product must be activated within 7 d.

[k]All formulations of cetazidime produce gas as CO_2 after reconstitution. Gas must be allowed to disperse before placing in syringes.

References

1. Trissel LA. ASHP's Interactive Handbook on Injectable Drugs. Bethesda, MD: American Society of Health-System Pharmacists. Accessed 2012 Jul.

2. Fortaz® Injection [prescribing information]. Research Triangle Park, NC: GlaxoSmithKline; February 2007.

continued on next page

Ceftazidime (cont'd)

3. Garrelts JC, Ast D, LaRocca J, et al. Postinfusion phlebitis after intravenous push versus intravenous piggyback administration of antimicrobial agents. *Clin Pharm.* 1988; 7:760–5.
4. *Drug Stability Data Using Elastomeric Infusion Systems.* B. Braun Medical Production Ltd. (Thailand); August 2011.
5. *Intermate/Infusor Drug Stability Information.* Deerfield, IL: Baxter Healthcare Corporation; 2008.
6. *Stability Data for Drugs Using Homepump Disposable Elastomeric Infusion Systems.* Lake Forest, CA: I-Flow Corporation; October 2009.
7. Rapp RP, Hatton J, Record K. *Drug Stability in Plastic Syringes.* HealthTek™ and University of KY Lexington. Chester, NY: Repro-Med Systems Inc.; 1998.
8. Tazicef® Injection [prescribing information]. Lake Forest, IL: Hospira Worldwide, Inc.; March 2007.
9. Fish JL [letter]. Research Triangle Park, NC: GlaxoSmithKline; January 2008.
10. Ceftazidime for Injection USP and Dextrose Injection USP in Duplex® Drug Delivery System [package insert]. Irvine, CA; B. Braun Medical Inc.; June 2011.
11. Drugs@FDA FDA Approved Drug Products. http://www.accessdata.fda.gov/scripts/cder/drugsatfda/index.cfm. Accessed 7/7/12.

Ceftriaxone Sodium

continued on next page

	Drug Manufacturer	Concentration	Diluents	Osmolality (mOsm/kg)	pH[f]	Temperature Room	Temperature Refrig	Temperature Frozen	Post-thaw Temp Room	Post-thaw Temp Refrig	Body Temp	Refer.
CONTAINER												
Ethyvinyl Acetate (EVA)	RC	10, 20 mg/mL	NS	n/a	f	5 d	30 d	n/a	n/a	n/a	n/a	1, 8
Polyvinyl Chloride (PVC)	unspec.	1 mg/mL	NS	n/a	f	10 d	n/a	n/a	n/a	n/a	n/a	1
	RC	2 mg/mL	D5W	n/a	f	14 d	14 d	n/a	n/a	n/a	n/a	1
	RC	10–40 mg/mL	NS, D5W	n/a	f	n/a	n/a	26 w	n/a	n/a	n/a	1
	RC	10, 20, 40 mg/mL	D5½S, D5S	n/a	f	2 d	n/a	n/a	n/a	n/a	n/a	1, 11
	RC	10, 20, 40 mg/mL	D5W, NS, W	n/a	f	2 d	10 d	n/a	n/a	n/a	n/a	1, 11
	RC	20 mg/mL	D5W	n/a	f	n/a	n/a	14 d	n/a	n/a	n/a	1
	RC	40 mg/mL	D5W	n/a	f	2 d	14 d	n/a	n/a	n/a	n/a	1
	RC	40 mg/mL	NS	n/a	f	3 d	30 d	n/a	n/a	n/a	n/a	1
	RC	50 mg/mL	NS	364	f	n/a	n/a	26 w	n/a	n/a	n/a	1
Syringes, Plastic	RC	8.33, 16.67, 33.33 mg/mL	NS	303, 335, 392	f	72 h	10 d	26 w	n/a	n/a	n/a	7
Syringes, Polypropylene	RC	10, 40 mg/mL	NS, D5W	n/a	f	48 h	48 h	10 d	48 h	48 h	n/a	1
	RC	100 mg/mL	W	n/a	f	72 h	40 d	180 d	3 d	30 d	n/a	1, 3
	RC	250 mg/mL	D5W	n/a	f	n/a	n/a	8 w	n/a	10 d	n/a	1
	RC	250, 450 mg/mL	d	n/a	f	n/a	n/a	168 d	n/a	n/a	n/a	1
OTHER INFUSION CONTAINERS												
AccuFlo™/ AccuFlux™	unspec.	10–40 mg/mL	D5W, NS	n/a	f	n/a	n/a	26 w[a]	n/a	n/a	n/a	4
	unspec.	10–100 mg/mL	NS	n/a	f	72 h[a]	10 d[a]	n/a	n/a	n/a	n/a	4
AccuRX® (B. Braun)	unspec.	20 mg/mL	NS	n/a	f	72 h[a]	n/a	n/a	n/a	n/a	n/a	4
AutoDose (Tandem Medical)	RC	10, 20 mg/mL	NS	n/a	f	5 d	30 d	n/a	n/a	n/a	n/a	1, 8

Ceftriaxone Sodium (cont'd)

Drug Manufacturer	Concentration	Diluents	Osmolality (mOsm/kg)	pH[f]	Temperature Room	Temperature Refrig	Temperature Frozen	Post-thaw Temp Room	Post-thaw Temp Refrig	Body Temp	Refer.
Homepump Eclipse® / Homepump C-Series (I-Flow Corp.)											
unspec.	10–40 mg/mL	NS, D5W	n/a	f	n/a	n/a	26 w[a]	n/a	n/a	n/a	6
unspec.	10, 20, 40 mg/mL	NS, D5W	n/a	f	3 d[a]	10 d[a]	n/a	n/a	n/a	n/a	6
unspec.	20 mg/mL	NS	n/a	f	72 h	n/a	n/a	n/a	n/a	n/a	6
INTERMATE (Baxter)											
RC	5 mg/mL	D5W, NS	n/a	f	24 h	28 d[i]	n/a	n/a	n/a	n/a	5
RC	5–40 mg/mL	NS, D5W	n/a	f	24 h	21 d[i]	n/a	n/a	n/a	n/a	5
RC	5–40 mg/mL	NS, D5W	n/a	f	n/a	10 d	30 d	24 h	n/a	n/a	5
RC	30 mg/mL	W	n/a	f	n/a	10 d	n/a	n/a	n/a	n/a	5
Polyolefin											
RC	10–40 mg/mL	D5W, NS	n/a	f	n/a	n/a	26 w	n/a	r/a	n/a	1
RC	20 mg/mL	D5W	n/a	f	n/a	n/a	14 w	n/a	44 d[i]	n/a	1
Unspecified											
unspec.	5, 40 mg/mL	D5W, NS	n/a	f	n/a	20 d	n/a	n/a	n/a	n/a	1
RC	10 mg/mL	NS	n/a	f	7 d	n/a	n/a	n/a	n/a	n/a	1
RC	10 mg/mL	NS	n/a	f	48 h	72 h	26 w	n/a	n/a	n/a	1
RC	10 mg/mL	D5½S	n/a	f	48 h	96 h	n/a	n/a	n/a	n/a	1
RC	10 mg/mL	D5W	n/a	f	72 h	96 h	n/a	n/a	n/a	n/a	1
RC	10 mg/mL	D5W	n/a	f	7 d	12 w	n/a	n/a	n/a	n/a	1
RC	50 mg/mL	NS	n/a	f	7 d	5 w	n/a	n/a	n/a	n/a	1
RC	50 mg/mL	D5W	351	f	24 h	8 w	26 w	n/a	n/a	n/a	1
RC	100 mg/mL	W	n/a	f	n/a	n/a	180 d	n/a	n/a	n/a	1
RC	100 mg/mL	W, NS, D5W	n/a	f	2 d	10 d	n/a	n/a	n/a	n/a	1
RC	100 mg/mL	BWFI[c,d]	n/a	f	24 h	10 d	n/a	n/a	n/a	n/a	1
RC	250, 350 mg/mL	W, NS, D5W, BWFI[c,d]	n/a	f	24 h	3 d	n/a	n/a	n/a	n/a	1

continued on next page

Ceftriaxone Sodium (cont'd)

COMMERCIAL PREPARATIONS (RTU)

	Drug Manufacturer	Concentration	Diluents	Osmolality (mOsm/kg)	pH[f]	Storage Conditions						Refer.
						Temperature			Post-thaw Temp		Body Temp	
						Room	Refrig	Frozen	Room	Refrig		
Duplex® Flexible Dual-Chambered Container (B. Braun)	BRN	20, 40 mg/mL	g	290	f	24 h[h]	7 d[h]	n/a	n/a	n/a	n/a	10
Galaxy Plastic Container (Baxter)	BA	20, 40 mg/mL	D	iso	6–8	n/a	n/a	e	48 h[e]	21 d[e]	n/a	2

Flush Compatibility: Heparin lock flush and normal saline.[1]

Special Considerations: Do not administer to neonates (≤28 days old) if they require or are expected to require treatment with calcium-containing IV solutions, including parenteral nutrition, because of the risk of precipitation of ceftriaxone-calcium. For all other patients, do not administer simultaneously with calcium-containing IV solutions (including continuous calcium-containing parenteral nutrition via Y-site); flush infusion line between infusions of ceftriaxone and any calcium-containing infusion. Do not use diluents containing calcium (such as Ringer's or Hartmann's solution) to reconstitute or further dilute ceftriaxone for administration.[9,11]

Notes

[a]Manufacturer(s) extrapolated data from other sources.

[b]Stable for 48 h at room temperature following 14 d refrigerated.

[c]Bacteriostatic water for injection contained benzyl alcohol 0.9% as a preservative.

[d]Lidocaine HCl 1% was also studied as a diluent.

[e]Frozen expiration date per manufacturer's label. Do not extrapolate commercial premix stability data to extemporaneously compounded solutions.

[f]pH of 1% reconstituted solution is 6.7.[2]

[g]Diluent in the Duplex® dual-chamber system is Hydrous Dextrose Injection at a concentration that renders the reconstituted solution iso-osmotic.

[h]Prior to activation, expiration date is per manufacturer's label. To avoid inadvertent activation, DUPLEX container should remain folded until intended activation time. Protect from light after removal of foil strip. If light-protecting foil strip is removed, product must be activated within 7 d.

[i]May be followed by 24 h at room temperature.

[j]Study showed 10% drug loss in 44–56 days depending on the power level used for thawing.

References

1. Trissel LA. ASHP's Interactive Handbook on Injectable Drugs. Bethesda, MD: American Society of Health-System Pharmacists. Accessed 2012 Jul.

2. Ceftriaxone Injection, USP in Dextrose in Galaxy Container [package insert]. Deerfield, IL: Baxter Healthcare; December 2010.

continued on next page

Ceftriaxone Sodium (cont'd)

3. Garrelts JC, Ast D, LaRocca J, et al. Postinfusion phlebitis after intravenous push versus intravenous piggyback administration of antimicrobial agents. *Clin Pharm.* 1988; 7:760–5.

4. *Drug Stability Data Using Elastomeric Infusion Systems.* B. Braun Medical Production Ltd. (Thailand); August 2011.

5. *Intermate/Infusor Drug Stability Information.* Deerfield, IL: Baxter Healthcare Corporation; 2008.

6. *Stability Data for Drugs Using Homepump Disposable Elastomeric Infusion Systems.* Lake Forest, CA: I-Flow Corporation; October 2009.

7. Rapp RP, Hatton J, Record K. *Drug Stability in Plastic Syringes.* HealthTek™ and University of KY Lexington. Chester, NY: Repro-Med Systems Inc.; 1998.

8. *AutoDose Stability Reference.* San Diego, CA: Tandem Medical Inc; 2002.

9. Rocephin® Important Clarification of Prescribing Information, Dear Healthcare Professional Letter. Nutley, NJ: Roche Laboratories, Inc.; May 2009.

10. CefTRIaxONE for Injection and Dextrose Injection in Duplex® Drug Delivery System [package insert]. Irvine, CA: B. Braun Medical Inc.; June 2010.

11. Rocephin® [prescribing information]. South San Francisco, CA: Genentech; November 2010.

Cefuroxime Sodium

Container	Drug Manufacturer	Concentration	Diluents	Osmolality (mOsm/kg)	pH[e]	Temperature Room	Temperature Refrig	Temperature Frozen	Post-thaw Temp Room	Post-thaw Temp Refrig	Body Temp	Refer.
CONTAINER												
Polyolefin Bags	unspec.	15 mg/mL	D5W	n/a	e	n/a	31 d	98 d	n/a	21 d	n/a	1
Polyvinyl Chloride (PVC)	GL	5, 10 mg/mL	NS, D5W	n/a	e	24 h	30 d	30 d	n/a	n/a	n/a	1
	unspec.	6 mg/mL	D5W, NS	n/a	e	24 h	24 h	n/a	n/a	n/a	n/a	1
	GSK	7.5, 15 mg/mL	NS, D5W	n/a	e	n/a	n/a	6 m	24 h	7 d	n/a	1, 2
	GSK	7.5, 15 mg/mL	NS, D5W	n/a	e	24 h	7 d	n/a	n/a	n/a	n/a	2
	GL	30 mg/mL	NS, D5W	314, 315	e	n/a	n/a	6 m	24 h	7 d	n/a	1
Syringes, Plastic	unspec.	12.5, 25, 50 mg/mL	NS	320, 379, n/a	e	24 h	7 d	6 m	n/a	n/a	n/a	8
	unspec.	12.5, 25, 50 mg/mL	D5W	305, 355, n/a	e	24 h	7 d	n/a	n/a	n/a	n/a	8
Syringes, Polypropylene	GL	50 mg/mL	NS	335	e	2 d	21 d	n/a	n/a	n/a	n/a	7
OTHER INFUSION CONTAINERS												
AccuFlo™/ AccuFlux™/ AccuRX® (B. Braun)	unspec.	1–30 mg/mL	NS, D5W	n/a	n/a	24 h[b]	7 d[b]	6 m[b]	n/a	n/a	n/a	4
ADD-Vantage® Flexible Container (Abbott)	BA	7.5, 15, 30 mg/mL	D5W, NS, ¹/₂S	n/a	n/a	24 h	7 d	n/a	n/a	n/a	n/a	2
CADD® Cassette (Pharmacia)	GL	22.5, 45 mg/mL	W	n/a	e	n/a	7 d	n/a	n/a	n/a	16 h[c]	1
	GL	30, 60 mg/mL	W	n/a	e	n/a	n/a	30 d	n/a	4 d	n/a	1
Glass	GL	15 mg/mL	D5W	n/a	e	n/a	11 d	n/a	n/a	n/a	n/a	1

Storage Conditions

continued on next page

Cefuroxime Sodium (cont'd)

Drug Manufacturer	Concentration	Diluents	Osmolality (mOsm/kg)	pHᵉ	Temperature			Post-thaw Temp			Refer.
					Room	Refrig	Frozen	Room	Refrig	Body Temp	
Homepump Eclipse®/ Homepump® C-Series (I-Flow Corp.)											
unspec.	1–30 mg/mL	NS, D5W	n/a	e	24 hᵇ	7 dᵇ	n/a	n/a	n/a	n/a	6
unspec.	5, 10 mg/mL	D5W, NS	n/a	e	n/a	n/a	30 dᵇ	n/a	n/a	n/a	6
INFUSOR (Baxter)											
GL	15–30 mg/mL	D5W	n/a	e	15 h	7 dᵃ	n/a	n/a	n/a	n/a	5
GL	15–30 mg/mL	D5W	n/a	n/a	n/a	14 d	n/a	n/a	n/a	n/a	5
INTERMATE (Baxter)											
LI	5–30 mg/mL	D5W, NS	n/a	e	n/a	10 d	30 d	24 h	n/a	n/a	5
Unspecified											
GSK, HSP	1–30 mg/mL	NS, D5W, D5S, D5½S, D5¼S	n/a	e	24 h	7 d	n/a	n/a	n/a	n/a	2, 3
COMMERCIAL PREPARATIONS (RTU)											
Duplex® Flexible Dual-Chambered Container (B. Braun)											
BRN	15, 30 mg/mL	f	290	4–6.5	24 hᵍ	7 dᵍ	n/a	n/a	n/a	n/a	9
Galaxy Plastic Container (Baxter)											
GSK	15 mg/mL	D	300	5–7.5	n/a	n/a	d	24 hᵈ	28 dᵈ	n/a	2
GSK	30 mg/mL	W	300	5–7.5	n/a	n/a	d	24 hᵈ	28 dᵈ	n/a	2

continued on next page

Flush Compatibility: Heparin lock flush and normal saline.[1]
Special Considerations: n/a

Notes

ᵃMay be followed by 15 h at room temperature.
ᵇManufacturer(s) extrapolated data from other sources.
ᶜEleven to twelve percent loss by HPLC in 16 h at 30°C; 4–6% loss in 8 h at 30°C.

Cefuroxime Sodium (cont'd)

[d] Frozen expiration date per manufacturer's label. Do not extrapolate commercial premix stability data to extemporaneously compounded solutions.
[e] pH of reconstituted solution is 6–8.5.[1,2]
[f] Diluent in the Duplex® dual-chamber system is Hydrous Dextrose Injection at a concentration that renders the reconstituted solution iso-osmotic.
[g] Prior to activation, expiration date is per manufacturer's label. To avoid inadvertent activation, DUPLEX container should remain folded until intended activation time. Protect from light after removal of foil strip. If light-protecting foil strip is removed, product must be activated within 7 d.

References

1. Trissel LA. ASHP's Interactive Handbook on Injectable Drugs. Bethesda, MD: American Society of Health-System Pharmacists. Accessed 2012 Jul.
2. Zinacef® [prescribing information]. Research Triangle Park, NC: GlaxoSmithKline; August 2010.
3. Cefuroxime for Injection [prescribing information]. Lake Forest, IL: Hospira, Inc.; January 2009.
4. Drug Stability Data Using Elastomeric Infusion Systems. B. Braun Medical Production Ltd. (Thailand); August 2011.
5. Intermate/Infusor Drug Stability Information. Deerfield, IL: Baxter Healthcare Corporation; 2008.
6. Stability Data for Drugs Using Homepump Disposable Elastomeric Infusion Systems. Lake Forest, CA: I-Flow Corporation; October 2009.
7. Gupta, VD. Chemical stability of cefuroxime sodium after reconstitution in 0.9% sodium chloride injection and storage in polypropylene syringes for pediatric use. Int J Pharm Compound. 2003:7(4); 310–2.
8. Rapp RP, Hatton J, Record K. Drug Stability in Plastic Syringes. HealthTek™ and University of KY Lexington. Chester, NY: Repro-Med Systems Inc.; 1998.
9. Cefuroxime for Injection USP and Dextrose Injection USP in Duplex® Drug Delivery System [package insert]. Irvine, CA: B. Braun Medical Inc.; October 2009.

Chlorpromazine Hydrochloride

	Drug Manufacturer	Concentration	Diluents	Osmolality (mOsm/kg)	pH[d]	Storage Conditions						Refer.
						Temperature			Post-thaw Temp		Body Temp	
						Room	Refrig	Frozen	Room	Refrig		
CONTAINER												
Polyvinyl Chloride (PVC)	MB	0.009 mg/mL	NS	n/a	d	7 d[a]	n/a	e	n/a	n/a	n/a	1
Syringes, Plastic	ES	6.25 mg/mL[b]	n/a	n/a	d	12 m[c]	12 m[c]	e	n/a	n/a	n/a	1
OTHER INFUSION CONTAINERS												
Glass Vials	SKF	1 mg/mL	NS	n/a	d	30 d[c]	n/a	e	n/a	n/a	n/a	1

Flush Compatibility: Normal saline.[1]
Special Considerations: n/a

Notes

[a]About 5% sorption during 1 w of storage in Travenol NS PVC bags. However, when buffered from pH 5 to pH 7.4, 86% of the drug was lost in 1 w due to sorption. During a 7 h simulated infusion through an infusion set (cellulose propionate burette chamber and PVC tubing by Travenol), 41% of the drug was lost to sorption. No appreciable loss occurred when infused through a polyethylene administration set (Tridilset) over 8 h at room temperature.

[b]With hydroxyzine HCl 12.5 mg/mL (Pfizer) and meperidine HCl 25 mg/mL (Winthrop).

[c]Protected from light.

[d]pH of undiluted solution is 3–5.4.[1]

[e]Do not freeze.

Reference

1. Trissel LA. ASHP's Interactive Handbook on Injectable Drugs. Bethesda, MD: American Society of Health-System Pharmacists. Accessed 2012 Jan.

Cidofovir

Storage Conditions

CONTAINER	Drug Manufacturer	Concentration	Diluents	Osmolality (mOsm/kg)	pH[b]	Temperature Room	Temperature Refrig	Temperature Frozen	Post-thaw Temp Room	Post-thaw Temp Refrig	Body Temp	Refer.
Polyolefin	GIL	0.085, 3.51 mg/mL	D5½S	n/a	6.7–7.0	24 h	24 h	n/a	n/a	n/a	24 h[c]	1
	GIL	0.2, 8.1 mg/mL	D5W	286	7.2–7.6	24 h	24 h	n/a	n/a	n/a	24 h[c]	1
	GIL	0.2, 8.1 mg/mL	NS	n/a	7.1–7.5	n/a	5 d[a]	5 d[a]	n/a	n/a	24 h[c]	1
	GIL	0.21, 8.12 mg/mL	NS	241	7.1–7.5	24 h	24 h	n/a	n/a	n/a	24 h[c]	1
Polyvinyl Chloride (PVC)	GIL	0.085, 3.51 mg/mL	D5½S	382, 392	6.7–7.0	24 h	24 h	n/a	n/a	n/a	24 h[c]	1
	GIL	0.2, 8.1 mg/mL	NS	n/a	7.1–7.5	24 h	5 d[a]	5 d[a]	n/a	n/a	24 h[c]	1
	GIL	0.21, 8.12 mg/mL	NS	275, 315	7.1–7.5	24 h	24 h	n/a	n/a	n/a	24 h[c]	1
	GIL	0.21, 8.12 mg/mL	D5W	241, 286	7.2–7.6	24 h	24 h	n/a	n/a	n/a	24 h[c]	1
Syringes, Plastic	GIL	6.25 mg/mL	NS	n/a	7.1–7.5	150 d	150 d[a]	n/a	n/a	n/a	n/a	1

Flush Compatibility: Normal saline. Compatibility with heparin has not been established.[2]

Special Considerations: Product labeling recommends dilution in 100 mL NS prior to administration. Compatibility with R, LR, or bacteriostatic fluids has not been evaluated.[2]

Notes

[a]Manufacturer does not recommend extending stability by refrigeration or freezing.[2]

[b]pH of undiluted solution is 7.4.[1]

[c]At 30°C.

References

1. Trissel LA. ASHP's Interactive Handbook on Injectable Drugs. Bethesda, MD: American Society of Health-System Pharmacists. Accessed 2012 Jun.

2. Vistide® [package insert]. Foster City, CA: Gilead Sciences, Inc.; September 2010.

Cimetidine Hydrochloride

	Drug Manufacturer	Concentration	Diluents	Osmolality (mOsm/kg)	pH[a]	Temperature Room	Temperature Refrig	Temperature Frozen	Post-thaw Temp Room	Post-thaw Temp Refrig	Body Temp	Refer.
CONTAINER												
Glass	SKB	0.6 mg/mL	NS	n/a	a	48 h	n/a	n/a	n/a	n/a	n/a	1
	SKF	1.2, 5 mg/mL	D5W, D10W	n/a	a	7 d	n/a	n/a	n/a	n/a	n/a	1
	SKF	15 mg/mL	W	n/a	a	28 d[f]	28 d	n/a	n/a	n/a	n/a	1
Polyvinyl Chloride (PVC)	SKF	1.2, 5 mg/mL	D5W, D10W, NS	n/a	a	7 d	n/a	n/a	n/a	n/a	n/a	1
	SKF	6 mg/mL	D5W	291	a	n/a	n/a	30 d	n/a	8 d	n/a	1
Syringes, Plastic	SKF	5 mg/mL[b]	NS, D5W	308, 285	a	24 h	8 d	28 d	n/a	n/a	n/a	2
Unspecified	SKF	1.2, 5 mg/mL	D5½S, D5¼S, D5LR, D5S, D10S, R, LR, NS	n/a	a	7 d	n/a	n/a	n/a	n/a	n/a	1
OTHER INFUSION CONTAINERS												
AccuFlo™/ AccuFlux™/ AccuRX® (B. Braun)	unspec.	6 mg/mL	D5W	n/a	n/a	48 h[e]	8 d[e]	4 w[e]	n/a	n/a	n/a	3
COMMERCIAL PREPARATIONS (RTU)												
Flexible Plastic Container (Hospira)	HSP	6 mg/mL	NS	356	5–7	30 d[c,d]	n/a	n/a	n/a	n/a	n/a	1, 4

Storage Conditions

Flush Compatibility: Heparin lock flush and normal saline.[1]
Special Considerations: n/a

Notes

[a]pH of the undiluted solution is 3.8–6.[1]
[b]Prepared in 60-mL syringes.

continued on next page

Cimetidine Hydrochloride (cont'd)

cExpiration date per manufacturer's label. Do not extrapolate commercial premix stability data to extemporaneously compounded preparations.
dDo not use beyond this date after removal of manufacturer's protective overwrap.
eManufacturer extrapolated data from other sources.
fStored in a closed cabinet.

References

1. Trissel LA. ASHP's Interactive Handbook on Injectable Drugs. Bethesda, MD: American Society of Health-System Pharmacists. Accessed 2012 Jun.
2. Rapp RP, Hatton J, Record K. Drug Stability in Plastic Syringes. HealthTek™ and University of KY Lexington; Repro-Med Systems Inc.; 1998.
3. Drug Stability Data Using Elastomeric Infusion Systems. B. Braun Medical Production Ltd. (Thailand); August 2011.
4. Chadha S. Lifecare® Flexible Containers [personal communication]. Lake Forest, IL: Medical Communications Department, Hospira Inc.; April 25. 2008.

Ciprofloxacin

Container	Drug Manufacturer	Concentration	Diluents	Osmolality (mOsm/kg)	pH[e]	Storage Conditions						Refer.
						Temperature			Post-thaw Temp			
						Room	Refrig	Frozen	Room	Refrig	Body Temp	
CONTAINER												
Ethyvinyl Acetate (EVA)	BAY	4 mg/mL	NS	n/a	e	7 d	30 d	n/a	n/a	n/a	n/a	1
Polyvinyl Chloride (PVC)	MI	2.86 mg/mL	NS, D5W	n/a	e	90 d	90 d	n/a	n/a	n/a	n/a	1
Unspecified	BED	0.5, 2 mg/mL	NS, D5W, D5½S, D5¼S, LR, W, D10W	n/a	e	14 d	14 d	n/a	n/a	n/a	n/a	2
OTHER INFUSION CONTAINERS												
AccuFlo™/ AccuFlux™/ AccuRx® (B. Braun)	unspec.	2 mg/mL	RTU/NS	n/a	n/a	24 h[b]	28 d[b]	n/a	n/a	n/a	n/a	3
AutoDose (Tandem Medical)	BAY	4 mg/mL	NS	n/a	e	7 d	30 d	n/a	n/a	n/a	n/a	1
Homepump Eclipse®/ Homepump® C-Series (I-Flow Corp.)	unspec.	2 mg/mL	RTU	n/a	e	24 h	27 d	n/a	n/a	n/a	n/a	5
INTERMATE (Baxter)	BAY	0.5–2 mg/mL	NS, D5W	n/a	n/a	30 d[c]	90 d[c]	n/a	n/a	n/a	n/a	4
	MI	0.5–6 mg/mL	NS, D5W, W	n/a	e	30 d[c]	90 d[c]	n/a	n/a	n/a	n/a	4
COMMERCIAL PREPARATIONS (RTU)												
Flexible Container[a] (Baxter)	BAY	2 mg/mL	D5W	n/a	3.5–4.6	d	n/a	n/a	n/a	n/a	n/a	2

continued on next page

119

Ciprofloxacin (cont'd)

Flush Compatibility: Normal saline. White precipitate forms immediately with heparin.[1]
Special Considerations: Protect from light. Do not freeze.[1]

Notes

[a]*Latex-free PVC bag.*
[b]*Manufacturer(s) extrapolated data from other sources.*
[c]*Stable for 14 d room temperature following 90 d refrigerated.*
[d]*Expiration date per manufacturer's label. Do not extrapolate commercial premix stability data to extemporaneously compounded solutions.*
[e]*pH of undiluted 1% solution is 3–3.9.*[2]

References

1. Trissel LA. ASHP's Interactive Handbook on Injectable Drugs. Bethesda, MD: American Society of Health-System Pharmacists. Accessed 2012 Jan.
2. Cipro® IV [prescribing information]. Wayne, NJ: Bayer Healthcare Pharmaceuticals, Inc.; November 2011.
3. Drug Stability Data Using Elastomeric Infusion Systems. B. Braun Medical Production Ltd. (Thailand); August 2011.
4. Intermate/Infusor Drug Stability Information. Deerfield, IL: Baxter Healthcare Corporation; 2008.
5. Stability Data for Drugs Using Homepump Disposable Elastomeric Infusion Systems. Lake Forest, CA: I-Flow Corporation; October 2009.

Cisplatin[a]

Container	Drug Manufacturer	Concentration	Diluents	Osmolality (mOsm/kg)	pH[g]	Storage Conditions						Refer.
						Temperature			Post-thaw Temp		Body Temp	
						Room	Refrig	Frozen	Room	Refrig		
CONTAINER												
Ethyvinyl Acetate (EVA)	BEL	0.5, 0.9 mg/mL	NS	n/a	g	28 d[b]	n/a	n/a	n/a	n/a	28 d[b,e]	1, 4
Polyvinyl Chloride (PVC)	WAS	0.167 mg/mL	NS	n/a	g	14 d	n/a	n/a	n/a	n/a	n/a	7
	BMS	0.485 mg/mL[c]	NS[c]	n/a	g	n/a	24 h[a,c,d]	n/a	n/a	n/a	7 d[c,d]	2, 4
	BEL	0.6 mg/mL	NS[b]	n/a	g	9 d[b]	n/a	n/a	n/a	n/a	n/a	4
	unspec.	1 mg/mL	NS	h	g	14 d	n/a	n/a	n/a	n/a	n/a	3
OTHER INFUSION CONTAINERS												
AccuFlo™/ AccuFlux™/ AccuRX® (B. Braun)	unspec.	0.2 mg/mL	NS	n/a	g	14 d[i]	14 d[a]	n/a	n/a	n/a	n/a	8
Cassette Reservoir (Pharmacia Deltec)	DB	1 mg/mL	W	h	g	14 d[b]	n/a	n/a	n/a	n/a	14 d[b]	4
Glass Bottles	WAS	0.167 mg/mL	NS	n/a	g	14 d	n/a	n/a	n/a	n/a	n/a	7
	unspec.	1 mg/mL[f]	undiluted	h	g	n/a	n/a	n/a	n/a	n/a	10 m[f]	4
Homepump®/ Homepump Eclipse® (I-Flow Corp.)	unspec.	0.5 mg/mL	NS	n/a	g	28 d[i]	n/a	n/a	n/a	n/a	n/a	5
INFUSOR (Baxter)	BEL	1.25 mg/mL	NS	n/a	g	4 d[b,j]	n/a	n/a	n/a	n/a	24 h[b,j]	6
Polyethylene Bag (Palex)	WAS	0.167 mg/mL	NS	n/a	g	14 d	n/a	n/a	n/a	n/a	n/a	7
Polypropylene Bag (ERN)	WAS	0.167 mg/mL	NS	n/a	g	14 d	n/a	n/a	n/a	n/a	n/a	7

continued on next page

Cisplatin (cont'd)

Flush Compatibility: Heparin lock flush and normal saline.[1]
Special Considerations: Protect from light if solution will not be used within 6 h.

Notes

[a]Manufacturer recommends not refrigerating because of danger of precipitation.
[b]Solution protected from light.
[c]With ondansetron (GL) 1.031 mg/mL.
[d]Solution was initially refrigerated for 24 h prior to storage at 30°C for 7 d. Solutions were protected from light.
[e]Stored at 35°C.
[f]With sodium chloride 9 mg/mL and mannitol 10 mg/mL, stored at 40°C in vials.
[g]pH range is 3.8–5.9.[4]
[h]Undiluted product is 285 mOsm/kg.[4]
[i]Extrapolated data.
[j]Stored 4 d at 25°C, followed by 24 h at 33°C.

References

1. Rochard E, Barthes D, Courtois P. Stability of cisplatin in ethylene vinylacetate portable infusion pump reservoirs. *J Clin Pharm Ther.* 1992; 17:315–8.
2. Henry DW, Marshall JL, Nazzaro D, et al. Stability of cisplatin and ondansetron hydrochloride in admixtures for continuous infusion. *Am J Health-Syst Pharm.* 1995; 52:2570–3.
3. Vyas HM, Baptista RJ, Mitrano FP, et al. Drug stability guidelines for a continuous infusion chemotherapy program. *Hosp Pharm.* 1987; 22:685–7.
4. Trissel LA. ASHP's Interactive Handbook on Injectable Drugs. Bethesda, MD: American Society of Health-System Pharmacists. Accessed 2012 Jul.
5. Stability Data for Drugs Using Homepump Disposable Elastomeric Infusion Systems. Lake Forest, CA: I-Flow Corporation; October 2009.
6. Intermate/Infusor Drug Stability Information. Deerfield, IL: Baxter Healthcare Corporaticn; October 2008.
7. Cubells MP, Aixela JP, Brumos VG, et al. Stability of cisplatin in sodium chloride 0.9% intravenous solution related to the container's material. *Pharm World Sci.* 1993; 15:34–6.
8. Drug Stability Data Using Elastomeric Infusion Systems. B. Braun Medical Production Ltd. (Thailand); August 2011.

Cladribine

Container	Drug Manufacturer	Concentration	Diluents	Osmolality (mOsm/kg)	pH[b]	Storage Conditions						
						Temperature			Post-thaw Temp		Body Temp	Refer.
						Room	Refrig	Frozen	Room	Refrig		
CONTAINER												
Polyvinyl Chloride (PVC)	JC	0.016 mg/mL	NS	c	b	30 d[a]	30 d[a]	n/a	n/a	n/a	n/a	1, 2
OTHER INFUSION CONTAINERS												
Cassette Reservoir (SIMS Deltec)	OB	unspec.[d]	NS[e]	c	b	n/a	n/a	n/a	n/a	n/a	n/a	1, 3
Glass	unspec.	0.024 mg/mL	NS	c	b	n/a	14 d	n/a	n/a	n/a	n/a	1

Flush Compatibility: Heparin lock flush and normal saline.[1]

Special Considerations: Store intact cladribine vials under refrigeration and protected from light. D5W is not recommended as a diluent because of increased cladribine degradation.[3]

Notes

[a]Solutions stored exposed to light and protected from light at both room temperature and refrigerated.

[b]pH of undiluted solution is 5.5–8.[1]

[c]Undiluted solution is isotonic.[1]

[d]Concentrations vary; calculated dose is diluted to a total volume of 100 mL.

[e]Bacteriostatic NS is specified by the manufacturer when preparing a 7 day continuous infusion. Both drug and diluent are added to the infusion reservoir through 0.22 micron filters. All air is aspirated from the reservoir.[1,3]

References

1. Trissel LA. ASHP's Interactive Handbook on Injectable Drugs. Bethesda, MD: American Society of Health-System Pharmacists. Accessed 2012 Jul.
2. Daouphars M, Vigneron J, Perrin A, et al. Stability of cladribine in either polyethylene containers or polyvinyl chloride bags. Eur Hosp Pharm. 1997; 3:154–6.
3. LEUSTATIN® (cladribine) Injection [prescribing information]. Raritan, NJ: Ortho Biotech; August 2007.

Clindamycin Phosphate

continued on next page

Container	Drug Manufacturer	Concentration	Diluents	Osmolality (mOsm/kg)	pH[d]	Temperature Room	Temperature Refrig	Temperature Frozen	Post-thaw Temp Room	Post-thaw Temp Refrig	Body Temp	Refer.
CONTAINER												
Ethyvinyl Acetate (EVA)	n/a	6, 12 mg/mL	NS	294, 309	d	7 d	30 d	n/a	n/a	n/a	n/a	1
Polyvinyl Chloride (PVC)	UP	6 mg/mL	D5W	268	d	n/a	n/a	30 d	24 h	n/a	n/a	1
	UP	6, 9, 12 mg/mL	D5W	268, n/a, 293	d	16 d	32 d	8 w	n/a	n/a	n/a	1
	UP	6, 9, 12 mg/mL	NS	294, n/a, 309	d	16 d	32 d	8 w	n/a	n/a	n/a	1
	QU	6, 12 mg/mL	D5W	n/a	d	22 d	54 d	68 d	n/a	n/a	n/a	1
	QU	6, 12 mg/mL	NS	294, 309	d	22 d	54 d	68 d	n/a	n/a	n/a	1
	UP	18 mg/mL	D5W, NS	n/a	d	n/a	n/a	28 d	n/a	n/a	n/a	1
Syringes, Plastic[a]	UP	5, 10 mg/mL	NS	302, 327	n/a	48 h	30 d	60 d	n/a	n/a	n/a	6
	UP	5, 10 mg/mL	D5W	279, 304	n/a	48 h	30 d	60 d	n/a	n/a	n/a	6
	UP	20, 40, 60, 120 mg/mL	W	n/a	d	30 d[a]	n/a	60 d[a]	n/a	n/a	n/a	1
Unspecified	unspec.	6 mg/mL	D5W	268	d	n/a	n/a	79 d	n/a	n/a	n/a	1
OTHER INFUSION CONTAINERS												
AccuFlo™/ AccuFlux™/ AccuRX® (B. Braun)	unspec.	6, 9, 12 mg/mL	NS, D5W	n/a	n/a	16 d[b]	32 d[b]	8 w[b]	n/a	n/a	n/a	3
	unspec.	10 mg/mL	NS	n/a	n/a	24 h[b]	10 d[b]	n/a	n/a	n/a	n/a	3
AutoDose (Tandem Medical)	n/a	6, 12 mg/mL	NS	294, 309	d	7 d	30 d	n/a	n/a	n/a	n/a	1
Homepump Eclipse®/	unspec.	6, 9, 12 mg/mL	D5W	268, n/a, 293	d	16 d[b]	32 d[b]	8 w[b]	n/a	n/a	n/a	5
Homepump® C-Series (I-Flow Corp.)	unspec.	6, 9, 12 mg/mL	NS	294, n/a, 309	d	16 d[b]	32 d[b]	8 w[b]	n/a	n/a	n/a	5
	unspec.	10 mg/mL	NS	n/a	d	24 h	10 d	n/a	n/a	n/a	n/a	5

Storage Conditions

Clindamycin Phosphate (cont'd)

	Drug Manufacturer	Concentration	Diluents	Osmolality (mOsm/kg)	pH[d]	Temperature Room	Temperature Refrig	Temperature Frozen	Post-thaw Temp Room	Post-thaw Temp Refrig	Body Temp	Refer.
INTERMATE (Baxter)	UP	2–12 mg/mL	D5W	n/a–293	d	24 h	10 d	30 d	24 h	n/a	n/a	4
	UP	2–12 mg/mL	NS	n/a–309	d	24 h	10 d	30 d	24 h	n/a	n/a	4
	UP	6 mg/mL	W	n/a	n/a	n/a	10 d	n/a	n/a	n/a	n/a	4
Polyolefin Container (McGaw)	UP	7.6 mg/mL	D5W	n/a	d	n/a	n/a	30 d	n/a	14 d	n/a	1
COMMERCIAL PREPARATIONS (RTU)												
Galaxy Bag (Baxter)	PF	6, 12, 18 mg/mL	D5W	296, 322, 339	d	c	n/a	n/a	n/a	n/a	n/a	2

Flush Compatibility: Heparin lock flush and normal saline.[1]

Special Considerations: When refrigerated or frozen, solutions form crystals which must be resolubilized before administration.[6]

Notes

[a]Clindamycin phosphate is incompatible with natural rubber closures because of the risk of crystalline particulate extraction. If clindamycin phosphate is repackaged in disposable syringes, storage at room temperature should be limited to a few days.[1]

[b]Manufacturer(s) extrapolated data from other sources.

[c]Expiration date per manufacturer label. Do not extrapolate commercial premix stability data to extemporaneously compounded solutions.

[d]pH range is 5.5–7, typically 6–6.3.[1]

References

1. Trissel LA. ASHP's Interactive Handbook on Injectable Drugs. Bethesda, MD: American Society of Health-System Pharmacists. Accessed 2012 Jul.
2. Cleocin® [product information]. New York, NY: Pfizer Inc.; April 2010.
3. Drug Stability Data Using Elastomeric Infusion Systems. B. Braun Medical Production Ltd. (Thailand); August 2011.
4. Intermate/Infusor Drug Stability Information. Deerfield, IL: Baxter Healthcare Corporation; 2008.
5. Stability Data for Drugs Using Homepump Disposable Elastomeric Infusion Systems. Lake Forest, CA: I-Flow Corporation; October 2009.
6. Rapp RP, Hatton J, Record K. Drug Stability in Plastic Syringes. HealthTek™ and University of KY Lexington. Chester, NY: Repro-Med Systems Inc.; 1998.

Clonidine Hydrochloride

Container	Drug Manufacturer	Concentration	Diluents	Osmolality (mOsm/kg)	pH[p]	Temperature Room	Temperature Refrig	Temperature Frozen	Post-thaw Temp Room	Post-thaw Temp Refrig	Body Temp	Refer.
CONTAINERS												
Polypropylene (Mark II Polybag)	BI	5 mcg/mL[i,j]	NS	n/a	p	30 d[i,j,k]	n/a	n/a	n/a	n/a	n/a	1, 5
	BI	50 mcg/mL[i]	NS	n/a	p	30 d[i,k]	n/a	n/a	n/a	n/a	n/a	1, 5
Polyvinyl Chloride (PVC)	BI	3 mcg/mL[b]	NS	n/a	p	21 d[b]	n/a	n/a	n/a	n/a	n/a	1
	BI	9 mcg/mL[g]	NS	n/a	p	24 d[c,g]	28 d[c,g]	n/a	n/a	n/a	n/a	1
Syringes, Plastic (BD)	ROX	100 mcg/mL	undiluted	n/a	p	7 d	n/a	n/a	n/a	n/a	n/a	1
Syringes, Polypropylene	BI	9 mcg/mL	NS	n/a	p	30 d	30 d	n/a	n/a	n/a	30 d	1, 4
	BI	9 mcg/mL[h]	NS	n/a	p	30 d[h]	30 d[h]	n/a	n/a	n/a	30 d[h]	1, 4
OTHER INFUSION CONTAINERS												
Epi-Cath (Abbott)	unspec.	100 mcg/mL	undiluted	n/a	p	n/a	n/a	n/a	n/a	n/a	7 d	1
Glass	SH	0.2 mg/mL[d]	NS	n/a	p	n/a	n/a	n/a	n/a	n/a	10 w[d]	1, 3
	FUJ	11 mcg/mL[f]	f	n/a	p	14 d[c]	n/a	n/a	n/a	n/a	n/a	1
	FUJ	50 mcg/mL[e]	e	n/a	p	14 d[c]	n/a	n/a	n/a	n/a	n/a	1
	ROX	100 mcg/mL	undiluted	n/a	p	7 d	n/a	n/a	n/a	n/a	n/a	1
Glass Vials	ASH	0.15 mg/mL	NS	n/a	p	24 m	24 m	n/a	n/a	n/a	3 m	2
	ASH	0.5 mg/mL	NS	n/a	p	24 m	24 m	n/a	n/a	n/a	3 m	2
	ASH	1.5 mg/mL	NS	n/a	p	24 m	24 m	n/a	n/a	n/a	3 m	2
PORT-A-CATH® (SIMS Deltec)	unspec.	100 mcg/mL	undiluted	n/a	p	n/a	n/a	n/a	n/a	n/a	7 d[q]	1
Pump Reservoir (Bard)	ROX	100 mcg/mL	undiluted	n/a	p	7 d	n/a	n/a	n/a	n/a	n/a	1

Storage Conditions

continued on next page

126

Clonidine Hydrochloride (cont'd)

Drug Manufacturer	Concentration	Diluents	Osmolality (mOsm/kg)	pH[p]	Temperature			Post-thaw Temp			Refer.
					Room	Refrig	Frozen	Room	Refrig	Body Temp	
Synchromed* Implantable Pump (Medtronic) BI	0.15 mg/mL[n]	W	n/a	p	n/a	n/a	n/a	n/a	n/a	35 d[q]	1
unspec.	0.2 mg/mL[o]	NS	n/a	p	n/a	n/a	n/a	n/a	n/a	10 w[q]	1
NVS	0.25, 0.5, 1 mg/mL[l]	NS	n/a	p	n/a	n/a	n/a	n/a	n/a	14 w[l]	6
unspec.	2 mg/mL[m]	W	n/a	p	n/a	n/a	n/a	n/a	n/a	90 d[q]	1

Flush Compatibility: Heparin lock flush and normal saline.[1]

Special Considerations: For epidural administration only.[7]

Notes

[a]Do not use products or diluents containing preservatives for epidural administration.

[b]With meperidine hydrochloride 8 mg/mL.

[c]Protected from light.

[d]Solutions contained clonidine alone, or combined with baclofen 1 mg/mL. Both solutions exhibited same stability.

[e]With bupivacaine 3.75 mg/mL or morphine sulfate 5 mg/mL.

[f]With bupivacaine 6.67 mg/mL.

[g]Solution also contained bupivacaine 1 mg/mL and fentanyl 35 mcg/mL.

[h]Combined with fentanyl citrate 35 mcg/mL and bupivacaine hydrochloride 1 mg/mL.

[i]Also contains ropivacaine 1 mg/mL.

[j]Also contains ropivacaine 2 mg/mL.

[k]Tested at 30°C.

[l]Combined with baclofen 0.25, 0.5, and 1 mg/mL, respectively.

[m]Combined with bupivacaine 25 mg/mL and morphine sulfate 50 mg/mL.

[n]Combined with hydromorphone 25 mcg/mL.

[o]Combined with baclofen 1 mg/mL.

[p]pH of the undiluted solution is 5–7.[1]

[q]Tested at 37°C.

References

1. Trissel LA. ASHP's Interactive Handbook on Injectable Drugs. Bethesda, MD: American Society of Health-System Pharmacists. Accessed 2012 Jul.
2. Trissel LA, Xu QA, Hassenbusch SJ. Development of clonidine hydrochloride injections for epidural and intrathecal administration. *Int J Pharm Compound*. 1997; 1:274–7.
3. Godwin DA, Kim NH, Zuniga R. Stability of a baclofen and clonidine hydrochloride admixture for intrathecal administration. *Hosp Pharm*. 2001; 36:950–4.
4. Jappinen A, Kokki H, Naaranlahti T. pH stability of injectable fentanyl, bupivacaine, or clonidine solution or a ternary mixture in 0.9% sodium chloride in two types of polypropylene syringes. *Int J Pharm Compound*. 2002; 6:471–4.
5. Svedberg KO, McKenzie EJ, Larrivee-Elkins C. Compatibility of ropivacaine with morphine, sufentanil, fentanyl or clonidine. *J Clin Pharm Ther*. 2002; 27:39–45.
6. Alvarez JC, Mazancourt P, Chartier-Kastler E, et al. Drug stability testing to support clinical feasibility investigations for intrathecal baclofen-clonidine admixture. *J Pain Symptom Manage*. 2004; 28:268–72.
7. Duraclon® Clonidine hydrochloride injection [prescribing information]. Lake Forest, IL: Bioniche Pharma USA; May 2010.

Coagulation Factor VIIa Recombinant[b]

Drug Manufacturer	Concentration	Diluents	Osmolality (mOsm/kg)	pH[d]	Storage Conditions						Refer.
					Temperature			Post-thaw Temp		Body Temp	
					Room	Refrig	Frozen	Room	Refrig		
CONTAINER											
Polyvinyl Chloride (PVC) NNO[c]	Various[a,e]	W	n/a	d	3 d	n/a	n/a	n/a	n/a	n/a	1
NNO[c]	Various[a,f]	NS	n/a	d	3 d	n/a	n/a	n/a	n/a	24 h	2
Syringes, Plastic NNO[c]	Various[a,e]	W	n/a	d	3 d	n/a	n/a	n/a	n/a	n/a	1
OTHER INFUSION CONTAINERS											
CADD® Plus Cassette NNO[c]	Various[a]	W	n/a	d	3 d	n/a	n/a	n/a	n/a	n/a	1
Glass Vial NNO[c]	0.6 mg/mL	W	n/a	d	3 h	3 h	n/a	n/a	n/a	n/a	3
NNO[c]	Various[a]	W	n/a	d	6 h	24 h	n/a	n/a	n/a	n/a	4

Flush Compatibility: Normal saline, D5W.

Special Considerations: Avoid exposure to direct sunlight. Do not freeze or store in syringes. Bring product and diluent to room temperature before preparation.[3]

Notes

[a]Concentration is at manufacturer's recommended dilution.

[b]Undiluted product stored at room temperature. Dating is up to (but not past) the manufacturer's expiration dating on the package.

[c]NovoSeven® Coagulation Factor VIIa recombinant.

[d]When reconstituted as recommended, the resulting solution is a clear, colorless, isotonic preparation of neutral pH.

[e]Evaluated alone, with a low molecular weight heparin (LMWH), concentrations unspecified, and with heparin 5–10 units/mL in W. Note that addition of heparin 5–10 units/mL caused a 50% decrease in FVII activity in 4 h, whereas the LMWH did not affect FVII activity.[1]

[f]Evaluated alone and with enoxapirin or heparin in NS. Addition of heparin at pH7, LMWH, and NS did not affect FVII activity.[2]

References

1. Schulman S, Bech Jensen M, Varon D, et al. Feasibility of using recombinant factor VIIa in continuous infusion. [Abstract.] Thromb Haemost. 1996; 75:432–6.
2. Bonde C, Jensen MB. Continuous infusion of recombinant activated factor VII: stability in infusion pump systems. [Abstract.] Blood Coagul Fibrinolysis 1998; 9(suppl1):S103–5.
3. Novo Seven® (Coagulation Factor VIIa Recombinant) [prescribing information]. Princeton, NJ: Novo Nordisk Inc.; August 2010.
4. Negergaard H, Vestergaard S, Jensen PT, et al. In vitro stability of lyophilized and reconstituted recombinant activated factor VII formulated for storage at room temperature. Clin Therapeutics 2008; 30(7):1309–15.

Coagulation Factor VIII

continued on next page

| Drug Manufacturer | Concentration[a] | Diluents | Osmolality[j] (mOsm/kg) | pH[l] | Storage Conditions | | | | | | Refer. |
| | | | | | Temperature | | | Post-thaw Temp | | | |
					Room	Refrig	Frozen	Room	Refrig	Body Temp	
CONTAINER											
Polyvinyl Chloride (PVC)											
BA[c]	Various	W	–	–	4 d	n/a	n/a	n/a	n/a	n/a	1
BA[c]	Various	W[m]	–	–	4 d	n/a	n/a	n/a	n/a	n/a	1
BA[g]	Various	W	–	–	4 d	n/a	n/a	n/a	n/a	n/a	5, 6
BA[g]	Various	W[m]	–	–	4 d	n/a	n/a	n/a	n/a	n/a	5, 6
BA[h]	Various	W	–	–	48 h	n/a	n/a	n/a	n/a	n/a	7
BA[h]	Various	W[n]	–	–	48 h	n/a	n/a	n/a	n/a	n/a	7
BA[h]	Various	NS, W, 1/2S, D51/2S[n]	–	–	48 h	n/a	n/a	n/a	n/a	n/a	8
BA[h]	Various	NS, W, 1/2S, D51/2S	–	–	48 h	n/a	n/a	n/a	n/a	n/a	8
BAY[d]	100 unit/mL	W	–	–	7 d	7 d	n/a	n/a	n/a	n/a	2
BAY[d]	100 unit/mL	W[o]	–	–	7 d	7 d	n/a	n/a	n/a	n/a	2
CSL[e]	Various	W	–	–	15 d	n/a	n/a	n/a	n/a	n/a	3
Syringes, Plastic											
BAY[d]	50, 80, 120 units/mL	W, NS, LR	–	–	72 h	n/a	n/a	n/a	n/a	n/a	9
BAY[d]	100 unit/mL	W	–	–	7 d	7 d	n/a	n/a	n/a	n/a	2
BAY[d]	100 unit/mL	W[o]	–	–	7 d	7 d	n/a	n/a	n/a	n/a	2
OTHER INFUSION CONTAINERS											
CADD® Plus Cassette (Deltec)											
BA[h]	Various	W	–	–	48 h	n/a	n/a	n/a	n/a	n/a	7
BA[h]	Various	NS, 1/2S, D51/2S, W[n]	–	–	48 h	n/a	n/a	n/a	n/a	n/a	8

Coagulation Factor VIII (cont'd)

| | | | | | Storage Conditions | | | | | | |
| | | | | | Temperature | | | Post-thaw Temp | | | |
Drug Manufacturer	Concentration[a]	Diluents	Osmolality[l] (mOsm/kg)	pH[l]	Room	Refrig	Frozen	Room	Refrig	Body Temp	Refer.
Glass Vial											
BA[c]	unspec.	W	–	–	3 h	n/a	n/a	n/a	n/a	n/a	13
BA[c]	unspec.	W[r]	–	–	4 w	>24 h	n/a	n/a	n/a	<24 h	1
BA[g]	n/a	n/a	n/a	n/a	90 d[b]	n/a	n/a	n/a	n/a	n/a	17
BA[g]	unspec.	W	n/a	n/a	3 h	n/a	n/a	n/a	n/a	n/a	19
BA[g]	unspec.	W[r]	–	–	4 w	4 w	n/a	n/a	n/a	<24 h	5
BA[h]	unspec.	W	–	–	3 h	n/a	n/a	n/a	n/a	n/a	11
BA[h]	unspec.	W	n/a	n/a	24 h	n/a	n/a	n/a	n/a	n/a	17
BA[h]	n/a	n/a	n/a	n/a	180 d[b]	n/a	n/a	n/a	n/a	n/a	11
BAY[d]	n/a	n/a	n/a	n/a	90 d[b]	n/a	n/a	n/a	n/a	n/a	16
BAY[d]	n/a	n/a	n/a	n/a	n/a	12 m[b]	n/a	n/a	n/a	n/a	16
BAY[d]	unspec.	W	–	–	3 h	n/a	n/a	n/a	n/a	n/a	16
CSL[e]	n/a	n/a	n/a	n/a	180 d[b]	n/a	n/a	n/a	n/a	n/a	18
CSL[e]	unspec.	W	–	–	3 h	n/a	n/a	n/a	n/a	n/a	18
CSL[p]	n/a	n/a	n/a	n/a	90 d[b]	n/a	n/a	n/a	n/a	n/a	10
CSL[p]	unspec.	W	–	–	3 h	n/a	n/a	n/a	n/a	n/a	10
CSL[q]	n/a	n/a	n/a	n/a	n/a	12 m[b]	n/a	n/a	n/a	n/a	10
CSL[q]	unspec.	W	–	–	3 h	n/a	n/a	n/a	n/a	n/a	14
CSL[q]	n/a	n/a	n/a	n/a	n/a	24 m[b]	n/a	n/a	n/a	n/a	14
GRI[i]	n/a	n/a	n/a	n/a	60 d[b]	n/a	n/a	n/a	n/a	n/a	12
GRI[i]	n/a	n/a	n/a	n/a	n/a	36 m[b]	n/a	n/a	n/a	n/a	12
GRI[i]	unspec.	W	–	–	3 h	n/a	n/a	n/a	n/a	n/a	12
OCT[f]	n/a	n/a	n/a	n/a	180 d[b]	n/a	n/a	n/a	n/a	n/a	4
TAL[j]	n/a	n/a	n/a	n/a	180 d[b]	n/a	n/a	n/a	n/a	n/a	15
TAL[j]	unspec.	W	–	–	3 h	n/a	n/a	n/a	n/a	n/a	15
WY[k]	n/a	n/a	n/a	n/a	90 d[b]	n/a	n/a	n/a	n/a	n/a	21
WY[k,s]	unspec.	NS	n/a	–	3 h	n/a	n/a	n/a	n/a	n/a	20, 21

continued on next page

Coagulation Factor VIII (cont'd)

Drug	Manufacturer	Concentration[a]	Diluents	Osmolality[l] (mOsm/kg)	pH[l]	Storage Conditions						Refer.
						Temperature			Post-thaw Temp		Body Temp	
						Room	Refrig	Frozen	Room	Refrig		
Polypropylene	BA[c-g]	unspec.	W[r]	–	–	4 w	4 w	n/a	n/a	n/a	2 w	1,5
	BA[h]	Various	W[n]	–	–	24 h	n/a	n/a	n/a	n/a	n/a	7

Flush Compatibility: NS, D5W.

Special Considerations: Avoid exposure to direct sunlight. Do not freeze or store in syringes. Bring product and diluent to room temperature before preparation.[3] Stability is defined as retaining >80% of baseline value indicated by one-state clotting assay. Several continuous Factor VIII infusion studies noted variation in the loss of Factor VIII activity in PVC or polyethylene tubing upon initial dilution or infusion. This was primarily due to initial adsorption, resolved relatively quickly, was less pronounced with higher flow rates, and the overall impact on a long duration continuous factor infusion was therapeutically negligible.[6]

Notes

[a]Concentration is at manufacturer's recommended dilution unless noted.
[b]Undiluted product stored at room temperature. Dating is up to (but not past) the manufacturer's expiration dating on the package.
[c]Hemofil® brand.
[d]Kogenate® brand.
[e]Monoclate® brand.
[f]Wilate® brand.
[g]Recombinate® brand.
[h]Advate® brand.
[i]Alphanate® brand.
[j]Koate® brand.
[k]Xyntha® brand.
[l]When reconstituted as recommended, the resulting solution is a clear, colorless, isotonic preparation of neutral pH.
[m]Combined with heparin 1 unit/mL.
[n]Combined with heparin 2 units/mL.
[o]Combined with heparin 4 units/mL.
[p]Helixate® brand.
[q]Humate® brand.
[r]Samples stored in the dark.
[s]Xyntha® Solofuse.™

continued on next page

Coagulation Factor VIII (cont'd)

References

1. Global Medical Affairs, Baxter Bioscience [written correspondence]. Westlake Village, CA: Baxter Bioscience; August 9, 2004.
2. Hurst D. Evaluation of recombinant factor VIII (Kogenate) stability for continuous infusion using a minipump infusion device. *Haemophilia* 1998; 4:785–9.
3. Schulman S. Monoclonally purified F VIII for continuous infusion: stability, microbiological safety and clinical experienced. *J Thromb Haemost.* 1994; 72:403–7.
4. Wilate® (von Willebrand Factor/Antihemophilic Factor Human) [prescribing information]. Hoboken, NJ: Octapharma USA; December 2009.
5. Global Medical Affairs, Baxter Bioscience [written correspondence]. Westlake Village, CA: Baxter Bioscience; February 21, 2005.
6. Parti R. In vitro stability of recombinant human factor VIII (recombinant). *Haemophilia* 2000; 6:513–22.
7. Global Medical Affairs, Baxter Bioscience [written correspondence]. Westlake Village, CA: Baxter Bioscience; February 9, 2005.
8. Fernandez M. Stability of Advate, antihemophilic factor (recombinant) plasma/albumin-free method, during simulated continuous infusion. *Blood Coagul Fibrinolysis* 2006; 17:165–71.
9. Rand M. Stability of dilutions of the recombinant factor VIII Kogenate FS stored in syringes. *J Thromb Haemostatis.* 2003; 1(suppl 1):1.
10. Helixate FS® (Antihemophilic Factor Recombinant) [prescribing information]. Tarrytown, NY: Bayer Healthcare; April 2011.
11. Advate® (Antihemophilic Factor Recombinant) [prescribing information]. Westlake Village, CA: Baxter Healthcare Corporation; December 2011.
12. Alphanate® (Antihemophilic Factor human) [prescribing information]. Los Angeles, CA: Grifols Biologicals, Inc.; June 2011.
13. Hemofil M® (Antihemophilic Factor Human) [prescribing information]. Westlake Village, CA: Baxter Healthcare Corporation; November 2010.
14. Humate-P® (Antihemophilic Factor/von Willebrand Factor Complex Human) [prescribing information]. Kankakee, IL: CSL Behring; January 2010.
15. Koate-DVI® (Antihemophilic Factor Human) [prescribing information]. Research Triangle Park, NC: Talecris Biotherapeutics; September 2006.
16. Kogenate FS® (Antihemophilic Factor Recombinant) [prescribing information]. Tarrytown, NY: Bayer Healthcare LLC; March 2011.
17. Trissel LA. ASHP's Interactive Handbook on Injectable Drugs. Bethesda, MD: American Society of Health-System Pharmacists. Accessed 2012 Jul.
18. Monoclate-P® (Antihemophilic Factor Human) [prescribing information]. Kankakee, IL: CSL Behring; October 2010.
19. Recombinate® (Antihemophilic Factor Recombinant) [prescribing information]. Westlake Village, CA: Baxter Healthcare Corporation; March 2010.
20. Xyntha® Solofuse™ (Antihemophilic Factor Recombinant) [prescribing information]. Philadelphia, PA: Wyeth; September 2011.
21. Xyntha® (Antihemophilic Factor Recombinant) [prescribing information]. Philadelphia, PA: Wyeth; June 2011.

Coagulation Factor IX

Coagulation Factor IX

Storage Conditions

| Drug Manufacturer | Concentration | Diluents | Osmolality (mOsm/kg) | pH | Temperature | | | Post-thaw Temp | | | Refer. |
					Room	Refrig	Frozen	Room	Refrig	Body Temp	
CONTAINER											
Syringes, Plastic (Polyethylene)											
WY[a]	100 units/mL[c]	W[l]	m	m	4 d	n/a	n/a	n/a	n/a	n/a	1
WY[a]	100 units/mL	W[l]	m	m	7 d	n/a	n/a	n/a	n/a	n/a	1
CSL[d]	100 units/mL	W[l]	m	m	28 d	n/a	n/a	n/a	n/a	n/a	2
OTHER INFUSION CONTAINERS											
Glass Vial											
GRI[b]	Various[e]	W[l]	m	m	3 h	n/a	n/a	n/a	n/a	n/a	3
GRI[b]	n/a	n/a	n/a	n/a	30 d[f]	n/a	n/a	n/a	n/a	n/a	3
WY[a]	Various[e]	1/4S[l]	m	m	3 h	n/a	n/a	n/a	n/a	n/a	4
WY[a]	n/a	n/a	n/a	n/a	180 d[f]	n/a	n/a	n/a	n/a	n/a	4
CSL[d]	Various[e]	W[l]	m	m	3 h	n/a	n/a	n/a	n/a	n/a	5
CSL[d]	n/a	n/a	n/a	n/a	30 d[f]	n/a	n/a	n/a	n/a	n/a	5
GRI[g]	Various[e]	W[l]	m	m	3 h	n/a	n/a	n/a	n/a	n/a	6
GRI[g]	n/a	n/a	n/a	n/a	90 d[f]	n/a	n/a	n/a	n/a	n/a	6
BA[h]	Various[e]	W[l]	m	m	3 h	n/a	n/a	n/a	n/a	n/a	7
BA[h]	n/a	n/a	n/a	n/a	14 d[i]	n/a	n/a	n/a	n/a	n/a	9
BA[j]	Various[e]	W[l]	m	m	3 h	n/a	n/a	n/a	n/a	n/a	8
BA[j]	n/a	n/a	n/a	n/a	12 m[k]	n/a	n/a	n/a	n/a	n/a	9

Flush Compatibility: NS, D5W.

Special Considerations: Stability is defined as retaining >80% of baseline value indicated by one-state clotting assay. All Factor IX products are labeled for refrigerated storage until prepared for patient use. Do not freeze.

continued on next page

Notes

[a]*BeneFIX® brand.*
[b]*AlphaNine SD® brand.*
[c]*Combined with heparin 4 units/mL.*
[d]*Mononine® brand.*
[e]*Dilution per manufacturer's instruction.*
[f]*Undiluted product stored at room temperature. Dating is up to (but not past) the manufacturer's expiration dating on the package.*
[g]*Profilnine SD® brand.*

Coagulation Factor IX (cont'd)

hProplex T® brand (Factor IX Complex, also contains Factors II, VII, and X).

iStored at 47.5°C to simulate brief unrefrigerated temperature excursions during warehousing or shipping. Manufacturer recommends minimizing such temperature excursions.

jBebulin VH® brand.

kStored at 30°C, protected from light, to simulated unrefrigerated temperature excursion during warehousing or shipping. Manufacturer recommends minimizing such temperature exposures.

lManufacturer-supplied diluent.

mWhen reconstituted as recommended, the resulting solution is a clear, colorless, isotonic preparation of neutral pH.

References

1. Chowdary P. Recombinant factor IX (Benefix®) by adjusted continuous infusion; a study of stability, sterility and clinical experience. Haemophilia. 2001; 7:140–5.
2. Schulman S. The feasibility of using concentrates containing factor IX for continuous infusion. Haemophilia 1995; 1:103–10.
3. Alphanine SD® (Coagulation Factor IX Human) [prescribing information]. Los Angeles, CA: Grifols Biologicals; August 2010.
4. BeneFIX® (Coagulation Factor IX Recombinant) [prescribing information]. Philadelphia, PA: Wyeth; November 2011.
5. Mononine® (Coagulation Factor IX Human) [prescribing information]. Kankakee, IL: CSL Behring; October 2011.
6. Profilnine SD® (Factor IX Complex) [prescribing information]. Los Angeles, CA: Grifols Biologicals; August 2010.
7. Proplex T® (Factor IX Complex) [prescribing information]. Westlake Village, CA: Baxter Healthcare; November 2002.
8. Bebulin VH® (Factor IX Complex) [prescribing information]. Westlake Village, CA. Baxter Healthcare Corporation; April 2011.
9. Global Medical Affairs, Baxter Bioscience [written correspondence]. Westlake Village, CA: Baxter Bioscience; April 14, 2008.

Coagulation Factor XIII

	Drug Manufacturer	Concentration	Diluents	Osmolality (mOsm/kg)	pH	Storage Conditions							Refer.
						Temperature			Post-thaw Temp			Body Temp	
						Room	Refrig	Frozen	Room	Refrig			
OTHER INFUSION CONTAINERS													
Glass Vial	CSL[a]	unspec.	W[b]	n/a	n/a	4 h	n/a	n/a	n/a	n/a	n/a	1
	CSL[a]	n/a	n/a	n/a	n/a	6 m[c]	c	n/a	n/a	n/a	n/a	1

Flush Compatibility: No information available.
Special Considerations: Store at 2–8°C. Avoid exposure to direct sunlight. Do not freeze. Do not store in syringes. Bring product and diluent to room temperature before preparation.

Notes

[a]*Cortifact® brand.*
[b]*Diluent provided with product.*
[c]*Undiluted product may be stored at room temperature up to 25°C for up to 6 months if within labeled manufacturer expiration date; do not return to refrigerator if stored at room temperature.*

Reference

1. Cortifact® (Factor XIII) [prescribing information]. Kankakee, IL: CSL Behring; February 2011.

Colistimethate Sodium

	Drug Manufacturer	Concentration	Diluents	Osmolality (mOsm/kg)	pH[a]	Storage Conditions							Refer.
						Temperature			Post-thaw Temp			Body Temp	
						Room	Refrig	Frozen	Room	Refrig	Body Temp		
CONTAINER													
Glass Vial	unspec.	75 mg/mL	W	n/a	7–8	7d	7d	n/a	n/a	n/a	n/a		1
Unspecified	unspec.	unspec.	NS, D5W D5¼S, LR, D5S, D5½S	n/a	a	24 h	n/a	n/a	n/a	n/a	n/a		1
OTHER INFUSION CONTAINERS													
INTERMATE (Baxter)	PX	1–3 mg/mL	NS, D5W	n/a	a	2 d[b]	30 d	n/a	2 d	n/a	n/a		2

Flush Compatibility: Normal saline and heparin.[1]
Special Considerations: n/a.

Notes

[a]*pH of reconstituted product is 7–8.[1]*
[b]*After 30 d refrigerated storage.*

References

1. Trissel LA. ASHP's Interactive Handbook on Injectable Drugs. Bethesda, MD: American Society of Health-System Pharmacists. Accessed 2012 Jan.
2. Intermate/Infusor Drug Stability Information. Deerfield, IL: Baxter Healthcare Corporation; October 2008.

Co-Trimoxazole (Trimethoprim–Sulfamethoxazole)[a,b]

Container	Drug Manufacturer	Concentration	Diluents	Osmolality (mOsm/kg)	pH[e]	Temperature			Post-thaw Temp		Body Temp	Refer.
						Room	Refrig	Frozen	Room	Refrig		
CONTAINER												
Polyvinyl Chloride (PVC)	ES	1.08 + 5.4 mg/mL, 1.6 + 8 mg/mL	D5W	n/a	e	24 h	n/a	n/a	n/a	n/a	n/a	1
Syringes, Plastic	ES	16 + 80 mg/mL	undiluted[b,c]	n/a	9.5–10.5	60 h	n/a	n/a	n/a	n/a	n/a	1
OTHER INFUSION CONTAINERS												
Glass	RC, BW	0.64 + 3.2 mg/mL	D5W, NS[d]	n/a	e	48 h	n/a	n/a	n/a	n/a	n/a	1
	RC	0.8 + 4 mg/mL	D5W	n/a	e	24 h	n/a	n/a	n/a	n/a	n/a	1
Unspecified	RC	0.64 + 3.2 mg/mL	D5½S, ½S D5W, NS[d]	n/a	e	24 h	n/a	n/a	n/a	n/a	n/a	1
	RC	0.8 + 4 mg/mL	D5½S, ½S D5W, NS[d]	n/a	e	24 h	n/a	n/a	n/a	n/a	n/a	1

Flush Compatibility: Heparin lock flush and normal saline.[1]
Special Considerations: n/a

Notes

[a]Co-trimoxazole should be stored at 15–25°C and not refrigerated. Concentrations cited are for trimethoprim + sulfamethoxazole in mg/mL.
[b]Because of the short stability of this drug, practitioners may elect to prefill and dispense syringes of undiluted drug so that the patient or caregiver can easily add this to the container(s) of diluent immediately prior to administration.
[c]In polypropylene syringes (BD).
[d]Manufacturer recommends only D5W for dilution and infusion.
[e]pH of undiluted solution is 9.5–10.5.[1]

Reference

1. Trissel LA. ASHP's Interactive Handbook on Injectable Drugs. Bethesda, MD: American Society of Health-System Pharmacists. Accessed 2012 Jan.

137

Cyclophosphamide

Cyclophosphamide[a,d]

Container	Drug Manufacturer	Concentration	Diluents	Osmolality (mOsm/kg)	pH[g]	Storage Conditions Temperature Room	Refrig	Frozen	Post-thaw Temp Room	Refrig	Body Temp	Refer.
CONTAINER												
Glass	unspec.	0.1, 3.1 mg/mL	D5S, D5W		g	8 h	6 d	n/a	n/a	n/a	n/a	5, 8
	unspec.	21 mg/mL	W		g	8 h	6 d	n/a	n/a	n/a	n/a	5, 8
Polyethylene Bag	ASM	1.8 mg/mL	D5W	i	g	6 h[f]	48 h[f]	n/a	n/a	n/a	n/a	6
	ASM	10.8 mg/mL	D5W	i	g	24 h[e]	72 h[e]	n/a	n/a	n/a	n/a	5, 6
Polyvinyl Chloride (PVC)	MJ	0.3, 2 mg/mL[b]	NS, D5W	i	g	5 d[b]	8 d[b]	n/a	n/a	n/a	n/a	1, 5
	CE	4 mg/mL	NS	i	g	n/a	19 w	19 w	n/a	n/a	n/a	2, 5
Syringes, Plastic	ES, BMS, AD	unspec.	NS, D5W	i	g	24 h	4 w	19 w[c]	n/a	n/a	n/a	10
Syringes, Polypropylene (BD)	CE	20 mg/mL	W[i]	i	g	n/a	4 w[c]	19 w[c]	n/a	n/a	n/a	2, 5
OTHER INFUSION CONTAINERS												
AccuFlo™/ AccuFlux™/ AccuRX® (B. Braun)	unspec.	4.5 mg/mL	NS	i	g	7 d	7 d	n/a	n/a	n/a	n/a	9
Homepump Eclipse®/ Homepump® C-Series (Block Medical)	unspec.	4.5 mg/mL	NS	i	g	7 d	7 d	n/a	n/a	n/a	n/a	4
INFUSOR (Baxter)	MJ	2–20 mg/mL	NS	i	g	2 d	48 d[h]	n/a	n/a	n/a	n/a	3, 7

Flush Compatibility: Heparin lock flush and normal saline.[5]
Special Considerations: Cyclophosphamide solutions should not be stored at temperatures above 25°C.[5] If frozen, avoid microwave thawing.[10]

continued on next page

Cyclophosphamide (cont'd)

Notes

[a] Do not use benzyl alcohol-preserved diluents.

[b] Combined with ondansetron (GL) 0.05 mg/mL and ondansetron (GL) 0.4 mg/mL, respectively.

[c] Solution in syringes precipitated after a microwave thaw and required vigorous shaking. Solutions may not precipitate if concentrations are <8 mg/mL. Frozen syringes exhibited a marked contraction of the plungers during cooling that allowed seepage of solution onto the syringe barrel.

[d] Do not store solutions at temperatures above 25°C.[5]

[e] Solution also contained mesna 3.2 mg/mL.

[f] Solution also contained mesna 0.54 mg/mL.

[g] pH of reconstituted solution is 3–9; 22 mg/mL is pH 6.87.[5]

[h] 48 d refrigerated followed by 12 h at room temp.[7]

[i] The osmolality of cyclophosphamide reconstituted with NS is 374 mOsm/kg. When reconstituted with W, the osmolality is 74 mOsm/kg, requiring further dilution in an appropriate IV solution for administration.[5]

References

1. Fleming RA, Olsen DJ, Savage PD, et al. Stability of ondansetron hydrochloride and cyclophosphamide in injectable solutions. *Am J Health-Syst Pharm*. 1995; 52:514–6.
2. Kirk B, Melia CD, Wilson JV, et al. Chemical stability of cyclophosphamide injection: effect of low temperature storage and microwave thawing. *Br J Parenter Ther*. 1984; 5:90, 2, 4, 6–7.
3. Akahoshi MP, Enriquez NC, Maki JK, et al. Safety and reliability of the travenol infusor in administering chemotherapy in the home. *J Pharm Technol*. 1987; (Mar–Apr):65–8.
4. *Stability Data for Drugs Using Homepump Disposable Elastomeric Infusion Systems*. Lake Forest, CA: I-Flow Corporation; October 2009.
5. Trissel LA. ASHP's Interactive Handbook on Injectable Drugs. Bethesda, MD: American Society of Health-System Pharmacists. Accessed 2012 Jul.
6. Menard C, Bourguignon C, Schlatter J, et al. Stability of cyclophosphamide and mesna admixtures in polyethylene infusion bags. *Ann Pharmacotherapy* 2003; 37:1789–92.
7. *Intermate/Infusor Drug Stability Information*. Deerfield, IL: Baxter Healthcare Corporation; October 2008.
8. Brooke D, Bequette RJ, Davis RE. Chemical stability of cyclophosphamide in parenteral solutions. *Am J Hosp Pharm*. 1973; 30:134–7.
9. *Drug Stability Data Using Elastomeric Infusion Systems*. B. Braun Medical Production Ltd. (Thailand); August 2011.
10. Rapp RP, Hatton J, Record K. *Drug Stability in Plastic Syringes*. HealthTek™ and University of KY Lexington. Chester, NY: Repro-Med Systems Inc.; 1998.

Cyclosporine[a]

Container / Drug Manufacturer	Concentration	Diluents	Osmolality (mOsm/kg)	pH	Storage Conditions Temperature Room	Refrig	Frozen	Post-thaw Temp Room	Refrig	Body Temp	Refer.
CONTAINER											
Polyvinyl Chloride (PVC)											
SZ	1 mg/mL	D5W	n/a	n/a	72 h[b]	n/a	n/a	n/a	n/a	n/a	1
SZ	2 mg/mL	NS	n/a	n/a	24 h[b]	n/a	n/a	n/a	n/a	n/a	1
OTHER INFUSION CONTAINERS											
AVIVA Bag (Baxter)[c]											
NVS	0.2, 2.5 mg/mL	D5W, NS	n/a	n/a	14 d	n/a	n/a	n/a	n/a	n/a	2
Glass Bottles											
SZ	2 mg/mL	D5W	n/a	n/a	48 h	48 h	n/a	n/a	n/a	n/a	1

Flush Compatibility: Normal saline.[1]

Special Considerations: Due to leaching of syringe plunger components, polypropylene syringes cannot be recommended for storage of cyclosporine solutions. Short term (less than 10 min) syringe use for preparation and transfer is considered safe.[2]

Notes

[a]Do not use DEHP-containing containers or tubing to administer cyclosporine.

[b]Although studies showed longer expiration dating, the manufacturer recommends 6 h expiration date in PVC due to the potential for DEHP leaching.

[c]Polypropylene–polyolefin bag.

References

1. Trissel LA. ASHP's Interactive Handbook on Injectable Drugs. Bethesda, MD: American Society of Health-System Pharmacists. Accessed 2012 Jan.
2. Li M, Forest JM, Coursol C, et al. Stability of cyclosporine solutions stored in polypropylene–polyolefin bags and polypropylene syringes. Am J Health-Syst Pharm. 2011; 68:1646–50.

Cytarabine

Container	Drug Manufacturer	Concentration	Diluents	Osmolality (mOsm/kg)	pH[e]	Temperature Room	Temperature Refrig	Temperature Frozen	Post-thaw Temp Room	Post-thaw Temp Refrig	Body Temp	Refer.
CONTAINER												
Ethyvinyl Acetate (EVA)	UP	1.25, 25 mg/mL	NS, D5W	n/a	e	28 d[a]	28 d[a]	n/a	n/a	n/a	7 d[a,c]	1, 6
Polyvinyl Chloride (PVC)	UP	8, 24, 32 mg/mL	D5W, NS D5¼S	n/a	e	7 d	7 d	7 d	n/a	n/a	n/a	6
	unspec.	20 mg/mL	BWFI, NS	n/a	e	8 d	n/a	n/a	n/a	n/a	n/a	2
Syringes, Plastic (BD)	UP	20, 50 mg/mL	W	n/a	e	29 d[a]	29 d[a]	n/a	n/a	n/a	n/a	3, 6
	unspec.	40, 80 mg/mL	W[d]	n/a	e	15 d	15 d	n/a	n/a	n/a	7 d	6
Unspecified	unspec.	0.5 mg/mL	D5W, NS, W	n/a	e	8 d	n/a	n/a	n/a	n/a	n/a	6
	unspec.	0.5–5 mg/mL	D5W, NS RL, W	n/a	e	14 d	n/a	n/a	n/a	n/a	n/a	6
	unspec.	20, 250 mg/mL[g]	W[d]	n/a	e	5 d[g]	n/a	n/a	n/a	n/a	n/a	6
OTHER INFUSION CONTAINERS												
Glass	UP	8, 24, 32 mg/mL	D5W, NS D5¼S	n/a	e	7 d	7 d	7 d	n/a	n/a	n/a	6
Infusaid (Metal Bellows Corp.)	UP	1 mg/mL	Elliott's B[b]	n/a	e	n/a	n/a	n/a	n/a	n/a	15 d	4, 6
INFUSOR (Baxter)	UP	5 mg/mL	D5W	n/a	e	7 d[a,f]	n/a	n/a	n/a	n/a	24 h[a,f]	5

Flush Compatibility: Heparin lock flush and normal saline.[6]
Special Considerations: Cytarabine 2.5 mg/mL in NS is 299 mOsm/kg; pH is 5.3.[6]

Notes

[a]Solutions stored in the dark.
[b]Artificial spinal fluid.
[c]Storage at 35°C.
[d]Bacteriostatic water for injection.

continued on next page

141

Cytarabine (cont'd)

[e]pH of reconstituted preparation is 4–6. pH of commercial injection 20 mg/mL is 7–9.[6]

[f]Stored at 25°C for 7 d, followed by 24 h at 33°C.

[g]Cytarabine has an aqueous solubility of 100 mg/mL. Precipitation from more concentrated solutions has been observed.[6]

References

1. Rochard EB, Barthes DMC, Courtois PY. Stability of fluorouracil, cytarabine, or doxorubicin hydrochloride in ethylene vinylacetete portable infusion-pump containers. *Am J Hosp Pharm.* 1992; 49:619–23.

2. Vyas HM, Baptista RJ, Mitrano FP, et al. Drug stability guidelines for a continuous infusion chemotherapy program. *Hosp Pharm.* 1987; 22:685–7.

3. Weir PJ, Ireland DS. Chemical stability of cytarabine and vinblastine injections. *Br J Pharm Pract.* 1990; 12:53–4, 60.

4. Keller JH, Ensminger WD. Stability of cancer chemotherapeutic agents in a totally implanted drug delivery system. *Am J Hosp Pharm.* 1982; 39:1321–3.

5. *Intermate/Infusor Drug Stability Information.* Deerfield, IL: Baxter Healthcare Corporation; October 2008.

6. Trissel LA. ASHP's Interactive Handbook on Injectable Drugs. Bethesda, MD: American Society of Health-System Pharmacists. Accessed 2012 Jun.

Dacarbazine[a]

CONTAINER	Drug Manufacturer	Concentration	Diluents	Osmolality (mOsm/kg)	pH[b]	Storage Conditions							Refer.
						Temperature			Post-thaw Temp			Body Temp	
						Room	Refrig	Frozen	Room	Refrig			
Polyvinyl Chloride (PVC)	AVE	1.4 mg/mL	D5W	n/a	b	48 h[c]	7 d[c]	n/a	n/a	n/a	n/a	n/a	1, 2

Flush Compatibility: Normal saline. Dacarbazine 10 mg/mL in NS and heparin sodium 100 units/mL.[1]
Special Considerations: Dacarbazine 25 mg/mL in NS formed an immediate precipitation when combined with heparin sodium 100 units/mL.[1]

Notes

[a]Manufacturer recommends protection from light.
[b]pH of reconstituted preparation 10 mg/mL in W is 3–4.[1]
[c]Protected from light.

References

1. Trissel LA. ASHP's Interactive Handbook on Injectable Drugs. Bethesda, MD: American Society of Health-System Pharmacists. Accessed 2012 Jun.
2. El Aatmani M, Poujol S, Astre C, et al. Stability of dacarbazine in amber glass vials and polyvinyl chloride bags. Am J Health-Syst Pharm. 2002; 59:1351–6.

Daclizumab

Storage Conditions

Container	Drug Manufacturer	Concentration	Diluents	Osmolality (mOsm/kg)	pH[e]	Temperature			Post-thaw Temp			Refer.
						Room	Refrig	Frozen	Room	Refrig	Body Temp	
CONTAINER												
Polyethylene Bag	RC	unspec.	NS	n/a	e	4 h	24 h	n/a	n/a	n/a	n/a	1
Polyvinyl Chloride (PVC)	RC	unspec.	NS	n/a	e	4 h	24 h	n/a	n/a	n/a	n/a	1, 2
OTHER INFUSION CONTAINERS												
Glass[a]	RC	5 mg/mL	a	n/a	e	7 d	12 m[b]	c	n/a	n/a	n/a	2
Glass	RC	5 mg/mL	a	n/a	e	14 d	6 m[d]	n/a	n/a	n/a	n/a	2

Flush Compatibility: Normal saline.[1]

Special Considerations: The calculated dosage of product must be diluted in 50 mL NS prior to administration over a 15 minute period by central or peripheral vein. To mix the solution, gently invert the bag to avoid foaming. Do not shake.[1]

Notes

[a]In original glass vial packaging.

[b]Product stored at room temperature, 30°C for 1 w, then 12 m at 2–8°C.

[c]Package insert states do not shake or freeze, store between 2–8°C. However, in accelerated studies conducted in original packaging, stability was maintained after freezing through 1–2 freeze/thaw cycles. The "avoid freezing" precaution is recommended to avoid unnecessary stress on the product.

[d]Product stored at room temperature, 30°C for 1 d, then 25°C for 13 d, then 6 m at 2–8°C.

[e]pH of undiluted concentrate is 6.9.[1]

References

1. Zenapax® [product insert]. Nutley, NJ: Roche Pharmaceuticals; September 2005.
2. Allison Bernkopf, Pharm.D. [personal communication]. Nutley, NJ: Roche Pharmaceuticals; April 1, 2008.

Daptomycin

Container	Drug Manufacturer	Concentration	Diluents	Osmolality (mOsm/kg)[b]	pH[b]	Temperature			Post-thaw Temp			Refer.
						Room	Refrig	Frozen	Room	Refrig	Body Temp	
CONTAINER												
Polyvinyl Chloride (PVC)	CUB	unspec.[a]	NS	n/a	n/a	12 h	48 h	n/a	n/a	n/a	n/a	1
	CUB	2.5, 10, 20 mg/mL	NS	n/a, n/a, & 323	n/a, n/a, & 4.5	n/a	10 d	n/a	n/a	n/a	n/a	2
Syringes, Plastic	CUB	20 mg/mL	NS	323	4.5	12 h	10 d	n/a	n/a	n/a	n/a	2
OTHER INFUSION CONTAINERS												
AccuFlo™/ AccuFlux™/ AccuRX® (B. Braun)	CUB	5 mg/mL	NS	304	4.5	7 d	14 d		n/a	n/a	n/a	4
Glass	CUB	50 mg/mL	NS	n/a	n/a	12 h	48 h	n/a	n/a	n/a	n/a	1
	CUB	50 mg/mL	W, LR	38–47, 307	4.8–5.0, 4.59	12 h	48 h	n/a	n/a	n/a	n/a	2
Homepump®/ Homepump Eclipse® (I-Flow Corp.)	CUB	20 mg/mL	NS	323	4.5	n/a	10 d	n/a	n/a	n/a	n/a	6
INTERMATE (Baxter)	CUB	20 mg/mL	NS	323	4.5	n/a	10 d	n/a	n/a	n/a	n/a	5

Storage Conditions

Flush Compatibility: Heparin lock flush and normal saline.[3]

Special Considerations: Manufacturer labeling states to administer intravenously over 2 or 30 min. Do not prepare in dextrose solutions. During reconstitution, avoid vigorous agitation or shaking of the vial to minimize foaming; slowly add 10 mL NS to vial and gently rotate vial to wet product. Allow to stand undisturbed for 10 min. Then gently rotate or swirl vial contents to completely reconstitute. Do not use with ReadyMED® elastomeric devices.[1]

Notes

[a]Appropriate volume of reconstituted (50 mg/mL) daptomycin is further diluted into 50 mL NS.[1]
[b]Osmolality figures are primarily due to the diluent. pH and osmolality data provided by manufacturer.[2]

continued on next page

Daptomycin (cont'd)

References

1. Cubicin® [product information]. Lexington, MA: Cubist Pharmaceuticals Inc.; November 2010.
2. Inguilizian A. Cubicin stability in syringes [personal communication]. Lexington, MA: Drug Information Department, Cubist Pharmaceuticals Inc.; February 2008.
3. Lai JJ, Brodeur SK. Physical and chemical compatibility of daptomycin with nine medications. *Ann Pharmacother*. 2004; 38(10):1612–6.
4. *Drug Stability Data Using Elastomeric Infusion Systems*. B. Braun Medical Production Ltd. (Thailand); August 2011.
5. Mitrano JA. Cubicin® Compatibility and Stability in Elastomeric Pumps [personal communication]. Lexington, MA: Drug Information Department, Cubist Pharmaceuticals Inc.; August 5, 2008.
6. *Stability Data for Drugs Using Homepump Disposable Elastomeric Infusion Systems*. Lake Forest, CA: I-Flow Corporation; October 2009.

Daunorubicin Hydrochloride (Daunomycin)

CONTAINER	Drug Manufacturer	Concentration	Diluents	Osmolality (mOsm/kg)	pH[c]	Storage Conditions						Refer.
						Temperature			Post-thaw Temp		Body Temp	
						Room	Refrig	Frozen	Room	Refrig		
Polyvinyl Chloride (PVC)	RP	0.1 mg/mL	NS, D5W	n/a	c	43 d[a]	43 d[a]	43 d[a,b]	n/a	n/a	n/a	1, 2
Syringes, Plastic	RP	0.1 mg/mL	D5W, NS, LR	n/a	c	28 d[a]	n/a	n/a	n/a	n/a	n/a	1, 3
Syringes, Polypropylene	RP	2 mg/mL	W	n/a	c	n/a	43 d[a]	n/a	n/a	n/a	n/a	1, 2

Flush Compatibility: Normal saline.[1]
Special Considerations: n/a

Notes

[a]All solutions stored in the dark.
[b]Frozen samples were subjected to 11 freeze/thaw cycles with no apparent loss in potency between cycles.
[c]pH of solutions is 4.5–6.5; maximum stability is at pH 4.2–5.5.[1]

References

1. Trissel LA. ASHP's Interactive Handbook on Injectable Drugs. Bethesda, MD: American Society of Health-System Pharmacists. Accessed 2012 Mar.
2. Wood MJ, Irwin WJ, Scott DK. Stability of doxorubicin, daunorubicin and epirubicin in plastic syringes and minibags. *J Clin Pharm Ther.* 1990; 15:279–89.
3. Beijnen JH, Rosing H, DeVries PA, et al. Stability of anthracycline antitumour agents in infusion fluids. *Bull Parenter Drug Assoc.* 1985; 39(Nov–Dec):220–2.

Deferoxamine Mesylate

continued on next page

	Drug Manufacturer	Concentration	Diluents	Osmolality[f] (mOsm/kg)	pH	Temperature Room	Temperature Refrig	Temperature Frozen	Post-thaw Temp Room	Post-thaw Temp Refrig	Body Temp	Refer.
CONTAINER												
Polypropylene Syringes (Pharmacia Deltec)	CG	250 mg/mL[d]	W	f	n/a	14 d[a]	n/a	n/a	n/a	n/a	n/a	1
OTHER INFUSION CONTAINERS												
AccuFlo™/ AccuFlux™/ AccuRX® (Medpro)	unspec.	5 mg/mL	NS	f	n/a	12 d	n/a	n/a	n/a	n/a	n/a	3
	unspec.	5–160 mg/mL	NS	f	n/a	n/a	28 d	n/a	n/a	n/a	n/a	3
	unspec.	73 mg/mL	NS	f	n/a	7 d	28 d	n/a	n/a	n/a	n/a	3
Homepump®/ Homepump Eclipse® (I-Flow Corp.)	unspec.	5 mg/mL	NS	f	n/a	12 d[b]	n/a	n/a	n/a	n/a	n/a	2
	unspec.	5–160 mg/mL	NS	f	n/a	n/a	28 d	n/a	n/a	n/a	n/a	2
	unspec.	73 mg/mL	NS	f	n/a	7 d[b]	28 d	n/a	n/a	n/a	n/a	2
INFUSOR (Baxter)	CG	0–83 mg/mL°	NS	f	n/a	3 d[g]	n/a	n/a	n/a	n/a	7 d[i]	4
	CG	0–83 mg/mL°	NS	f	n/a	6 d[h]	n/a	n/a	n/a	n/a	5 d[i]	4
	CG	0–83 mg/mL°	NS	f	n/a	14 d[g]	n/a	n/a	n/a	n/a	7 d[i]	4
	CG	0–83 mg/mL°	NS	f	n/a	3 d	15 d[i]	n/a	n/a	n/a	7 d[i]	4
	CG	0–83 mg/mL°	NS	f	n/a	3 d	35 d[p]	n/a	n/a	n/a	6 d[i]	4
	CG	0–83 mg/mL°	NS	f	n/a	17 d[h]	n/a	n/a	n/a	n/a	5 d[i]	4
	CG	0–83 mg/mL°	NS	f	n/a	21 d[k]	n/a	n/a	n/a	n/a	2 d[i]	4
	CG	25 mg/mL°	NS	f	n/a	3 d	15 d[i]	n/a	n/a	n/a	7 d[i]	4
	CG	83.3 mg/mL°	W	f	n/a	4 d	31 d[q]	n/a	n/a	n/a	3 d[i]	4
	CG	83.3 mg/mL°	W	f	n/a	3 d	35 d[e]	n/a	n/a	n/a	3 d[i]	4
	CG	83.3 mg/mL°	W	f	n/a	15 d	n/a	n/a	n/a	n/a	n/a	4
	CG	83.3 mg/mL°	W	f	n/a	20 d	n/a	n/a	n/a	n/a	n/a	4
	CG	83–160 mg/mL°	W	f	n/a	3 d	35 d[p]	n/a	n/a	n/a	6 d[i]	4
	CG	83–160 mg/mL°	W	f	n/a	3 d[g]	n/a	n/a	n/a	n/a	7 d[i]	4

148

Drug Manufacturer	Concentration	Diluents	Osmolality[f] (mOsm/kg)	pH	Storage Conditions						Refer.
					Temperature			Post-thaw Temp		Body Temp	
					Room	Refrig	Frozen	Room	Refrig		
INFUSOR (Baxter) *continued*											
CG	83–160 mg/mL[o]	W	f	n/a	14 d[l]	n/a	n/a	n/a	n/a	1 d[i]	4
CG	83–160 mg/mL[o]	W	f	n/a	12 d[k]	n/a	n/a	n/a	n/a	2 d[i]	4
CG	83–160 mg/mL[o]	W	f	n/a	6 d[h]	n/a	n/a	n/a	n/a	5 d[i]	4
CG	83–160 mg/mL[o]	W	f	n/a	3 d	15 d[j]	n/a	n/a	n/a	7 d[i]	4
CG	90 mg/mL[o]	W	f	n/a	3 d	15 d[j]	n/a	n/a	n/a	7 d[i]	4
CG	100–200 mg/mL[o]	W	f	n/a	10 d	n/a	n/a	n/a	n/a	n/a	4
FAU	160–200 mg/mL[o]	W	f	n/a	3 d[n]	n/a	n/a	n/a	n/a	4 d[i]	4
FAU	160–200 mg/mL[o]	W	f	n/a	3 d	35 d[m]	n/a	n/a	n/a	5 d[i]	4
FAU	175–212 mg/mL[o]	W	f	n/a	3 d	15 d[c]	n/a	n/a	n/a	4 d[i]	4
FAU	200–210 mg/mL[o]	W	f	n/a	3 d	15 d[c]	n/a	n/a	n/a	4 d[i]	4
FAU	200–210 mg/mL[o]	W	f	n/a	3 d[n]	n/a	n/a	n/a	n/a	4 d[i]	4

continued on next page

Flush Compatibility: Normal saline.[1]
Special Considerations: Precipitate may form at high concentrations and over longer time periods.[1] Turbid solutions should not be used.[1]

Notes

[a]Stored at 30°C.
[b]Room temperature range not specified.
[c]Followed by 3 d at 25°C, followed by 4 d at 33°C.
[d]Packaged as 3 mL in 10 mL syringes.
[e]Followed by 3 d at 25°C, followed by 3 d at 33°C.
[f]Reconstituted deferoxamine 95 mg/mL is isotonic.[1]
[g]Followed by 7 d at 33°C.
[h]Followed by 5 d at 33°C.
[i]Near body temperature, 33°C.
[j]Followed by 3 d at 25°C, followed by 7 d at 33°C.
[k]Followed by 2 d at 33°C.
[l]Followed by 1 d at 33°C.
[m]Followed by 3 d at 25°C, followed by 5 d at 33°C.
[n]Followed by 4 d at 33°C.
[o]Up to 100 mg/mL, reconstituted with W and diluted with NS. Above 100 mg/mL reconstituted and diluted with W.

pFollowed by 3 d at 25°C, followed by 6 d at 33°C.
qFollowed by 4 d at 25°C, followed by 3 d at 33°C.

References

1. Trissel LA. ASHP's Interactive Handbook on Injectable Drugs. Bethesda, MD: American Society of Health-System Pharmacists. Accessed 2012 Jul.

2. Stability Data for Drugs Using Homepump Disposable Elastomeric Infusion Systems. Lake Forest, CA: I-Flow Corporation; October 2009.

3. Drug Stability Data Using Elastomeric Infusion Systems. B. Braun Medical Production Ltd. (Thailand); August 2011.

4. Intermate/Infusor Drug Stability Data. Deerfield, IL: Baxter Healthcare Corporation; October 2008.

Dexamethasone Sodium Phosphate

Dexamethasone Sodium Phosphate

CONTAINER	Drug Manufacturer	Concentration	Diluents	Osmolality (mOsm/kg)	pH[g]	Temperature Room	Temperature Refrig	Temperature Frozen	Post-thaw Temp Room	Post-thaw Temp Refrig	Body Temp	Refer.
Polyvinyl Chloride (PVC)	MSD	0.009 mg/mL	NS	n/a	g	7 d	n/a	n/a	n/a	n/a	n/a	1
	AMR	0.092, 0.66 mg/mL	NS	n/a	g	14 d[b]	n/a	n/a	n/a	n/a	n/a	1
	AMR	0.092, 0.66 mg/mL	D5W, NS	n/a	g	14 d[b,d]	14 d[b,d]	n/a	n/a	n/a	n/a	1
	AMR	0.094, 0.658 mg/mL	D5W	n/a	g	14 d[b]	n/a	n/a	n/a	n/a	n/a	1
	ES	0.2, 0.4 mg/mL	NS	n/a	g	n/a	30 d[c]	n/a	n/a	n/a	n/a	1
	MSD	0.43 mg/mL[a]	NS, D5W	n/a	g	28 d	28 d	n/a	n/a	n/a	n/a	3
Syringes, Plastic	SI	10 mg/mL	undiluted	n/a	g	35 d[e]	n/a	n/a	n/a	n/a	n/a	1
	SI	10 mg/mL	undiluted	n/a	g	55 d[f]	n/a	n/a	n/a	n/a	n/a	1
Syringes, Polypropylene	OR[q]	0.07 mg/mL[l,m]	NS[n]	n/a	5.29–5.40[l] 4.26–4.37[m]	8 d	8 d	n/a	n/a	n/a	8 d	1, 4
	APP	0.1, 1 mg/mL	NS	n/a	g	22 d[j]	n/a	n/a	n/a	n/a	n/a	1
	ME	0.33, 1.33, 1.67, 3.33 mg/mL[o]	NS	n/a	n/a	5 d[b]	n/a	n/a	n/a	n/a	n/a	1, 5
	ME	0.33–3.33 mg/mL[p]	NS	n/a	n/a	5 d	5 d	n/a	n/a	n/a	n/a	1, 6
OTHER INFUSION CONTAINERS												
AccuFlo™/ AccuFlux™/ AccuRX® (B. Braun)	unspec.	0.8 mg/mL	D5W	n/a	g	24 h[k]	48 h[k]	n/a	n/a	n/a	n/a	7
Glass Vials	LY	1 mg/mL	NS	n/a	g	28 d	28 d	n/a	n/a	n/a	n/a	1
Glaspak Syringes (Becton Dickinson)	OR	10 mg/mL	undiluted	n/a	g	91 d	91 d	n/a	n/a	n/a	n/a	1
PVC Cassette (Pharmacia Deltec)	AMR	0.4 mg/mL[h]	NS	n/a	g	14 d	14 d	n/a	n/a	n/a	n/a	1
	unspec.	0.02 mg/mL[i]	unspec.	n/a	g	7 d	n/a	n/a	n/a	n/a	n/a	2

continued on next page

151

Dexamethasone Sodium Phosphate (cont'd)

Flush Compatibility: Heparin lock flush and normal saline.[1]

Special Considerations: Osmolality of 4 mg/mL (ES) is 356 mOsm/kg. Dilutions of 0.5, 1, and 2 mg/mL in NS were 265, 260, 238 mOsm/kg.[1]

Notes

[a]With ondansetron (GL) 0.15 mg/mL.

[b]Stored protected from light.

[c]30 d refrigerated followed by 2 d at room temperature.

[d]With granisetron (SKB) 0.01 and 0.04 mg/mL.

[e]In 1-mL monoject syringe.

[f]In 3-mL monoject syringe.

[g]pH of undiluted solutions is 7–8.5. Dilutions of 0.5, 1, and 2 mg/mL in NS are 7.3, 7.3, and 7.5.[1]

[h]With 200 mg diphenhydramine, 4 mg lorazepam, and 400 mg metoclopramide in 100 mL NS. Above stability pertains to dexamethasone, diphenhydramine, and metoclopramide only.

[i]With morphine sulfate 15 mg/mL.

[j]Tested using Becton-Dickinson 3- and 5-mL syringes.

[k]Manufacturer(s) extrapolated data from other sources.

[l]With ketamine (Ketalar®, PF) 3.6 mg/mL, exposed to normal fluorescent light.

[m]With ketamine (Ketalar®, PF) 42.9 mg/mL, exposed to normal fluorescent light.

[n]Parkfield Pharmaceuticals.

[o]With tramadol (Grunenthal) 8.3, 16.66, 33.33 mg/mL, protected from light.

[p]With furosemide (HO) 3.33–10 mg/mL.

[q]Organon Labs.

References

1. Trissel LA. ASHP's Interactive Handbook on Injectable Drugs. Bethesda, MD: American Society of Health-System Pharmacists. Accessed 2012 May.
2. Swanson G, Smith J, Bulich R, et al. Patient-controlled analgesia for chronic cancer pain in the ambulatory setting: a report of 117 patients. *J Clin Oncol.* 1989; 7(12):1903–8.
3. Evrard B, Ceccato A, Gaspard O, et al. Stability of ondansetron hydrochloride and dexamethasone sodium phosphate in 0.9% sodium chloride injection and 5% dextrose injection. *Am J Health Syst Pharm.* 1997; 54(May 1):1065–8.
4. Watson DG, Lin M, Morton A, et al. Compatibility and stability of dexamethasone sodium phosphate and ketamine hydrochloride subcutaneous infusions in polypropylene syringes. *Journal of Pain and Symptom Management* 2005; 30(1):80–6.
5. Negro S, Salama A, Sanchez Y, et al. Compatibility and stability of tramadol and dexamethasone in solution and its use in terminally ill patients. *J Clin Pharm Ther.* 2007; 32(5):441–4.
6. Negro S, Randon AL, Azuara ML, et al. Compatibility and stability of furosemide and dexamethasone combined in infusion solutions. *Arzeneimittelforschung* 2006; 56(10):714–20.
7. Drug Stability Data Using Elastomeric Infusion Systems. B. Braun Medical Production Ltd. (Thailand); August 2011.

Dimenhydrinate

Dimenhydrinate

Drug Manufacturer	Concentration	Diluents	Osmolality (mOsm/kg)	pH	Storage Conditions Temperature Room	Refrig	Frozen	Post-thaw Temp Room	Refrig	Body Temp	Refer.
OTHER INFUSION CONTAINERS											
Unspecified	unspec.	D5W, NS, W	n/a	a	10 d	n/a	n/a	n/a	n/a	n/a	1

Flush Compatibility: Heparin lock flush and normal saline.[1]
Special Considerations: n/a

Note
aThe pH of undiluted solution is 6.4–7.2.[1]

Reference
1. Trissel LA. ASHP's Interactive Handbook on Injectable Drugs. Bethesda, MD: American Society of Health-System Pharmacists. Accessed 2012 Jan.

153

Diphenhydramine

	Drug Manufacturer	Concentration	Diluents	Osmolality (mOsm/kg)	pH[c]	Storage Conditions							Refer.
						Temperature			Post-thaw Temp			Body Temp	
						Room	Refrig	Frozen	Room	Refrig			
CONTAINER													
Polyvinyl Chloride (PVC)	PD	0.25, 0.5, 1 mg/mL	D5W, NS	n/a	n/a	91 d[b]	91 d[b]	n/a	r/a	n/a	n/a	n/a	2
Syringes, Plastic	PD	1.25, 2.5, 5 mg/mL	NS	n/a	n/a	28 d[b]	28 d[b]	n/a	n/a	n/a	n/a	n/a	2
OTHER INFUSION CONTAINERS													
PVC Cassette (Pharmacia Deltec)	ES	2 mg/mL[a]	NS	n/a	n/a	14 d[d]	14 d	n/a	n/a	n/a	n/a	n/a	1

Flush Compatibility: Heparin lock flush and normal saline.[1]
Special Considerations: Protect from light; avoid freezing.[1]

Notes

[a]With 40 mg dexamethasone, 4 mg lorazepam, and 400 mg metoclopramide in 100 mL NS. Above stability pertains to dexamethasone, diphenhydramine, and metoclopramide only.
[b]Protected from light.
[c]pH of undiluted solution is 4–6.5.[1]
[d]At 23°C and 30°C.

References

1. Trissel LA. ASHP's Interactive Handbook on Injectable Drugs. Bethesda, MD: American Society of Health-System Pharmacists. Accessed 2012 May.
2. Donnelly RF. Chemical stability of diphenhydramine hydrochloride in minibags and polypropylene syringes. Can J Hosp Pharm. 1999; 52:150–5.

DOBUTamine Hydrochloride

DOBUTamine Hydrochloride

| Drug Manufacturer | Concentration | Diluents | Osmolality (mOsm/kg) | pH[c] | Storage Conditions | | | | | | Refer. |
| | | | | | Temperature | | | Post-thaw Temp | | Body Temp | |
					Room	Refrig	Frozen	Room	Refrig		
CONTAINERS											
Polyvinyl Chloride (PVC)											
LI	0.25 mg/mL	NS, D5W	n/a	c	48 h	7 d	n/a	n/a	n/a	n/a	1
LI	1 mg/mL	D5W	n/a	c	48 h	234 d[a]	n/a	n/a	n/a	n/a	1
LI	1 mg/mL	NS	n/a	c	48 h	n/a	n/a	n/a	n/a	n/a	1
AB	4 mg/mL	D5W	n/a	c	30 d[a]	30 d[a]	n/a	n/a	n/a	n/a	1, 3
LI	5 mg/mL	D5W	361	c	n/a	100 d[a]	n/a	n/a	n/a	n/a	1
Syringes, Polypropylene											
LI	5 mg/mL	D5W	361	c	48 h	48 h	n/a	n/a	n/a	n/a	1
COMMERCIAL PREPARATIONS (RTU)											
Flexible CR3 Container (Hospira)											
HSP, BRN[e]	1, 2, 4 mg/mL	D5W	260–284	c	14 d[b,d]	n/a	n/a	n/a	n/a	n/a	2, 4
Viaflex (Baxter)											
BA	1, 2, 4 mg/mL	D5W	260–284	c	7 d[b,d]	n/a	n/a	n/a	n/a	n/a	5

Flush Compatibility: Heparin lock flush (several studies show heparin and dobutamine combinations to be incompatible in D5W).[1]
Special Considerations: n/a

Notes

[a]Stored protected from light.
[b]Expiration date per manufacturer's label when stored in the protective overwrap or overpouch under labeled storage conditions.
[c]pH of premixed solution and undiluted solutions is 2.5–5.5.[1]
[d]Do not use beyond this date after removal of manufacturer's protective overwrap.
[e]The B. Braun product is purchased for distribution only; it is manufactured by and under the labeling of Hospira.

References

1. Trissel LA. ASHP's Interactive Handbook on Injectable Drugs. Bethesda, MD: American Society of Health-System Pharmacists. Accessed 2012 Apr.
2. DOBUTamine in Dextrose [package insert]. Lake Forest, IL: Hospira; June 2006.
3. Webster AA, English BA, McGuire JM, et al. Stability of dobutamine hydrochloride 4 mg/mL in 5% dextrose injection at 5 and 23°C. Int J Pharm Compound. 1999; 3(5):412–4.
4. Medical Communications Department [personal communication]. Lake Forest, IL: Hospira; April 25, 2008.
5. Product Information Center [personal communication]. Round Lake, IL: Baxter Healthcare Corporation; April 1, 2008.

Docetaxel

	Drug Manufacturer	Concentration	Diluents	Osmolality (mOsm/kg)	pH	Storage Conditions								
						Temperature			Post-thaw Temp		Body Temp	Refer.		
						Room	Refrig	Frozen	Room	Refrig				
CONTAINERS														
Glass	RPR	0.3, 0.9 mg/mL	D5W, NS	n/a	n/a	28 d[a]	n/a	n/a	n/a	n/a	n/a	1		
Polyethylene	RPR	0.3, 0.9 mg/mL	NS	n/a	n/a	28 d[a]	n/a	n/a	n/a	n/a	n/a	1		
Polypropylene	RPR	0.3, 0.9 mg/mL	D5W	n/a	n/a	28 d[a]	n/a	n/a	n/a	n/a	n/a	1		
Polypropylene-Polyethylene Copolymer Bag[b] (B. Braun)	AVE	0.4, 0.8 mg/mL	NS	n/a	n/a	35 d	35 d	n/a				1, 2		
OTHER INFUSION CONTAINERS														
Glass (Vial)	AVE	10 mg/mL	c	n/a	n/a	21 d	21 d	n/a	n/a	n/a	n/a	2		

Flush Compatibility: Heparin lock flush and normal saline.[1]

Special Considerations: Do not admix in PVC containers, inline filtration is not required.

Notes

[a]Protected from light.
[b]Partial Additive Bag (PAB).
[c]Ethanol-Polysorbate 80 provided by the manufacturer with the undiluted product.

References

1. Trissel LA. ASHP's Interactive Handbook on Injectable Drugs. Bethesda, MD: American Society of Health-System Pharmacists. Accessed 2012 Mar.
2. Walker SE, Charbonneau F, Law S. Stability of docetaxel solution after dilution in ethanol and storage in vials and after dilution in normal saline and storage in bags. Can J Hosp Pharm. 2007; 60:231–7.

Dolasetron Mesylate

CONTAINER	Drug Manufacturer	Concentration	Diluents	Osmolality (mOsm/kg)	pH[a]	Storage Conditions						Refer.
						Temperature			Post-thaw Temp		Body Temp	
						Room	Refrig	Frozen	Room	Refrig		
Polyvinyl Chloride (PVC)	SAV	unspec.[b]	D5W, NS, D5½S, LR M10, D5LR	n/a	[a]	24 h	48 h	n/a	n/a	n/a	n/a	1, 2
Syringes, Plastic	SAV	20 mg/mL	undiluted	n/a	3.2–3.8	240 d	n/a	n/a	n/a	n/a	n/a	2
Syringes, Polypropylene	HMR	10 mg/mL	D5W, NS	n/a	[a]	31 d	31 d	n/a	n/a	n/a	n/a	2
	unspec.	12.5 mg/mL	NS	n/a	[a]	31 d	n/a	n/a	n/a	n/a	n/a	2

Flush Compatibility: Normal saline.[1,2] Flush the infusion line before and after administration.[1,2] Not compatible with heparin. Precipitation occurs when dolasetron mesylate 2 mg/mL in NS is administered by y-site with heparin sodium 50 units/mL in NS.[3]

Special Considerations: Maximum rate for administration of undiluted intravenous administration is 100 mg in 30 seconds. When diluted in 50 mL of a compatible solution, infuse over 15 min. Do not mix with other drugs.[1,2]

Notes

[a]pH of undiluted solution is 3.2–3.8.[1]
[b]Unspecified concentration diluted for infusion.

References

1. Anzemet® Injection [prescribing information]. Bridgewater, NJ: Sanofi-Aventis; September 2011.
2. Trissel LA. ASHP's Interactive Handbook on Injectable Drugs. Bethesda, MD: American Society of Health-System Pharmacists. Accessed 2012 May.
3. Montgomery K. Anzemet® Compatibility and Stability Information Request [personal communication]. Medical Information Center, Bridgewater, NJ: Sanofi-Aventis; January 2008.

DOPamine Hydrochloride

	Drug Manufacturer	Concentration	Diluents	Osmolality (mOsm/kg)	pH[e]	Temperature Room	Temperature Refrig	Temperature Frozen	Post-thaw Temp Room	Post-thaw Temp Refrig	Body Temp	Refer.
CONTAINERS												
Polyvinyl Chloride (PVC)	ES	0.4 mg/mL	D5W, NS	n/a	e	48 h	n/a	n/a	n/a	n/a	n/a	1
	AS	0.8 mg/mL	NS	n/a	e	48 h	n/a	n/a	n/a	n/a	n/a	1
	AS	0.8 mg/mL	D5W	n/a	e	24 h	7 d	n/a	n/a	n/a	n/a	1
	DB, ES	3.2 mg/mL	D5W	n/a	e	48 h	14 d[a]	n/a	n/a	n/a	n/a	1
	ES	3.2 mg/mL	D5W, NS	n/a	e	48 h	n/a	n/a	n/a	n/a	n/a	1
Syringes, Plastic	TLP	4 mg/mL	D5W	n/a	e	48 h	48 h	n/a	n/a	n/a	n/a	1
Syringes, Polypropylene	NY	0.5 mg/mL	D5W	n/a	e	7 d[c]	3 m[c]	6 m[c,d]	n/a	n/a	n/a	3
COMMERCIAL PREPARATIONS (RTU)												
Flexible CR3 Container (Hospira)	HSP	0.8, 1.6, 3.2 mg/mL	D5W	g	e	7 d[b,f]	n/a	n/a	n/a	n/a	n/a	4, 5
Viaflex Plus Bag (Baxter)	BA	0.8, 1.6, 3.2 mg/mL	D5W	n/a	e	7 d[b,f]	n/a	n/a	n/a	n/a	n/a	2

Flush Compatibility: Heparin lock flush.[1]

Special Considerations: Temperature excursions up to 38°C for up to 4 weeks showed no drug loss.[1]

Notes

[a]Stability reported as 14.75 d, protected from light.
[b]Expiration date per manufacturer's label when stored in the protective overwrap or overpouch under labeled storage conditions.
[c]Protected from light.
[d]Frozen stability data was only consistent in Codan syringes. Do not use Braun syringes if preparation will be frozen.
[e]pH of premixed solution range is 2.5–4.5 and undiluted solution is 2.5–5.[1]
[f]Do not use beyond this date after removal of manufacturer's protective overwrap.
[g]Osmolarlity is 261, 269, 286 mOsmol/liter (calc.)[4]

References

1. Trissel LA. ASHP's Interactive Handbook on Injectable Drugs. Bethesda, MD: American Society of Health-System Pharmacists. Accessed 2012 Jun.
2. Product Information Center [personal communication]. Round Lake, IL: Baxter Healthcare Corporation; April 1, 2008.
3. Braenden JU, Stendal TL, Fagernaes CB. Stability of dopamine hydrochloride 0.5 mg/mL in polypropylene syringes. J Clin Pharm Ther. 2003; 28:471–4.
4. DOPamine in Dextrose [package insert]. Lake Forest, IL: Hospira Inc.; April, 2007.
5. Medical Communications Department [personal communication]. Lake Forest, IL: Hospira Inc.; April 25, 2008.

Doripenem

Container	Drug Manufacturer	Concentration	Diluents	Osmolality (mOsm/kg)	pH	Temperature Room	Temperature Refrig	Temperature Frozen	Post-thaw Temp Room	Post-thaw Temp Refrig	Body Temp	Refer.
CONTAINER												
Bag, Polyethylene	OMN	1, 10 mg/mL	NS	n/a	n/a	12 h	72 h	n/a	n/a	n/a	n/a	7
	OMN	1, 10 mg/mL	D5W	n/a	n/a	8 h	48 h	n/a	n/a	n/a	n/a	7
	OMN	5 mg/mL	NS	n/a	4.81–5.24[i]	12 h	72 h	n/a	n/a	n/a	n/a	2
	OMN	5 mg/mL	D5W	n/a	4.74–4.99[i]	4 h	48 h	n/a	n/a	n/a	n/a	2
Polyvinyl Chloride (PVC)	OMN	1, 10 mg/mL	NS	n/a	n/a	12 h	72 h	n/a	n/a	n/a	n/a	7
	OMN	1, 10 mg/mL	D5W	n/a	n/a	8 h	48 h	n/a	n/a	n/a	n/a	7
	OMN	5 mg/mL	D5W	n/a	n/a	16 h	10 d	n/a	n/a	n/a	n/a	5
	OMN	5 mg/mL	D5W	n/a	4.74–4.99	4 h	48 h	n/a	n/a	n/a	n/a	2
	OMN	5 mg/mL	NS	n/a	4.81–5.24	12 h	72 h	n/a	n/a	n/a	n/a	2
	OMN	5, 10 mg/mL	NS	n/a	n/a	24 h	10 d	14 d[b]	16 h[d]	n/a	n/a	5
	OMN	5, 10 mg/mL	NS	n/a	n/a	n/a	n/a	28 d[b]	16 h[e]	24 h[e]	n/a	5
	OMN	10 mg/mL	D5W	n/a	n/a	16 h	7 d	n/a	n/a	n/a	n/a	5
Unspecified Infusion Bag	OMN	2.3–4.5 mg/mL[c]	NS	n/a	n/a	12 h[a]	72 h[a]	b	n/a	n/a	n/a	1
	OMN	2.3–4.5 mg/mL[c]	D5W	n/a	n/a	4 h[a]	24 h[a]	b	n/a	n/a	n/a	1
	OMN	5 mg/mL	D5W	n/a	n/a	4 h	48 h	b	n/a	n/a	n/a	6
	OMN	5 mg/mL	NS	n/a	n/a	12 h	72 h	b	n/a	n/a	n/a	6
	OMN	5 mg/mL	NS	n/a	n/a	16 h[g]	n/a	n/a	n/a	n/a	8–12 h[h]	3
OTHER INFUSION CONTAINERS												
Glass	JN	10 mg/mL	W	n/a	n/a	24 h	n/a	n/a	n/a	n/a	12 h[f]	4
Homepump®/Homepump Eclipse® (I-Flow Corp.)	OMN	5 mg/mL	D5W	n/a	n/a	16 h	10 d	n/a	n/a	n/a	n/a	5
	OMN	5, 10 mg/mL	NS	n/a	n/a	24 h	10 d	14 d[b]	16 h[d]	n/a	n/a	5
	OMN	5, 10 mg/mL	NS	n/a	n/a	n/a	n/a	28 d[b]	16 h[e]	24 h[e]	n/a	5
	OMN	10 mg/mL	D5W	n/a	n/a	16 h	7 d	n/a	n/a	n/a	n/a	5

Storage Conditions (Temperature; Post-thaw Temp)

continued on next page

Doripenem (cont'd)

Flush Compatibility: Normal saline, heparin flush.[6]

Special Considerations: After constitution with SW or NS, suspension in vial may be held for 1 h prior to transfer and dilution in infusion bag.[1]

Notes

[a]Includes the storage and infusion time.[1]

[b]Prescribing information states not to freeze constituted suspension or diluted solutions.[1] In this study, after thawing, a white precipitate was observed which returned to the solution after vigorous shaking for 3–12 min; to avoid potential for patient injury, do not infuse a previously frozen solution until all the precipitate has been fully redissolved.[5]

[c]Final concentration when prepared per prescribing information.[1]

[d]Thawed at 25°C.

[e]Thawed at 4°C for 24 h and then at 25°C for 2 h.

[f]Approximately 12 h.

[g]Stored at 30°C.

[h]12 h stability at 35°C; 8 h stability at 40°C

[i]Acceptable pH range was 4.5–6.0; all samples met this criteria.

References

1. Doribax® (doripenem for injection) [prescribing information]. Raritan, NJ: Ortho-McNeil Division of Ortho-McNeil-Janssen Pharmaceuticals, Inc.; October 2010.
2. Psathas P, Kuzmission A, Ikeda K, et al. Stability of doripenem in vitro in representative infusion solutions and infusion bags. Clin Ther. 2008; 30:2075–87.
3. Keel R, Sutherland C, Crandon J, et al. Stability of doripenem, imipenem and meropenem at elevated room temperatures. Int J Antimicrob Agents 2011; 37:174–85.
4. Berthoin K, LeDuff C, Marchand-Brynaert J, et al. Stability of meropenem and doripenem solutions for administration by continuous infusion. J Antimicrob Chemother. February 2010; 21:1073–5.
5. Crandon J, Sutherland C, Nicolau D. Stability of doripenem in polyvinyl chloride bags and elastomeric pumps. Am J Health-Syst Pharm. 2010; 67:1539–44.
6. Trissel LA. ASHP's Interactive Handbook on Injectable Drugs. Bethesda, MD: American Society of Health-System Pharmacists. Accessed 2012 Jan.
7. Psathas P, Gilmor T, Schaufelberger D, et al. Stability of high and low concentrations of doripenem (500 mg) for injection in representative infusion fluids and containers. Poster presentation at ASHP Summer Meeting and Exhibition. Seattle, WA; June 8–11, 2008.

Doxorubicin Hydrochloride

Doxorubicin Hydrochloride

Container	Drug Manufacturer	Concentration	Diluents	Osmolality (mOsm/kg)	pH	Room	Refrig	Frozen	Room	Refrig	Body Temp	Refer.
Ethylvinyl Acetate (EVA)	BEL	0.5, 1.25 mg/mL	D5W	n/a	j	28 d[g]	28 d[g]	n/a	n/a	n/a	7 d[g]	1, 2
	BEL	0.5 mg/mL	NS	n/a	j	14 d[g]	14 d[g]	n/a	n/a	n/a	7 d[g]	2
	BEL	1.25 mg/mL	NS	n/a	j	28 d[g]	28 d[g]	n/a	n/a	n/a	7 d[g]	2
Polyolefin	BMS	0.12 mg/mL[l]	NS	n/a	j	n/a	124 h[l]	n/a	n/a	n/a	124 h[l]	2, 8
	BMS	0.24 mg/mL[m]	NS	n/a	j	n/a	124 h[m]	n/a	n/a	n/a	124 h[m]	2, 8
	BMS	0.4 mg/mL[n]	NS	n/a	j	n/a	124 h[n]	n/a	n/a	n/a	124 h[n]	2, 8
Polyvinyl Chloride (PVC)	unspec.	0.04 mg/mL	NS, D5W	n/a	j	n/a	7 d[g]	n/a	n/a	n/a	n/a	2
	FA	0.1 mg/mL	NS, D5W	n/a	j	43 d[a]	43 d[a]	43 d[a,b]	n/a	n/a	n/a	2
	unspec.	1 mg/mL	NS	n/a	j	n/a	n/a	35 d[k]	n/a	n/a	n/a	2
	FA	1.4 mg/mL	NS	n/a	j	n/a	n/a	30 d	n/a	n/a	n/a	2
Syringes, Plastic, Monoject, Terumo®	AD	1, 2 mg/mL	NS	n/a	j	124 d[c]	124 d[c]	n/a	n/a	n/a	n/a	2
Syringes, Polypropylene	FA	2 mg/mL	undiluted	n/a	3.0	n/a	43 d	n/a	n/a	n/a	n/a	2
AccuFlo™/ AccuFlux™/ AccuRX® (Medpro)	unspec.	2 mg/mL	NS	n/a	j	24 h	14 d	n/a	n/a	n/a	n/a	9
CADD® Cassette (Pharmacia Deltec)	NY	1.67 mg/mL[d]	NS	n/a	j	n/a	7 d[q]	n/a	n/a	n/a	4 d[c]	2, 3
	CET	2 mg/mL	NS	n/a	j	14 d	14 d	n/a	n/a	n/a	28 d[h]	2, 4
Graseby™ 9000 Cassette (Graseby Medical)	FA	2 mg/mL[i]	W[i]	n/a	j	n/a	14 d	4 w	n/a	n/a	7 d	2, 7

continued on next page

161

Doxorubicin Hydrochloride (cont'd)

Drug Manufacturer	Concentration	Diluents	Osmolality (mOsm/kg)	pH[i]	Temperature			Post-thaw Temp		Body Temp	Refer.
					Room	Refrig	Frozen	Room	Refrig		
Homepump Eclipse®/ Homepump® C-Series (I-Flow Corp.)	2 mg/mL	NS	n/a	j	n/a	48 h	n/a	n/a	n/a	n/a	6
Implantable Pump — FA	1.4 mg/mL°	NS, 1/2S, D2.5	n/a	j	14 d°	n/a	n/a	n/a	n/a	14 d°	2
Implantable Pump DAD (Medtronic) — unspec.	3, 5 mg/mL	NS	n/a	j	n/a	n/a	n/a	n/a	n/a	2 w	2
INFUSOR (Baxter) — AD	0.2 mg/mL	NS	n/a	j	n/a	47 d	n/a	n/a	n/a	n/a	5
AD	0.2–1 mg/mL	NS	n/a	j	9 d	n/a	n/a	n/a	n/a	n/a	5
AD	0.2–2 mg/mL	NS	n/a	j	5 d	42 d[p]	n/a	n/a	n/a	n/a	5
AD	0.2–5 mg/mL	NS	n/a	j	9 d[f]	34 d[e,f]	n/a	n/a	n/a	n/a	5
AD	1 mg/mL	NS	n/a	j	9 d	96 d	n/a	n/a	n/a	n/a	5

First row drug manufacturer: unspec.

Flush Compatibility: Normal saline, heparin 40 units/mL.[2]
Special Considerations: Heparin at 1,000 units/mL caused immediate precipitation when injected into Y site with no flush.[2]

Notes

aSolutions stored in dark.
bFrozen samples were subjected to 11 freeze/thaw cycles with no apparent loss in potency between cycles.
cSolutions not protected from light.
dSolutions also contained vincristine sulfate 0.036 mg/mL (LI).
eFollowed by 9 d at 25°C.
fManufacturer extrapolated data from other sources.
gProtected from light.
hMeasured at 30°C.
iSolution also contained vincristine sulfate (FAU) 0.2 mg/mL.
jpH of lyophilized product reconstituted in NS is 3.8–6.5. pH of undiluted solution product is 3.0.[2]
kFrozen and thawed after 14 d, refrozen and thawed at room temperature 21 d later.

continued on next page

Doxorubicin Hydrochloride (cont'd)

_l_Also contains etoposide phosphate (BMS) 0.6 mg/mL and vincristine sulfate (LI) 5 mcg/mL.

_m_Also contains etoposide phosphate (BMS) 1.2 mg/mL and vincristine sulfate (LI) 10 mcg/mL.

_n_Also contains etoposide phosphate (BMS) 2 mg/mL and vincristine sulfate (LI) 16 mcg/mL.

_o_Also contains vincristine sulfate (LI) 33 mcg/mL; stored at 25°C, 30°C, and 37°C.

_p_Followed by 5 d at 25°C.

_q_Followed by 4 d at 35°C.

References

1. Rochard EB, Barthes DMC, Courtois PY. Stability of fluorouracil, cytarabine, or doxorubicin hydrochloride in ethylene vinylacetete portable infusion-pump containers. _Am J Hosp Pharm._ 1992; 49:619–23.

2. Trissel LA. ASHP's Interactive Handbook on Injectable Drugs. Bethesda, MD: American Society of Health-System Pharmacists. Accessed 2012 Jul.

3. Nyhammar EK, Johansson SG, Seiving BE. Stability of doxorubicin hydrochloride and vincristine sulfate in two portable infusion-pump reservoirs. _Am J Health-Syst Pharm._ 1996; 53:1171–3.

4. Stiles ML, Allen LV. Stability of doxorubicin hydrochloride in portable pump reservoirs. _Am J Hosp Pharm._ 1991; 48:1976–7.

5. Intermate/Infusor Drug Stability Information. Deerfield, IL: Baxter Healthcare Corporation; October 2008.

6. Stability Data for Drugs Using Homepump Disposable Elastomeric Infusion Systems. Lake Forest, CA: I-Flow Corporation; October 2009.

7. Priston MJ. Sewell GJ. Stability of three cytotoxic drug infusions in the Graseby 900 ambulatory infusion pump. _J Oncol Pharm Practice._ 1998; 4(3):143–9.

8. Yuan P, Grimes GJ, Shankman SE, et al. Compatibility and stability of vincristine sulfate, doxorubicin hydrochloride, and etoposide phosphate in 0.9% sodium chloride injection. _Am J Health-Syst Pharm._ 2001; 58:594–8.

9. Drug Stability Data Using Elastomeric Infusion Systems. B. Braun Medical Production Ltd. (Thailand); August 2011.

Doxycycline Hyclate[a]

Container	Drug Manufacturer	Concentration	Diluents	Osmolality (mOsm/kg)	pH[e]	Storage Conditions Temperature Room	Temperature Refrig	Temperature Frozen	Post-thaw Temp Room	Post-thaw Temp Refrig	Body Temp	Refer.
CONTAINER												
Polyvinyl Chloride (PVC)	PF	0.1–1 mg/mL	NS, D5W	n/a	e	48 h[a]	72 h[b]	n/a	n/a	n/a	n/a	1, 2
	PF	0.8, 1 mg/mL	NS, D5W	n/a	e	96 h	7 d	n/a	n/a	n/a	n/a	1
	PF	1 mg/mL	D5W	292	e	n/a	n/a	8 w	n/a	n/a	n/a	1
OTHER INFUSION CONTAINERS												
AccuFlo™/ AccuFlux™/ AccuRX® (B. Braun)	unspec.	0.1 to 1 mg/mL	NS, D5W	n/a	n/a	48 h[c]	3 d[c]	n/a	n/a	n/a	n/a	4
	unspec.	1 mg/mL	D5W	n/a	n/a	n/a	n/a	8 w[c]	n/a	n/a	n/a	4
Glass Vials	PF	10 mg/mL	W	507	e	n/a	n/a	8 w	n/a	n/a	n/a	1, 2
Homepump Eclipse®/ Homepump® C-Series (I-Flow Corp.)	unspec.	0.1–1 mg/mL	D5W, NS	n/a	e	48 h[c]	3 d[c]	n/a	n/a	n/a	n/a	3
	unspec.	1 mg/mL	D5W	292	e	n/a	n/a	8 w[c]	n/a	n/a	n/a	3
Portable Pump Reservoir (Pharmacia Deltec)	ES	2 mg/mL	NS	n/a	e	n/a	n/a	n/a	n/a	n/a	24 h[d]	1

Flush Compatibility: Normal saline. Incompatible with heparin.[1]
Special Considerations: Administer by slow intravenous infusion over 1–4 h. Avoid extravasation.[1,3]

Notes

[a]Protect from direct sunlight.
[b]When protected from artificial light and sunlight, and stored under refrigeration for 72 h, solution is stable for an additional 12 h at room temperature.[3]
[c]Manufacturer's extrapolated data from other sources.
[d]Simulated administration with portable pump reservoir at 30°C.
[e]pH of reconstituted solution is 1.8–3.3.[1]

continued on next page

Doxycycline Hyclate (cont'd)

References

1. Trissel LA. ASHP's Interactive Handbook on Injectable Drugs. Bethesda, MD: American Society of Health-System Pharmacists. Accessed 2012 Jan.
2. Vibramycin® Intravenous [prescribing information.] New York, NY: Pfizer Inc.; November 2001.
3. Stability Data for Drugs Using Homepump Disposable Elastomeric Infusion Systems. Lake Forest, CA: I-Flow Corporation; October 2009.
4. Drug Stability Data Using Elastomeric Infusion Systems. B. Braun Medical Production Ltd. (Thailand); August 2011.

Enoxaparin Sodium

<table>
<tr><th rowspan="3">CONTAINER</th><th rowspan="3">Drug Manufacturer</th><th rowspan="3">Concentration</th><th rowspan="3">Diluents</th><th rowspan="3">Osmolality (mOsm/kg)</th><th rowspan="3">pH</th><th colspan="6">Storage Conditions</th><th rowspan="3">Refer.</th></tr>
<tr><th colspan="3">Temperature</th><th colspan="3">Post-thaw Temp</th></tr>
<tr><th>Room</th><th>Refrig</th><th>Frozen</th><th>Room</th><th>Refrig</th><th>Body Temp</th></tr>
<tr><td>Polyvinyl Chloride (PVC)</td><td>RPR</td><td>1.2 mg/mL</td><td>NS</td><td>n/a</td><td>n/a</td><td>48 h</td><td>n/a</td><td>n/a</td><td>n/a</td><td>n/a</td><td>n/a</td><td>1</td></tr>
<tr><td rowspan="2">Syringes, Plastic</td><td>RPR</td><td>100 mg/mL</td><td>undiluted</td><td>n/a</td><td>5.5–7.51</td><td>n/a</td><td>10 d</td><td>n/a</td><td>n/a</td><td>n/a</td><td>n/a</td><td>1</td></tr>
<tr><td>RPR</td><td>100 mg/mL</td><td>undiluted</td><td>n/a</td><td>5.5–7.51</td><td>5 d</td><td>n/a</td><td>n/a</td><td>n/a</td><td>n/a</td><td>n/a</td><td>1</td></tr>
<tr><td rowspan="2">Syringes, Polypropylene</td><td>RPR</td><td>20 mg/mL</td><td>W</td><td>n/a</td><td>n/a</td><td>14 d</td><td>14 d</td><td>n/a</td><td>n/a</td><td>n/a</td><td>n/a</td><td>1</td></tr>
<tr><td>SAV[a]</td><td>20 mg/mL</td><td>NS</td><td>n/a</td><td>n/a</td><td>42 d[b,c]</td><td>42 d[c]</td><td>n/a</td><td>n/a</td><td>n/a</td><td>n/a</td><td>2</td></tr>
</table>

Flush Compatibility: Normal saline.[1]
Special Considerations: n/a

Notes

[a]Clexane®, SAV, Macquarie Park NSW, Australia.
[b]Under natural light and in the dark.
[c]In the dark.

References

1. Trissel LA. ASHP's Interactive Handbook on Injectable Drugs. Bethesda, MD: American Society of Health-System Pharmacists. Accessed 2012 Feb.
2. Summerhayes R, Chan M, Ignajatovic V, et al. Stability and sterility of diluted enoxaparin under three different storage conditions. *J Paediatr Child Health*. 2011; 47(5):299–301.

Epirubicin Hydrochloride

Storage Conditions

CONTAINER	Drug Manufacturer	Concentration	Diluents	Osmolality (mOsm/kg)	pH[c]	Temperature Room	Refrig	Frozen	Post-thaw Temp Room	Refrig	Body Temp	Refer.
Polyethylene	FA	0.05 mg/mL	D5W	n/a	c	n/a	30 d[a]	n/a	n/a	n/a	n/a	1
	FA	0.05 mg/mL	NS	n/a	c	n/a	25 d[a]	n/a	n/a	n/a	n/a	1
Polyvinyl Chloride (PVC)	FA	0.04 mg/mL	D5W, NS	n/a	c	n/a	7 d[a]	n/a	n/a	n/a	n/a	1
	FA	0.05 mg/mL	D5W	n/a	c	n/a	30 d[a]	n/a	n/a	n/a	n/a	1
	FA	0.05 mg/mL	NS	n/a	c	n/a	25 d[a]	n/a	n/a	n/a	n/a	1
	FA	0.1 mg/mL	D5W, NS	n/a	c	43 d[a]	43 d[a]	43 d	n/a	n/a	n/a	1
	unspec.	1 mg/mL	NS	n/a	c	n/a	n/a	4 w	n/a	n/a	n/a	1
Syringes, Polypropylene (BD)	unspec.	0.5 mg/mL	NS	n/a	c	28 d	28 d	n/a	n/a	n/a	n/a	1
	PH	1 mg/mL	NS	n/a	c	n/a	84 d[b]	n/a	n/a	n/a	n/a	1, 3
	FA	2 mg/mL	NS	n/a	c	14 d	180 d[a]	n/a	n/a	n/a	n/a	1, 2
	unspec.	2 mg/mL	W	n/a	c	n/a	43 d	n/a	n/a	n/a	n/a	1
OTHER INFUSION CONTAINERS												
Glass	FA	0.05 mg/mL	D5W	n/a	c	n/a	30 d[a]	n/a	n/a	n/a	n/a	1
	FA	0.05 mg/mL	NS	n/a	c	n/a	25 d[a]	n/a	n/a	n/a	n/a	1
INFUSOR (Baxter)	unspec.	0.2–1 mg/mL	NS	n/a	c	n/a	91 d[d]	n/a	n/a	n/a	7 d[d]	4

Flush Compatibility: Normal saline.[1] Epirubicin is not compatible with heparin.
Special Considerations: Per product labeling, do not use a filter to administer this medication. One study determined that the loss of drug via filtration was negligible.[1]

Notes

[a] Protected from light.
[b] Storage at 8°C.
[c] pH of undiluted preparation is 3.0.[1]
[d] Solutions <0.5 mg/mL should be protected from light. Dating valid for unbuffered solutions only.[4]

References

1. Trissel LA. ASHP's Interactive Handbook on Injectable Drugs. Bethesda, MD: American Society of Health-System Pharmacists. Accessed 2012 Jun.
2. Pujol M, Munoz M, Prat Jet al. Stability study of epirubicin in NaCl 0.9% injection. Ann Pharmacother. 1997; 31:992–5.
3. Sewell GJ, Rigby-Jones AE, Priston MJ. Stability of intravesical epirubicin infusion: a sequential temperature study. J Clin Pharm Ther. 2003; 28:349–53.
4. Intermate/Infusor Drug Stability Information. Deerfield, IL: Baxter Healthcare Corporation; October 2008.

Epoetin Alfa

Container	Drug Manufacturer	Concentration	Diluents	Osmolality (mOsm/kg)	pH	Storage Conditions						Refer.
						Temperature			Post-thaw Temp			
						Room	Refrig	Frozen	Room	Refrig	Body Temp	
Syringes, Plastic	ORT	0.1 units/mL[a]	D10W	n/a	n/a	24 h	n/a	n/a	n/a	n/a	n/a	1
	unspec.	2,000, 10,000 units/mL	undiluted	iso	e,f	14 d[c]	14 d[c]	n/a	n/a	n/a	n/a	1
	AMG	20,000 units/mL	undiluted	iso	e,f	n/a	6 w	n/a	n/a	n/a	n/a	1
OTHER INFUSION CONTAINERS												
Glass Vials	ORT	4,000 units/mL	NS[b]	n/a	n/a	12 w[d]	12 w[d]	n/a	n/a	n/a	n/a	1

Flush Compatibility: n/a: Not used intravenously.
Special Considerations: n/a

Notes

[a]Samples also contained a final concentration of albumin 0.5% or albumin 0.1%.
[b]NS preserved with 0.9% benzyl alcohol was added to epoetin vials at a dilution of 1.5:1.
[c]Due to lack of preservative in manufacturer's formulation, use shortly after drawing up in syringes is recommended.
[d]The solution is stable and bacteriostatic for up to 12 w, but literature recommends limiting the use of this dilution as a multiple dose vial to 28 d after initial vial entry.
[e]The pH of undiluted epoetin alfa from single use vials is 6.6–7.2.[1]
[f]The pH of undiluted epoetin alfa from multidose vials is 5.8–6.4.[1]

Reference

1. Trissel LA. ASHP's Interactive Handbook on Injectable Drugs. Bethesda, MD: American Society of Health-System Pharmacists. Accessed 2012 Jan.

Epoprostenol Sodium

Container	Drug Manufacturer	Concentration	Diluents	Osmolality (mOsm/kg)	pH[e]	Temperature			Post-thaw Temp		Body Temp	Refer.
						Room	Refrig	Frozen	Room	Refrig		
CONTAINER												
Glass	ACT[f]	300,000 ng/mL (0.3 mg/mL)	W, NS	n/a	>11.0	48 h[d]	5 d[d]	n/a	n/a	n/a	n/a	4
	GSK[k]	3,000–15,000 ng/mL	a,j	n/a	10.2–10.8	8 h[b,d]	48 h[c,d]	n/a	n/a	n/a	n/a	1, 2, 3
	TE[i]	Various	a,j	n/a	11.0–11.8	n/a	48 h[d]	n/a	n/a	n/a	n/a	5
OTHER INFUSION CONTAINERS												
Ambulatory Infusion Pump Reservoir (Polyvinyl Chloride, Polypropylene, or Glass)	ACT[f]	≥15,000 ng/mL	W, NS	n/a	>11.0	24 h[g]	n/a	n/a	n/a	n/a	n/a	4
		<15,000 ng/mL	W, NS	n/a	>11.0	12 h[g]	n/a	n/a	n/a	n/a	n/a	4
		≥3,000 <6,000 ng/mL	W, NS	n/a	>11.0	12 h[h]	n/a	n/a	n/a	n/a	n/a	4
		≥6,000–30,000 ng/mL	W, NS	n/a	>11.0	24 h[h]	n/a	n/a	n/a	n/a	n/a	4
		≥30,000 ng/mL	W, NS	n/a	>11.0	72 h[h]	n/a	n/a	n/a	n/a	n/a	4
		≥6,000 <12,000 ng/mL	W, NS	n/a	>11.0	12 h[l]	n/a	n/a	n/a	n/a	n/a	4
		≥12,000 <30,000 ng/mL	W, NS	n/a	>11.0	24 h[l]	n/a	n/a	n/a	n/a	n/a	4
		≥30,000 ng/mL	W, NS	n/a	>11.0	48 h[l]	n/a	n/a	n/a	n/a	n/a	4
		≥9,000 <12,000 ng/mL	W, NS	n/a	>11.0	12 h[m]	n/a	n/a	n/a	n/a	n/a	4
		≥12,000 <30,000 ng/mL	W, NS	n/a	>11.0	12 h[m]	n/a	n/a	n/a	n/a	n/a	4
		≥30,000 ng/mL	W, NS	n/a	>11.0	24 h[m]	n/a	n/a	n/a	n/a	n/a	4
	GSK[k]	3,000–15,000 ng/mL	a,j	n/a	10.2–10.8	8 h[b,d]	48 h[c,d]	n/a	n/a	n/a	n/a	1, 2, 3
	TE[i]	3,000–15,000 ng/mL	a,j	n/a	11.0–11.8	8 h[c,d]	48 h[c,d]	n/a	n/a	n/a	n/a	5

Flush Compatibility: Infusion should not be interrupted.

Special Considerations: Protect from light. DO NOT FREEZE.[2,4,5] Stability is formulation dependent. Do not extrapolate stability data across brands.

Notes

[a]Sterile diluent provided by manufacturer contains 94 mg glycine, 73.3 mg sodium chloride, and sodium hydroxide (to adjust pH) in 50 mL of sterile water for injection.

[b]If administered in a cold pouch with frozen gel packs, may be administered over 24 h. Pouch must be capable of maintaining temperature between 2°C to 8°C for 12 h.

[c]Inclusive of administration time. Protect reconstituted product from temperatures >20°C and <0°C. Do not freeze.

[d]Protect reconstituted product from light.

continued on next page

Epoprostenol Sodium (cont'd)

e pH of reconstituted preparation is 10.2–10.8[k], >11.0[f], 11.0–11.8[i], and is increasingly unstable at lower pH.[2,4,5]

f Veletri®.

g Used after storage of the reconstituted solution for up to 5 d at 2–8°C or up to 48 h at 25°C.

h Used after reconstitution and immediate dilution to final concentration and immediate administration.

i Epoprostenol Sodium for Inj [Teva].

j Do not reconstitute or mix with other solutions or medications.

k Flolan®.

l Used after reconstitution and immediate dilution to final concentration and storage for 1 d at 2–8°C.

m Used after reconstitution and immediate dilution to final concentration and storage for 7 d at 2–8°C.

References

1. Trissel LA. ASHP's Interactive Handbook on Injectable Drugs. Bethesda, MD: American Society of Health-System Pharmacists. Accessed 2012 Jul.
2. Flolan® [prescribing information]. Research Triangle Park, NC: Glaxo Smith Kline; March 2011.
3. Medical Information, Respiratory Division [personal communication]. Research Triangle Park, NC: GlaxoSmithKline; August 2002.
4. Veletri® [prescribing information]. South San Francisco, CA: Actelion Pharmaceuticals; March 2011.
5. Epoprostenol Sodium for Injection [prescribing information]. Irvine, CA: Teva; March 2008.

Ertapenem

Container	Drug Manufacturer	Concentration	Diluents	Osmolality (mOsm/kg)	pH[a]	Temperature Room	Temperature Refrig	Temperature Frozen	Post-thaw Temp Room	Post-thaw Temp Refrig	Body Temp	Refer.
CONTAINER												
Unspecified	ME	10 mg/mL	NS	n/a	a	20 h	6 d[b]	n/a	n/a	n/a	n/a	3
	ME	20 mg/mL	NS	n/a	a	6 h	5 d[b]	n/a	n/a	n/a	n/a	3
OTHER INFUSION CONTAINERS												
AccuFlo™/AccuFlux™/AccuRX® (B. Braun)	unspec.	10 mg/mL	NS	n/a	a	24 h	7 d	n/a	n/a	n/a	n/a	1
Homepump®/Homepump Eclipse® (I-Flow Corp.)	ME	10 mg/mL	NS	n/a	a	24 h	7 d	n/a	n/a	n/a	n/a	2
	ME	20 mg/mL	NS	n/a	a	18 h	5 d	n/a	n/a	n/a	n/a	2
INTERMATE (Baxter)	ME	10 mg/mL	NS	n/a	a	30 h	8 d	n/a	n/a	n/a	n/a	3
	ME	20 mg/mL	NS	n/a	a	24 h	7 d	n/a	n/a	n/a	n/a	3

Flush Compatibility: Heparin lock flush and normal saline.[3]

Special Considerations: Ertapenem should not be reconstituted or mixed with solutions containing dextrose.[3] Do not freeze.[3]

Notes

[a]pH of reconstituted solution is 7.5.[3]

[b]Incompatible by conventional standards, however, this is recommended for dilution in shorter periods of time.[3]

References

1. *Drug Stability Data Using Elastomeric Infusion Systems.* B. Braun Medical Production Ltd. (Thailand); August 2011.
2. *Stability Data for Drugs Using Homepump Disposable Elastomeric Infusion Systems.* Lake Forest, CA: I-Flow Corporation; October 2009.
3. Trissel LA. ASHP's Interactive Handbook on Injectable Drugs. Bethesda, MD: American Society of Health-System Pharmacists. Accessed 2012 Jan.

Erythromycin Lactobionate

Erythromycin Lactobionate[a]

	Drug Manufacturer	Concentration	Diluents	Osmolality (mOsm/kg)	pH[d]	Storage Conditions Temperature Room	Refrig	Frozen	Post-thaw Temp Room	Refrig	Body Temp	Refer.
CONTAINER												
Glass	AB	1 mg/mL	NS, D5W, D5S	n/a	d	n/a	24 h	n/a	n/a	n/a	n/a	1
Polyvinyl Chloride (PVC)	AB	1 mg/mL	NS, D5W, D5S	n/a	d	n/a	24 h	n/a	n/a	n/a	n/a	1
	AB	4 mg/mL	NS	n/a	d	24 h	n/a	n/a	n/a	n/a	n/a	1
	AB	4.55 mg/mL	NS	n/a	d	n/a	n/a	12 m	n/a	n/a	n/a	1
	AB	8.3 mg/mL	NS	n/a	d	n/a	60 d	n/a	n/a	n/a	n/a	1
Unspecified	AB	2 mg/mL	NS	n/a	d	24 h	20 d	n/a	n/a	n/a	n/a	1
OTHER INFUSION CONTAINERS												
AccuFlo™/ AccuFlux™/ AccuRX® (B. Braun)	unspec.	5 mg/mL	D5W	n/a	n/a	8 h[c]	1 d[c]	4 w[c]	n/a	n/a	n/a	2
CADD® Cassette (Pharmacia Deltec)	ES	20 mg/mL	NS, W	n/a	d	n/a	24 h[b]	n/a	n/a	n/a	24 h[b]	1
INTERMATE/ INFUSOR (Baxter)	AB	2.5–10 mg/mL	NS	n/a	d	24 h[e]	10 d[e]	n/a	n/a	n/a	n/a	3
	AB	2.5–10 mg/mL	D5W	n/a	d	n/a	10 d[e]	n/a	n/a	n/a	n/a	3
	AB	10 mg/mL	D5W	n/a	d	24 h[e]	10 d[e]	n/a	n/a	n/a	n/a	3

Flush Compatibility: Incompatible with heparin; forms precipitate.[1]
Special Considerations: n/a

Notes

[a]Do not use normal saline or other solutions containing inorganic ions to reconstitute regular vials; precipitate will result.
[b]Stable for 24 h at 30°C after 24 h refrigerated.
[c]Manufacturer(s) extrapolated data from other sources.
[d]pH of reconstituted product is 6.5–7.5 in W; pH of 5 mg/mL dilution is 6.8 in D5W and 7.15 in NS.[1]
[e]Diluents were used as is. D5W was not neutralized as instructed by drug insert; therefore, allocated shelf life is worst case.

continued on next page

Erythromycin Lactobionate (cont'd)

References

1. Trissel LA. ASHP's Interactive Handbook on Injectable Drugs. Bethesda, MD: American Society of Health-System Pharmacists. Accessed 2012 Jan.
2. Drug Stability Data Using Elastomeric Infusion Systems. B. Braun Medical Production Ltd. (Thailand); August 2011.
3. Intermate/Infusor Drug Stability Information. Deerfield, IL: Baxter Healthcare Corporation; October 2008.

Ethanol (Catheter Lock)

| | | | | | Storage Conditions | | | | | | |
| | | | | | Temperature | | | Post-thaw Temp | | Body Temp | |
Drug Manufacturer	Concentration	Diluents	Osmolality (mOsm/kg)	pH	Room	Refrig	Frozen	Room	Refrig		Refer.
CONTAINER											
Syringes, Polypropylene											
AMR	70%	W	n/a	n/a	14 d	n/a	n/a	n/a	n/a	n/a	2
AMR	70%	BWFI[a]	n/a	n/a	14 d	n/a	n/a	n/a	n/a	n/a	2
b	50%[c]	W	n/a	n/a	28 d	n/a	n/a	n/a	n/a	n/a	4

Flush Compatibility: Normal saline.[3] Incompatible with heparin.[1,2]

Special Considerations: Ethanol concentrations above 40% are required to inhibit bacterial growth in established biofilms.[3] Ethanol may cause deterioration of certain plastic materials, including polyurethane catheters; check with the device manufacturer to verify compatibility or potential for degradation due to extended exposure to ethanol catheter lock.[5]

Notes

[a]BWFI containing benzyl alcohol as a preservative.
[b]AAPER Alcohol and Chemical, Shelbyville, KY.
[c]Diluted solution was filtered through two 0.22 micron filters.

References

1. Trissel LA. ASHP's Interactive Handbook on Injectable Drugs. Bethesda, MD: American Society of Health-System Pharmacists. Accessed 2012 Feb.
2. Cober MP, Johnson CE. Stability of 70% alcohol solutions in polypropylene syringes for use in ethanol-lock therapy. Am J Health-Syst Pharm. 2007; 64:2480–2.
3. Cober MP, Kovacevich DS, Teitelbaum DH. Ethanol-lock therapy for the prevention of central venous access device infections in pediatric patients with intestinal failure. J Parent Enteral Nutr. 2011; 35:67–73.
4. Pomplun M, Johnson JJ, Johnston S, et al. Stability of a heparin-free 50% ethanol lock solution for central venous catheters. J Oncol Pharm Practice. 2007; 13:33–7.
5. Bing CM, Ross KL. Antibiotic and ethanol lock therapy. Home Infusion Continuum 2008; 1(2):1,10–1.

Etoposide

Container	Drug Manufacturer	Concentration	Diluents	Osmolality (mOsm/kg)	pH[i]	Storage Conditions						Refer.
						Temperature			Post-thaw Temp		Body Temp	
						Room	Refrig	Frozen	Room	Refrig		
CONTAINER												
Polyvinyl Chloride (PVC)	SZ	0.157 mg/mL[j]	D5W	n/a	i	48 h	48 h	n/a	n/a	n/a	n/a	6
	unspec.	0.2 mg/mL	NS, D5W	n/a	i	72 h	72 h	n/a	n/a	n/a	n/a	6
	BR	0.4 mg/mL[f]	NS	n/a	i	4 d	n/a	n/a	n/a	n/a	n/a	1, 6
Syringes, Plastic	unspec.	1 mg/mL[a]	NS	n/a	i	28 d[a]	28 d[a]	n/a	n/a	n/a	n/a	2
Unspecified	unspec.	0.2 mg/mL	NS	n/a	i	22 d	22 d	n/a	n/a	n/a	n/a	6
OTHER INFUSION CONTAINERS												
AccuFlo™/ AccuFlux™/ AccuRX® (B. Braun)	unspec.	0.1–0.4 mg/mL	NS	n/a	i	9 d	n/a	n/a	n/a	n/a	n/a	7
Excel® Container§ (MG Canada)	BMS	0.125, 0.175 mg/mL[e]	NS[e]	n/a	i	4 d	n/a	n/a	n/a	n/a	n/a	4, 6
	BMS	0.2 mg/mL[d]	NS[d]	n/a	i	72 h[b,c]	n/a	n/a	n/a	n/a	n/a	4, 6
Glass	NOV	0.2 mg/mL	NS	n/a	i	22 d	14 d	n/a	n/a	n/a	n/a	5, 6
	NOV	0.3 mg/mL	NS	n/a	i	2 d	7 d	n/a	n/a	n/a	n/a	5, 6
	BR	0.4 mg/mL	NS, D5W, LR	n/a	i	4 d	n/a	n/a	n/a	n/a	n/a	1, 6
	NOV	10 mg/mL[h]	NS	n/a	i	5 d[h]	7 d	n/a	n/a	n/a	n/a	5, 6
	NOV	10.5 mg/mL[h]	NS	n/a	i	14 d[h]	22 d	n/a	n/a	n/a	n/a	5
	NOV	11 mg/mL[h]	NS	n/a	i	7 d[h]	22 d	n/a	n/a	n/a	n/a	5, 6
	NOV	12 mg/mL[h]	NS	n/a	i	7 d[h]	14 d	n/a	n/a	n/a	n/a	5, 6
Homepump Eclipse®/ Homepump® C-Series (I-Flow Corp.)	unspec.	0.1–0.4 mg/mL	NS	n/a	i	9 d	n/a	n/a	n/a	n/a	n/a	3

continued on next page

Etoposide (cont'd)

Flush Compatibility: Heparin lock flush and normal saline.[6]

Special Considerations: Precipitation of etoposide may be exacerbated by the use of peristaltic pumps, especially at concentrations of 0.4 mg/mL or above. Volumetric pumps may reduce this problem.[6]

Notes

[a] Manufacturer recommends against using solutions more concentrated than 0.4 mg/mL. Etoposide crystallization is unpredictable. Some syringes in the study showed precipitate of drug. At least one syringe seized during administration because of crystallization at a concentration of 1 mg/mL. The author noted that etoposide syringes prepared at a concentration of 0.5 and 1 mg/mL have remained stable and free of precipitate for over 1 y stored in laboratory refrigerator.

[b] Protected from light.

[c] Sample storage temperature 31–33°C.

[d] Sample also contained vincristine 1.6 mcg/mL and doxorubicin 40 mcg/mL.

[e] 0.125 mg/mL etoposide solution also contained vincristine 1 mcg/mL and doxorubicin 25 mcg/mL. 0.175 mg/mL etoposide solution also contained vincristine 1.4 mcg/mL and doxorubicin 35 mcg/mL.

[f] DEHP is leached from PVC due to the polysorbate 80 in the etoposide formulation (Sandoz.) 12 mcg/mL DEHP was leached in 8 h and 50 mcg/mL at 96 h at room temperature. Refrigeration reduced but did not eliminate DEHP leaching.

[g] Excel® containers are polyolefin-lined.

[h] Authors recommended that room temperature storage of etoposide solutions in NS ≥10 mg/mL not exceed 5 d to ensure that at least 94% of the drug concentration is retained.

[i] pH of undiluted solution is 3–4.[6]

[j] Also contains cytarabine (UP) 0.157 mg/mL and daunorubicin HCl (BEL) 15.7 mcg/mL.

References

1. Beijnen JH, Beijnen-Bandhoe AU, Dubbelman AC, et al. Chemical and physical stability of etoposide and teniposide in commonly used infusion fluids. *J Parenter Sci Technol.* 1991; 45:108–12.

2. Adams PS, Haines-Nutt RF, Bradford E, et al. Pharmaceutical aspects of home infusion therapy for cancer patients. *Pharm J.* 1987; 238:476–8.

3. *Stability Data for Drugs Using Homepump Disposable Elastomeric Infusion Systems.* Lake Forest, CA: I-Flow Corporation; October 2009.

4. Wolfe JL, Thoma LA, Du C, et al. Compatibility and stability of vincristine sulfate, doxorubicin hydrochloride, and etoposide in 0.9% sodium chloride injection. *Am J Health-Syst Pharm.* 1999; 56:985–9.

5. Lepage R, Walker SE, Godin J. Stability and compatibility of etoposide in normal saline. *Can J Hosp Pharm.* 2000; 53:338–45.

6. Trissel LA. ASHP's Interactive Handbook on Injectable Drugs. Bethesda, MD: American Society of Health-System Pharmacists. Accessed 2012 Jul.

7. *Drug Stability Data Using Elastomeric Infusion Systems.* B. Braun Medical Production Ltd. (Thailand); August 2011.

Etoposide Phosphate[c]

CONTAINER	Drug Manufacturer	Concentration	Diluents	Osmolality (mOsm/kg)	pH[d]	Temperature Room	Temperature Refrig	Temperature Frozen	Post-thaw Temp Room	Post-thaw Temp Refrig	Body Temp	Refer.
Polyolefin	BMS	0.6 mg/mL[e]	NS	n/a	d	124 h[e]	n/a	n/a	n/a	n/a	124 h[e]	1, 2
	BMS	1.2 mg/mL[f]	NS	n/a	d	124 h[f]	n/a	n/a	n/a	n/a	124 h[f]	1, 2
	BMS	2 mg/mL[g]	NS	n/a	d	124 h[g]	n/a	n/a	n/a	n/a	124 h[g]	1, 2
Polyvinyl Chloride (PVC)	BR	0.1, 10 mg/mL	NS, D5W	n/a	d	31 d	31 d	n/a	n/a	n/a	7 d[a]	1
Syringes, Polypropylene	BR	10, 20 mg/mL	BWFI[b]	n/a	d	31 d	31 d	n/a	n/a	n/a	7 d[a]	1

Flush Compatibility: Heparin lock flush and normal saline.[1]

Notes

[a]Storage at 32°C.
[b]Preserved with benzyl alcohol.
[c]Unlike etoposide, the phosphate ester etoposide phosphate is very water soluble and is suitable for administration via multiple-day ambulatory infusion devices.[1]
[d]pH when reconstituted with W to 1 mg/mL is ~2.9.[1]
[e]Also contains vincristine sulfate (LI) 5 mcg/mL and doxorubicin HCl (PHU) 120 mcg/mL.
[f]Also contains vincristine sulfate (LI) 10 mcg/mL and doxorubicin HCl (PHU) 240 mcg/mL.
[g]Also contains vincristine sulfate (LI) 16 mcg/mL and doxorubicin HCl (PHU) 400 mcg/mL.

References

1. Trissel LA. ASHP's Interactive Handbook on Injectable Drugs. Bethesda, MD: American Society of Health-System Pharmacists. Accessed 2012 Jul.
2. Yuan P, Grimes GJ, Shankman SE, et al. Compatibility and stability of vincristine sulfate, doxorubicin hydrochloride, and etoposide phosphate in 0.9% sodium chloride injection. Am J Health-Syst Pharm. 2001; 58:594–8.

Famotidine

Container	Drug Manufacturer	Concentration	Diluents	Osmolality (mOsm/kg)	pH[b]	Temperature			Post-thaw Temp			Refer.
						Room	Refrig	Frozen	Room	Refrig	Body Temp	
CONTAINER												
Polyvinyl Chloride (PVC)	MSD	0.2 mg/mL	D5W, NS	n/a	b	n/a	14 d	28 d	r/a	14 d	n/a	1
	unspec.	0.2 mg/mL	D5W, NS	n/a	b	15 d	63 d	n/a	n/a	n/a	n/a	1
Syringes, Plastic	MSD	2 mg/mL	D5W, NS, W	n/a	b	n/a	14 d	n/a	n/a	n/a	n/a	1
	MSD	2 mg/mL	D5W	n/a	b	n/a	n/a	3 w	n/a	n/a	n/a	2
	MSD	2 mg/mL	D5W, NS, W	n/a	b	n/a	n/a	8 w	n/a	n/a	n/a	1, 2
Syringes, Polypropylene	MSD	0.2 mg/mL	D5W, NS	n/a	b	15 d	n/a	n/a	n/a	n/a	n/a	1
Unspecified	MSD	0.2 mg/mL	D5W, NS, W, D10W, LR	n/a	b	7 d	n/a	n/a	n/a	n/a	n/a	3
COMMERCIAL PREPARATIONS (RTU)												
Galaxy Bag (Baxter)	MSD	0.4 mg/mL	NS	iso	5.7–6.4	a	n/a	n/a	n/a	n/a	n/a	4

Flush Compatibility: Heparin lock flush and normal saline.[1]
Special Considerations: n/a

Notes

[a]Expiration date per manufacturer's label. Do not extrapolate commercial premix stability data to extemporaneously compounded solutions.
[b]pH of undiluted solution is 5–5.6.[1]

References

1. Trissel LA. ASHP's Interactive Handbook on Injectable Drugs. Bethesda, MD: American Society of Health-System Pharmacists. Accessed 2012 Jan.
2. Shea BF, Souney PF. Stability of famotidine frozen in polypropylene syringes. Am J Hosp Pharm. 1990; 47:2073–4.
3. Famotidine injection [package insert]. Schaumburg, IL: APP Pharmaceuticals LLC; August 2011.
4. Famotidine Injection in Galaxy container (PL2501 Plastic) [package insert]. Deerfield, IL: Baxter Healthcare Corporation; February 2010.

CONTAINER	Drug Manufacturer	Concentration	Diluents	Osmolality (mOsm/kg)	pH[n]	Temperature			Post-thaw Temp		Body Temp	Refer.
						Room	Refrig	Frozen	Room	Refrig		
Ethyvinyl Acetate (EVA)	CUR	3 mcg/mL[o]	NS	n/a	[n]	51 d[o]	51 d[o]	n/a	n/a	n/a	n/a	1
Non-DEHP Bags (INTRAVIA, Baxter)	SZ	0.15 mcg/mL[r]	NS	n/a	4.1–4.7	n/a	28 d[h,r]	n/a	n/a	n/a	n/a	8
	SZ	0.15, 25 mcg/mL[q]	NS	n/a	4.0–5.6	n/a	28 d[h,q]	n/a	n/a	n/a	n/a	8
	SZ	0.15, 43 mcg/mL[p]	NS	n/a	4.1–5.6	n/a	28 d[h,p]	n/a	n/a	n/a	n/a	8
Polypropylene (Mark II Polybag)	JN	1 mcg/mL[m]	NS	n/a	[n]	30 d[f,h,m]	n/a	n/a	n/a	n/a	n/a	1, 5
	JN	1, 10 mcg/mL[l]	NS	n/a	[n]	30 d[f,h,l]	n/a	n/a	n/a	n/a	n/a	1, 5
Polyvinyl Chloride (PVC)	JN	2 mcg/mL[j]	NS	n/a	[n]	30 d[j]	30 d[j]	n/a	n/a	n/a	n/a	1
	JN	2, 20 mcg/mL[i]	NS	n/a	[n]	30 d[i]	30 d[i]	n/a	n/a	n/a	n/a	1
	CUR	3 mcg/mL[o]	NS	n/a	[n]	7 d[o]	7 d[o]	n/a	n/a	n/a	n/a	1
	JN	10 mcg/mL[s]	NS	n/a	[n]	30 d[s]	30 d[s]	n/a	n/a	n/a	n/a	1
	JN	20 mcg/mL	NS	n/a	[n]	30 d	30 d	n/a	n/a	n/a	n/a	1
	JN	20 mcg/mL[a]	NS	n/a	[n]	30 d	30 d	n/a	n/a	n/a	n/a	1
	JN	35 mcg/mL	NS	n/a	[n]	24 d[k]	28 d[k]	n/a	n/a	n/a	n/a	1
	AB	50 mcg/mL	undiluted	n/a	5.43	28 d	28 d[h]	n/a	n/a	n/a	n/a	1, 6
Syringes, Polypropylene	SZ	0.15 mcg/mL[r]	NS	n/a	4.6–5.0	n/a	28 d[h,r]	n/a	n/a	n/a	n/a	8
	SZ	0.15, 25 mcg/mL[q]	NS	n/a	4.5–5.3	n/a	28 d[h,q]	n/a	n/a	n/a	n/a	8
	SZ	0.15, 43 mcg/mL[p]	NS	n/a	4.4–5.8	n/a	28 d[h,p]	n/a	n/a	n/a	n/a	8
	HSP	5 mcg/mL	NS	n/a	4.0–7.0	90 d	n/a	n/a	n/a	n/a	n/a	7
	DB	12.5, 33 mcg/mL	NS	n/a	[n]	7 d	7 d	n/a	n/a	n/a	7 d	1
	JN	35 mcg/mL	NS	n/a	[n]	30 d[t]	30 d[t]	n/a	n/a	n/a	30 d[t]	1, 4
	JN	35 mcg/mL[k]	NS	n/a	[n]	30 d[k,t]	30 d[k,t]	n/a	n/a	n/a	30 d[k,t]	4
	AB	50 mcg/mL	undiluted	n/a	5.43	28 d	28 d[h]	n/a	n/a	n/a	n/a	1, 6

continued on next page

Fentanyl Citrate (cont'd)

continued on next page

Drug Manufacturer	Concentration	Diluents	Osmolality (mOsm/kg)	pH[n]	Storage Conditions						Refer.
					Temperature			**Post-thaw Temp**		**Body Temp**	
					Room	Refrig	Frozen	Room	Refrig		
OTHER INFUSION CONTAINERS											
CADD® Cassette (SIMS Deltec)											
JN	1.25 mcg/mL[e]	[e]	n/a	n	20 d	20 d	n/a	n/a	n/a	48 h[f]	1
JN	20 mcg/mL	NS	n/a	n	30 d	30 d	n/a	n/a	n/a	n/a	1, 2
ME	30, 50 mcg/mL	NS	n/a	n	14 d	14 d	n/a	n/a	n/a	n/a	1
Glass											
CUR	3 mcg/mL[o]	NS	n/a	n	51 d[o]	51 d[o]	n/a	n/a	n/a	n/a	1
INFUSOR (Baxter)											
JN	1–5 mcg/mL	NS, D5W	n/a	n	30 d[b]	n/a	n/a	n/a	n/a	7 d[b]	1, 3
JN	1–5 mcg/mL	NS, D5W	r/a	n	14 d[c]	90 d[c]	n/a	n/a	n/a	7 d[c]	1, 3
JN	1–5 mcg/mL	NS, D5W	n/a	n	n/a	90 d[d]	n/a	n/a	n/a	7 d[d]	3

Flush Compatibility: Heparin lock flush and normal saline.[1]
Special Considerations: n/a

Notes

[a] Combined in a solution of bupivacaine 1.25 mg/mL in NS. Bupivacaine is frequently co-administered with intraspinal fentanyl; it should not be used as a diluent without physician orders.

[b] Storage for 30 d at room temperature followed by 7 d at 33°C.

[c] Storage for 90 d refrigerated, followed by 14 d room temperature, followed by 7 d at 33°C.

[d] Storage for 90 d refrigerated, followed by 7 d at 33°C.

[e] Also contained bupivacaine 0.44 mg/mL and epinephrine 0.69 mcg/mL.

[f] Tested at 30°C. (Near body temperature.)

[g] Combined with ropivacaine 1 mg/mL.

[h] Protected from light.

[i] Combined with bupivacaine 600 mcg/mL and 1.25 mg/mL.

[j] Combined with lidocaine 2.5 mg/mL.

[k] Combined with bupivacaine hydrochloride 1 mg/mL and clonidine hydrochloride 9 mcg/mL.

[l] Combined with ropivacaine 2 mg/mL.

[m] Combined with ropivacaine 1 mg/mL.

[n] pH range of undiluted solutions is 4–7.5.[1]

[o] Combined with ropivacaine 1.5 mg/mL.

[p] With 0.01 mg/mL bupivacaine hydrochloride (HSP).

[q] With 20 mg/mL bupivacaine hydrochloride (HSP).

Fentanyl Citrate (cont'd)

rWith 37.5 mg/mL bupivacaine hydrochloride (HSP).

sWith 50 mcg/mL droperidol (JN) and 1 mg/mL ketamine hydrochloride (JN).

tAlthough pH remained within stability range for the drug, this does not definitively demonstrate stability.[1]

References

1. Trissel LA. ASHP's Interactive Handbook on Injectable Drugs. Bethesda, MD: American Society of Health-System Pharmacists. Accessed 2012 Jul.
2. Allen LV, Stiles ML, Tu YH. Stability of fentanyl citrate in 0.9% sodium chloride solution in portable infusion pumps. Am J Health-Syst Pharm. 1990; 47:1572–4.
3. Intermate/Infusor Drug Stability Information. Deerfield, IL: Baxter Healthcare Corporation; October 2008.
4. Jappinen A, Kokki H, Naaranlahti T. pH stability of injectable fentanyl, bupivacaine, or clonidine solution or a ternary mixture in 0.9% sodium chloride in two types of polypropylene syringes. Int J Pharm Compound. 2002; 6:471–4.
5. Svedberg KO, McKenzie EJ, Larrivee-Elkins C. Compatibility of ropivacaine with morphine, sufentanil, fentanyl or clonidine. J Clin Pharm Ther. 2002; 27:39–45.
6. Donnelly RF. Chemical stability of fentanyl in polypropylene syringes and polyvinyl chloride bags. Int J Pharm Compound. 2005; 9(6):482–3.
7. McCluskey SV, Graner KK, Kemp J, et al. Stability of fentanyl 5 mcg/mL diluted with 0.9% sodium chloride injection and stored in polypropylene syringes. Am J Health-Syst Pharm. 2009; 6:860–3.
8. Donnelly RF, Wong K, Spencer J. Physical compatibility of high-concentration bupivacaine with hydromorphone, morphine, and fentanyl. Can J Hosp Pharm. 2010; 63:154–5.

Filgrastim[a]

CONTAINER	Drug Manufacturer	Concentration	Diluents	Osmolality (mOsm/kg)	pH[c]	Storage Conditions							Refer.
						Temperature			Post-thaw Temp			Body Temp	
						Room	Refrig	Frozen	Room	Refrig			
Polyvinyl Chloride (PVC)	AMG	2–15 mcg/mL[a,b]	D5W	n/a	c	24 h	7 d	n/a	n/a	n/a		n/a	1
	AMG	>15 mcg/mL	D5W	n/a	c	24 h	7 d	n/a	n/a	n/a		n/a	1
Syringes, Plastic	AMG	2–15 mcg/mL[a,b]	D5W	n/a	c	24 h	7 d	n/a	n/a	n/a		n/a	1
	AMG	>15 mcg/mL	D5W	n/a	c	24 h	7 d	n/a	n/a	n/a		n/a	1
	AMG	300 mcg/mL	undiluted	n/a	c	24 h	7 d	n/a	n/a	n/a		n/a	1

Flush Compatibility: D5W or use small volume of W. Incompatible with sodium chloride, and therefore with heparin lock flush (heparinized saline).[1]

Special Considerations: Stable at pH 3.8 to 4.2; stability is limited at neutral pH.[1]

Notes

[a]At filgrastim concentrations between 2 and 15 mcg/mL, add human albumin to a final concentration of 0.2% to minimize adsorption to containers.

[b]The manufacturer does not recommend dilutions less than 5 mcg/mL.

[c]pH is 4.

Reference

1. Trissel LA. ASHP's Interactive Handbook on Injectable Drugs. Bethesda, MD: American Society of Health-System Pharmacists. Accessed 2012 Jan.

Floxuridine

	Drug Manufacturer	Concentration	Diluents	Osmolality (mOsm/kg)	pH[c]	Storage Conditions						Refer.
						Temperature			Post-thaw Temp		Body Temp	
						Room	Refrig	Frozen	Room	Refrig		
CONTAINER												
Syringes, Polypropylene	RC	1, 50 mg/mL	NS	n/a	c	n/a	n/a	n/a	n/a	n/a	21 d[a]	1, 2
OTHER INFUSION CONTAINERS												
Implantable Pump (Fresenius)	unspec.	10 mg/mL	unspec.	n/a	c	n/a	n/a	n/a	n/a	n/a	6 w	1
Implantable Pump (Infusaid)	RC	2.58–12.2 mg/mL[b]	NS	n/a	c	n/a	n/a	n/a	n/a	n/a	12 d	1, 3
Unspecified	unspec.	5–10 mg/mL	D5W, NS, W	n/a	c	14 d	n/a	n/a	n/a	n/a	n/a	1

Flush Compatibility: Normal saline.[3]

Special Considerations: Store reconstituted solution under refrigeration and use within 2 weeks.[1]

Notes

[a]Stored at 30°C.

[b]Solution also contained 200 units/mL heparin sodium in bacteriostatic saline.

[c]pH of reconstituted preparation is 4–5.5.[1]

References

1. Trissel LA. ASHP's Interactive Handbook on Injectable Drugs. Bethesda, MD: American Society of Health-System Pharmacists. Accessed 2012 Jul.
2. Stiles ML, Allen LV, Prince SJ. Stability of deferoxamine mesylate, floxuridine, fluorouracil, hydromorphone hydrochloride, lorazepam, and midazolam hydrochloride in polypropylene infusion-pump syringes. Am J Health-Syst Pharm. 1996; 53:1583–8.
3. Keller JH, Ensminger WD. Stability of cancer chemotherapeutic agents in a totally implanted drug delivery system. Am J Hosp Pharm. 1982; 39:1321–3.

Fluconazole

Fluconazole[a]

Drug	Manufacturer	Concentration	Diluents	Osmolality (mOsm/kg)	pH[e]	Temperature Room	Temperature Refrig	Temperature Frozen	Post-thaw Temp Room	Post-thaw Temp Refrig	Body Temp	Refer.
CONTAINER												
Polyvinyl Chloride (PVC)	BA	1 mg/mL	D5W	n/a	n/a	24 h	n/a	a	n/a	n/a	n/a	1
OTHER INFUSION CONTAINERS												
AccuFlo™/AccuFlux™/AccuRx® (B. Braun)	unspec.	2 mg/mL	RTU[f]	n/a	n/a	24 h[b]	14 d[b]	n/a	n/a	n/a	n/a	5
Homepump Eclipse®/Homepump® C-Series (I-Flow Corp.)	unspec.	2 mg/mL	RTU[f]	iso	e	24 h	14 d	n/a	n/a	n/a	n/a	4
INTERMATE (Baxter)	PF	2 mg/mL	NS	iso	4–8	n/a	15 d	n/a	n/a	n/a	n/a	3
COMMERCIAL PREPARATIONS (RTU)												
Flexible Plastic Container (Hospira)	HSP	2 mg/mL	Dextrose[d]	iso	3.5–6.5	c	n/a	n/a	n/a	n/a	n/a	6
	HSP	2 mg/mL	NS	iso	4–8	c	n/a	n/a	n/a	n/a	n/a	6
INTRAVIA Plastic Container (Baxter)	BA	2 mg/mL	NS	iso	4–6.5	c	n/a	n/a	n/a	n/a	n/a	7
Viaflex® Plus Bag (Baxter)	PF	2 mg/mL	NS, Dextrose[d]	iso	4–8, 3.5–6.5	c	n/a	n/a	n/a	n/a	n/a	2

Flush Compatibility: Heparin lock flush and normal saline.[1]
Special Considerations: Administer intravenously at a maximum rate of 200 mg/h.[1]

continued on next page

Fluconazole (cont'd)

Notes

[a] Do not freeze solutions containing fluconazole.

[b] Manufacturer(s) extrapolated data from other sources. Do not extrapolate commercial premix stability data to extemporaneously prepared solutions.

[c] Expiration date per manufacturer's label. Do not remove from overwrap moisture barrier until ready to use.

[d] Each mL of RTU solution also contains 56 mg of dextrose, hydrous.

[e] pH of RTU solution is 3.5–6.5 in dextrose diluent; 4.0–8.0 in sodium chloride diluent.[2]

[f] RTU diluent is unspecified.

References

1. Trissel LA. ASHP's Interactive Handbook on Injectable Drugs. Bethesda, MD: American Society of Health-System Pharmacists. Accessed 2012 Jan.
2. Diflucan® Injection [product information]. New York, NY: Pfizer Inc.; November 2011.
3. Intermate/Infusor Drug Stability Information. Deerfield, IL: Baxter Healthcare Corporation; October 2008.
4. Stability Data for Drugs Using Homepump Disposable Elastomeric Infusion Systems. Lake Forest, CA: I-Flow Corporation; October 2009.
5. Drug Stability Data Using Elastomeric Infusion Systems. B. Braun Medical Production Ltd. (Thailand); August 2011.
6. Fluconazole Injection [package insert]. Lake Forest, IL: Hospira Inc.; April 2010.
7. Fluconazole Injection in Intravia Plastic Container [product information]. Deerfield, IL: Baxter Healthcare, Inc.; October 2010.

Fludarabine Phosphate

Container	Drug Manufacturer	Concentration	Diluents	Osmolality (mOsm/kg)	pH[b]	Temperature			Post-thaw Temp		Body Temp	Refer.
						Room	Refrig	Frozen	Room	Refrig		
CONTAINER												
Polyvinyl Chloride (PVC)	BX	0.04 mg/mL	NS, D5W	n/a	b	48 h[a]	48 h[a]	n/a	n/a	n/a	n/a	1
OTHER INFUSION CONTAINERS												
Glass Vials	BX	0.04 mg/mL	NS, D5W	n/a	b	48 h[a]	48 h[a]	n/a	n/a	n/a	n/a	1
	BX	1 mg/mL	NS, D5W	n/a	b	16 d[a]	n/a	n/a	n/a	n/a	n/a	1
INTERMATE (Baxter)	SC	0.1–1.5 mg/mL	NS, D5W	n/a	b	35 d	n/a	n/a	n/a	n/a	n/a	2

Flush Compatibility: Heparin lock flush and normal saline.[1]
Special Considerations: n/a

Notes

[a]Solution exposed to normal room light.
[b]pH of solutions is 7.2–8.2.[1]

References

1. Trissel LA. ASHP's Interactive Handbook on Injectable Drugs. Bethesda, MD: American Society of Health-System Pharmacists. Accessed 2012 Jul.
2. Intermate/Infusor Drug Stability Information. Deerfield, IL: Baxter Healthcare Corporation; October 2008.

Fluorouracil

Container	Drug Manufacturer	Concentration	Diluents	Osmolality (mOsm/kg)	pH[e]	Storage Conditions						Refer.
						Temperature			Post-thaw Temp		Body Temp	
						Room	Refrig	Frozen	Room	Refrig		
CONTAINER												
Ethyvinyl Acetate (EVA)	RC	10 mg/mL	NS, D5W	n/a	e	28 d[a]	28 d[a]	n/a	n/a	n/a	28 d[a,g]	8, 9
	RC	15, 45 mg/mL	NS	n/a	e	72 h[a]	n/a	n/a	n/a	n/a	n/a	9
	RC	50 mg/mL	undiluted	n/a	8.6–9.4	28 d[a]	28 d[a]	n/a	n/a	n/a	28 d[a,g]	8, 9
Polyvinyl Chloride (PVC)	RC	1, 10 mg/mL	D5W, NS	n/a	e	14 d	14 d	n/a	n/a	n/a	n/a	9
	RC	1.5 mg/mL	D5W, NS	n/a	e	8 w[d]	n/a	n/a	n/a	n/a	n/a	9
	FA, RC	5, 50 mg/mL	NS, undil.	n/a	e	7 d[a]	91 d[a,h,j]	n/a	n/a	n/a	n/a	9
	TE	8 mg/mL	NS	n/a	e	n/a	n/a	79 d	n/a	28 d	n/a	11
	DB	25 mg/mL	unspec.	n/a	e	n/a	14 d	n/a	n/a	n/a	14 d	9
	unspec.	50 mg/mL	undiluted	n/a	8.6–9.4	14 d	n/a	n/a	n/a	n/a	n/a	2
Syringes, Plastic	DB	24.04 mg/mL	b	n/a	e	14 d	n/a	n/a	n/a	n/a	7 d	5
Syringes, Polypropylene	Abic	10 mg/mL	NS	n/a	e	n/a	n/a	8 w[d]	n/a	n/a	n/a	9
	RC	12, 40 mg/mL	NS, D5W	n/a	e	72 h[a]	n/a	n/a	n/a	n/a	n/a	9
	unspec.	25 mg/mL	unspec.	n/a	e	28 d	28 d	n/a	n/a	n/a	n/a	6, 9
	RC	50 mg/mL	undiluted	n/a	8.6–9.4	21 d[i]	n/a	n/a	n/a	n/a	n/a	3, 9
OTHER INFUSION CONTAINERS												
AccuFlo™/ AccuFlux™/ AccuRX® (B. Braun)	unspec.	1–25 mg/mL	NS	n/a	e	45 d	45 d	n/a	n/a	n/a	n/a	12
	unspec.	50 mg/mL	undiluted	n/a	8.6–9.4	8 w	n/a	n/a	n/a	n/a	n/a	12
CADD® Cassette	LY, RC, SO	50 mg/mL	undiluted	n/a	8.6–9.4	7 d[i]	n/a	n/a	n/a	n/a	7 d[i]	9
Cormed II Model 10500	LY, RC, SO	50 mg/mL	undiluted	n/a	8.6–9.4	7 d[i]	n/a	n/a	n/a	n/a	7 d[i]	9

continued on next page

Fluorouracil (cont'd)

Drug	Manufacturer	Concentration	Diluents	Osmolality (mOsm/kg)	pH[e]	Temperature Room	Temperature Refrig	Temperature Frozen	Post-thaw Temp Room	Post-thaw Temp Refrig	Body Temp	Refer.
Dosi-Fuser (Leventon)	unspec.	1, 10 mg/mL	NS	n/a	e	90 d	n/a	n/a	n/a	n/a	n/a	7
	unspec.	5, 15, 30 mg/mL	NS	n/a	e	30 d	n/a	n/a	n/a	n/a	n/a	7
	unspec.	10 mg/mL	D5W	n/a	e	90 d	n/a	n/a	n/a	n/a	n/a	7
	unspec.	50 mg/mL	undiluted	n/a	8.6–9.4	30 d	n/a	n/a	n/a	n/a	n/a	7
Easypump (Braun)	ICN	25 mg/mL	NS, D5W	n/a	e	21 d	14 d	n/a	n/a	n/a	21 d[c]	9, 10
	ICN	50 mg/mL	undiluted	n/a	8.6–9.4	21 d	n/a	n/a	n/a	n/a	21 d[c]	9, 10
Fresenius VIP 30 Implantable	unspec.	50 mg/mL	undiluted	n/a	8.6–9.4	n/a	n/a	n/a	n/a	n/a	8 w	9
Homepump Eclipse/ Homepump C-Series (I-Flow Corp.)	unspec.	1–25 mg/mL	NS	n/a	e	45 d	45 d	n/a	n/a	n/a	n/a	1
	RC	50 mg/mL	undiluted	n/a	8.6–9.4	8 w	n/a	n/a	n/a	n/a	n/a	1
	unspec.	50 mg/mL	undiluted	n/a	8.6–9.4	45 d	n/a	n/a	n/a	n/a	n/a	1
INFUSOR (Baxter)	Various	0.1–25 mg/mL	NS, D5W	n/a	e	n/a	123 d[f]	n/a	n/a	n/a	7 d	4
	Various	0.1–50 mg/mL	NS, D5W	n/a	e	38 d[f]	n/a	n/a	n/a	n/a	7 d	4
Medfusion Infumed 200	LY, RC, SO	50 mg/mL	undiluted	n/a	8.6–9.4	7 d[j]	n/a	n/a	n/a	n/a	7 d[j]	9
Pancreatec Provider 2000	LY, RC, SO	50 mg/mL	undiluted	n/a	8.6–9.4	7 d[j]	n/a	n/a	n/a	n/a	7 d[j]	9
Polyvinyl Chloride (PVC) Drug Reservoir	RC	10 mg/mL	D5W	n/a	e	7 d	16 w	n/a	n/a	n/a	n/a	9

Flush Compatibility: Heparin lock flush and normal saline.[9]
Special Considerations: n/a

continued on next page

Fluorouracil (cont'd)

Notes

[a]Solutions protected from light.

[b]Diluted to a concentration of 961.54 units/mL of heparin.

[c]Stored at 31°C.

[d]Stability was not affected by re-freezing and further storage at −20°C for two additional weeks (total of 10 w).

[e]pH of the undiluted solution is 8.6–9.4.[9]

[f]Followed by 7 d at 33°C.

[g]Stored at 35°C: concentrations increased due to water evaporation.

[h]Followed by 7 d at 25°C in the dark.

[i]Stored at 30°C.

[j]Fine precipitation was observed with the Roche product in the tubing and bags.

References

1. Stability Data for Drugs Using Homepump Disposable Elastomeric Infusion Systems. Lake Forest, CA: I-Flow Corporation; October 2009.

2. Vyas HM, Baptista RJ, Mitrano FP, et al. Drug stability guidelines for a continuous infusion chemotherapy program. Hosp Pharm. 1987; 22:685–7.

3. Stiles ML, Allen LV, Prince SJ. Stability of deferoxamine mesylate, floxuridine, fluorouracil, hydromorphone hydrochloride, lorazepam, and midazolam hydrochloride in polypropylene infusion-pump syringes. Am J Health-Syst Pharm. 1996; 53:1583–8.

4. Intermate/Infusor Drug Stability Information. Deerfield, IL: Baxter Healthcare Corporation; October 2008.

5. Sewell GJ, Allsopp M, Collinson MP, et al. Stability studies on admixtures of 5-fluorouracil with carboplatin and 5-fluorouracil with heparin for administration in continuous infusion regimens. J Clin Pharm Ther. 1994; 19:127–33.

6. Adams PS, Haines-Nutt RF, Bradford E, et al. Pharmaceutical aspects of home infusion therapy for cancer patients. Pharm J. 1987; 238:476–8.

7. Drug Stability Chart for Dosi-Fuser® Portable Elastomeric Infuser. Barcelona, Spain: Leventon SAU; 2006.

8. Rochard EB, Barthes DMC, Courtois PY. Stability of fluorouracil, cytarabine, or doxorubicin hydrochloride in ethylene vinylacetate portable infusion-pump reservoirs. Am J Hosp Pharm. 1992; 49:619–23.

9. Trissel LA. ASHP's Interactive Handbook on Injectable Drugs. Bethesda, MD: American Society of Health-System Pharmacists. Accessed 2012 Jul.

10. Roberts S, Sewell GJ. Stability and compatibility of 5-fluorouracil infusions in the Braun Easypump. J Oncol Pharm Practice. 2003; 9:109–12.

11. Galanti L, Lebitasy MP, Hecq JD, et al. Long term stability of 5-fluorouracil in 0.9% sodium chloride after freezing, microwave thawing and refrigeration. Can J Hosp Pharm. 2009; 62:34–8.

12. Drug Stability Data Using Elastomeric Infusion Systems. B. Braun Medical Production Ltd. (Thailand); August 2011.

Foscarnet Sodium

Container	Drug Manufacturer	Concentration	Diluents	Osmolality (mOsm/kg)	pH[d]	Temperature			Post-thaw Temp		Body Temp	Refer.
						Room	Refrig	Frozen	Room	Refrig		
CONTAINER												
Polyvinyl Chloride (PVC)	AST	12 mg/mL	D5W, NS	n/a	d	35 d	35 d	n/a	n/a	n/a	n/a	1
	AST	12 mg/mL	NS	n/a	d	30 d	30 d	n/a	n/a	n/a	n/a	1
OTHER INFUSION CONTAINERS												
AccuFlo™/ AccuFlux™/ AccuRX® (B. Braun)	unspec.	12 mg/mL	NS	n/a	d	7 d[e]	14 d[e]	n/a	n/a	n/a	n/a	2
	unspec.	24 mg/mL	undiluted	n/a	d	7 d[e]	14 d[e]	n/a	n/a	n/a	n/a	2
Homepump®/ Homepump Eclipse® (I-Flow Corp.)	AST	12 mg/mL	NS, D5W	n/a	d	7 d	14 d	n/a	n/a	n/a	n/a	4
	AST	24 mg/mL	undiluted[a]	n/a	7.4[l]	7 d	14 d	n/a	n/a	n/a	n/a	4
INTERMATE (Baxter)	AST	2–20 mg/mL	D5W, NS	n/a	d	4 d	14 d[b]	n/a	n/a	n/a	n/a	3
	AST	2–20 mg/mL	NS, D5W	n/a	d	7 d	n/a	n/a	n/a	n/a	n/a	3
	AST	12 mg/mL	NS, D5W	n/a	d	10 d[f]	16 d	n/a	n/a	n/a	n/a	3
	AST	12 mg/mL	NS, D5W	n/a	d	16 d	n/a	n/a	n/a	n/a	n/a	3
	AST	24 mg/mL	undiluted	n/a	d	16 d	n/a	n/a	n/a	n/a	n/a	3
COMMERCIAL PREPARATIONS (RTU)												
Glass Bottle (Hospira)	HSP	24 mg/mL	undiluted	iso	7.4	c	n/a	n/a	n/a	n/a	n/a	5

Flush Compatibility: Heparin lock flush and normal saline.[1]

Special Considerations: Do not give by rapid injection. Administer IV at ≤ 60 mg/kg/h. For peripheral administration, dilute to 12 mg/mL with D5W or NS. Administer with an infusion pump.[1] Precipitation may occur during storage of 24 mg/mL solution at 2–8°C; visually inspect all solutions before administration.[3]

Notes

[a]Foscarnet is available as an isotonic 24 mg/mL solution.[5]

[b]Room temperature stability 4 d following 14 d refrigerated.

[c]Expiration date per manufacturer's label, and must be used within 24 h of initial entry into the bottle.[5]

[d]pH of undiluted solution is 7.4.[1,5]

continued on next page

Foscarnet Sodium (cont'd)

eManufacturer extrapolated data from other source(s).
f10 d room temperature after 16 d refrigerated.

References

1. Trissel LA. ASHP's Interactive Handbook on Injectable Drugs. Bethesda, MD: American Society of Health-System Pharmacists. Accessed 2012 May.
2. Drug Stability Data Using Elastomeric Infusion Systems. B. Braun Medical Production Ltd. (Thailand); August 2011.
3. Intermate/Infusor Drug Stability Information. Deerfield, IL: Baxter Healthcare Corporation; October 2008.
4. Stability Data for Drugs Using Homepump Disposable Elastomeric Infusion Systems. Lake Forest, CA: I-Flow Corporation; October 2009.
5. Foscarnet sodium in Water for Injection [product information]. Lake Forest, IL: Hospira Inc; July 2008.

Fosphenytoin Sodium

Fosphenytoin Sodium[a]

Container	Drug Manufacturer	Concentration	Diluents	Osmolality (mOsm/kg)	pH	Temperature			Post-thaw Temp		Body Temp	Refer.
						Room	Refrig	Frozen	Room	Refrig		
CONTAINER												
Polyvinyl Chloride (PVC)	PD	1 mg PE/mL	D5W, NS	n/a	n/a	30 d	30 d	30 d	7 d	7 d	n/a	1
	PD	1 mg PE/mL	D5LR, LR, D5½S D10W	n/a	n/a	7 d	n/a	n/a	n/a	n/a	n/a	1
	PD	8 mg PE/mL	D5W, NS	n/a	n/a	30 d	30 d	30 d	7 d	7 d	n/a	1
	PD	8 mg PE/mL	D5LR, LR, D5½S D10W	n/a	n/a	7 d	n/a	n/a	n/a	n/a	n/a	1
	PD	20 mg PE/mL	D5W, NS	n/a	n/a	30 d	30 d	30 d	30 d	7 d	7 d	1
	PD	20 mg PE/mL	D5LR, LR, D5½S D10W	n/a	n/a	7 d	n/a	n/a	n/a	n/a	n/a	1
Syringes, Polypropylene (BD)	PD	50 mg PE/mL	undiluted	n/a	8.6–9.0	30 d	30 d	30 d	7 d	7 d	n/a	1

Flush Compatibility: Normal saline.[1]
Special Considerations: n/a

Note

[a]*PE = phenytoin equivalent.*

Reference

1. Trissel LA. ASHP's Interactive Handbook on Injectable Drugs. Bethesda, MD: American Society of Health-System Pharmacists. Accessed 2012 Jan.

Furosemide

Furosemide[a]

Container	Drug Manufacturer	Concentration	Diluents	Osmolality (mOsm/kg)	pH	Temperature			Post-thaw Temp		Body Temp	Refer.
						Room	Refrig	Frozen	Room	Refrig		
CONTAINER												
Polyvinyl Chloride (PVC)	HO	1 mg/mL	NS	n/a	n/a	24 h	26 d[b]	n/a	n/a	n/a	n/a	1
	AB	1.2, 2.4, 3.2 mg/mL	NS	n/a	n/a	84 d	84 d[c]	n/a	n/a	n/a	n/a	1
Syringes, Polypropylene	AB	1, 2, 4, 8 mg/mL	NS	n/a	n/a	84 d	84 d[c]	n/a	n/a	n/a	n/a	1
	HO	3.33–10 mg/mL	NS[a]	n/a	n/a	5 d	5 d	n/a	n/a	n/a	n/a	1, 3
	HO	10 mg/mL	undiluted	287	8–9.3	24 h	n/a	n/a	n/a	n/a	n/a	1
OTHER INFUSION CONTAINERS												
AccuFlo™/ AccuFlux™/ AccuRX® (B. Braun)	unspec.	0.5–10 mg/mL	NS	n/a	n/a	4 d[d]	7 d[d]	n/a	n/a	n/a	n/a	4
Homepump Eclipse®/ Homepump® C-Series (I-Flow Corp.)	unspec.	0.5–10 mg/mL	NS	n/a	n/a	4 d	7 d	n/a	n/a	n/a	n/a	2

Flush Compatibility: Heparin lock flush and normal saline.[1]

Special Considerations: Refrigeration may result in precipitation or crystallization. Resolubilize at room temperature without affecting drug stability. Protection from light is recommended. Do not use if solution has a yellow color.[1]

Notes

[a]With dexamethasone (ME) 0.33–3.33 mg/mL.

[b]10% furosemide loss at 6°C.

[c]Followed by an additional 7 d at room temperature.

[d]Manufacturer extrapolated data from other sources.

References

1. Trissel LA. ASHP's Interactive Handbook on Injectable Drugs. Bethesda, MD: American Society of Health-System Pharmacists. Accessed 2012 Jan.
2. Stability Data for Drugs Using Homepump Disposable Elastomeric Infusion Systems. Lake Forest, CA: I-Flow Corporation; October 2009.
3. Negro S, Rendon AL, Azuara ML, et al. Compatibility and stability of furosemide and dexamethasone combined in infusion solutions. Arzeneimittelforschung. 2006; (56)10:714–20.
4. Drug Stability Data Using Elastomeric Infusion Systems. B. Braun Medical Production Ltd. (Thailand); August 2011.

Ganciclovir Sodium

continued on next page

Container	Drug Manufacturer	Concentration	Diluents	Osmolality (mOsm/kg)	pH[a]	Temperature Room	Temperature Refrig	Temperature Frozen	Post-thaw Temp Room	Post-thaw Temp Refrig	Body Temp	Refer.
CONTAINER												
Polyvinyl Chloride (PVC)	SY	0.28, 1.4 mg/mL	NS	n/a	a	7 d	80 d	364 d	n/a	n/a	n/a	1
	SY	1, 5 mg/mL	D5W, NS	n/a	a	35 d	35 d	n/a	n/a	n/a	n/a	1
	SY	1, 5, 10 mg/mL	D5W	n/a	a	n/a	35 d[c]	n/a	n/a	n/a	n/a	1
	SY	2.44 mg/mL	D5W	n/a	a	5d	5d[c]	n/a	n/a	n/a	n/a	1
	SY	2.59 mg/mL	NS	n/a	a	5d	5d[c]	n/a	n/a	n/a	n/a	1
	RC	<10 mg/mL	NS	n/a	a	24 h	14 d	n/a	n/a	n/a	n/a	6
Syringes, Polypropylene	SY	1.4, 4, 7 mg/mL	NS	n/a	a	7 d	80 d	364 d	n/a	n/a	n/a	1
	SY	5.8 mg/mL	NS	n/a	a	12 h	10 d	n/a	n/a	n/a	n/a	1
	SY	8.33 mg/mL	NS	336	a	24 h	10 d	n/a	n/a	n/a	n/a	4
	SY	8.33 mg/mL	D5W	313	a	24 h	n/a	n/a	n/a	n/a	n/a	4
OTHER INFUSION CONTAINERS												
AccuFlo™/ AccuFlux™/ AccuRX® (B. Braun)	unspec.	1 mg/mL	NS	n/a	a	24 h	14 d	n/a	n/a	n/a	n/a	3
	unspec.	2–5 mg/mL	NS	n/a	a	7 d[b]	n/a	n/a	n/a	n/a	n/a	3
	unspec.	5 mg/mL	NS	n/a	a	24 h[b]	15 d[b]	n/a	n/a	n/a	n/a	3
Homepump Eclipse®/ Homepump® C-Series (I-Flow Corp.)	unspec.	2–5 mg/mL	NS	n/a	a	7 d	n/a	n/a	n/a	n/a	n/a	5
	unspec.	5 mg/mL	NS	n/a	a	24 h	15 d	n/a	n/a	n/a	n/a	5
INTERMATE (Baxter)	SY	1 mg/mL	D5W	n/a	a	7 d[d]	28 d[f]	n/a	n/a	n/a	n/a	2
	RC	1, 5 mg/mL	NS	n/a	a	n/a	35 d[c]	n/a	n/a	n/a	n/a	1
	SY	1–6 mg/mL	D5W, NS	n/a	a	7 d[e]	n/a	63 d	n/a	n/a	n/a	2
	SY	1–6 mg/mL	D5W, NS	n/a	a	3 d[d]	28 d[f]	n/a	n/a	n/a	n/a	2
	SY	1–6 mg/mL	D5W, NS	n/a	a	7 d	n/a	n/a	n/a	n/a	n/a	2
	RC	1–6 mg/mL	D5W, NS	n/a	a	42 d	42 d[f]	n/a	n/a	n/a	n/a	2

Ganciclovir Sodium (cont'd)

Flush Compatibility: Normal saline.[1]

Special Considerations: Do not use if discoloration is noted. Ganciclovir sodium is incompatible with solutions containing parabens. Do not reconstitute with bacteriostatic water for injection containing parabens; precipitation may result.[1] Administer by IV infusion only. Reconstituted solution (50 mg/mL) should not be refrigerated.[6]

Notes

[a]pH of 50 mg/mL reconstituted solution is ~11.[1]
[b]Manufacturer extrapolated data from other sources.
[c]Protected from light.
[d]Following 28 d refrigerated.
[e]Following 63 d frozen.
[f]Inspect for possible crystal formation in D5W; redissolves with gentle shaking and warming to ambient room temperature.

References

1. Trissel LA. ASHP's Interactive Handbook on Injectable Drugs. Bethesda, MD: American Society of Health-System Pharmacists. Accessed 2012 May.
2. Intermate/Infusor Drug Stability Information. Deerfield, IL: Baxter Healthcare Corporation; October 2008.
3. Drug Stability Data Using Elastomeric Infusion Systems. B. Braun Medical Production Ltd. (Thailand); August 2011.
4. Rapp RP, Hatton J, Record K. Drug Stability in Plastic Syringes. HealthTek™ and University of KY Lexington; Repro-Med Systems Inc.; 1998.
5. Stability Data for Drugs Using Homepump Disposable Elastomeric Infusion Systems. Lake Forest, CA: I-Flow Corporation; October 2009.
6. Cytovene® [product information]. Nutley, NJ: Roche Laboratories Inc.; February 2010.

Gemcitabine Hydrochloride

	Drug Manufacturer	Concentration	Diluents	Osmolality (mOsm/kg)	pH[c]	Temperature			Post-thaw Temp		Body Temp	Refer.
						Room	Refrig	Frozen	Room	Refrig		
CONTAINER												
Polyvinyl Chloride (PVC)	LI	0.1, 10 mg/mL	D5W, NS	n/a	c	35 d	35 d[a,b]	n/a	n/a	n/a	n/a	1, 2
	LI	0.1, 10, 38 mg/mL	D5W, NS	n/a	c	n/a	n/a	n/a	n/a	n/a	7 d[a,d]	1, 2
	LI	7.5, 25 mg/mL	NS	n/a	c	27 d	n/a	n/a	n/a	n/a	n/a	2
Syringes, Polypropylene (BD)	LI	38 mg/mL	NS	n/a	c	35 d	b	n/a	n/a	n/a	n/a	1, 2
OTHER INFUSION CONTAINERS												
Glass	LI	38 mg/mL	NS, W	n/a	c	35 d	7 d[a,b]	n/a	n/a	n/a	n/a	1, 2
INTERMATE (Baxter)	LI	3–40 mg/mL	NS	n/a	c	7 d	n/a	n/a	n/a	n/a	n/a	3

Flush Compatibility: Heparin lock flush and normal saline.[2]
Special Considerations: Avoid refrigeration due to the potential for crystallization.

Notes

[a]Protected from light.
[b]Reconstituted solution may develop non-redissolving crystals when stored at 4°C.[1,2]
[c]pH of reconstituted solution is 2.7–3.3.[1]
[d]Stored at 32°C in the dark to simulate ambulatory infusion conditions.

References

1. Xu Q, Zhang Y, Trissel LA. Physical and chemical stability of gemcitabine hydrochloride solutions. *J Am Pharm Assoc.* 1999; 39:509–13.
2. Trissel LA. ASHP's Interactive Handbook on Injectable Drugs. Bethesda, MD: American Society of Health-System Pharmacists. Accessed 2012 May.
3. Intermate/Infusor Drug Stability Information. Deerfield, IL: Baxter Healthcare Corporation: October 2008.

Gentamicin Sulfate

Gentamicin Sulfate

Container	Drug Manufacturer	Concentration	Diluents	Osmolality (mOsm/kg)	pH[c]	Storage Conditions						Refer.
						Temperature			Post-thaw Temp		Body Temp	
						Room	Refrig	Frozen	Room	Refrig		
CONTAINER												
Ethyvinyl Acetate (EVA)	APP	0.85 mg/mL	NS	n/a	c	7 d	30 d	n/a	n/a	n/a	n/a	1
Polyvinyl Chloride (PVC)	SC	0.8 mg/mL	D5W	n/a	c	n/a	n/a	30 d	24 h	n/a	n/a	1
	SC	1 mg/mL	D5W, NS	n/a	c	n/a	n/a	30 d	n/a	n/a	n/a	1
	UP	1.2 mg/mL	D5W, NS	n/a	c	48 h	48 h	n/a	n/a	n/a	n/a	1
	ES	2.4 mg/mL	NS, D5W	n/a	c	n/a	n/a	28 d	n/a	n/a	n/a	1
Syringes, Glass	ES	10 mg/mL	NS	n/a	c	n/a	12 w	n/a	n/a	n/a	n/a	1
Syringes, Plastic	unspec.	1.3 mg/mL	NS, D5W	280, 257	c	30 d	30 d	30 d	n/a	n/a	n/a	6
Syringes, Polypropylene	ES	40 mg/mL	undiluted	160	c	30 d	30 d	n/a	n/a	n/a	n/a	1
OTHER INFUSION CONTAINERS												
AccuFlo™/ AccuFlux™/ AccuRX® (B. Braun)	unspec.	0.8 mg/mL	NS, D5W	n/a	c	n/a	n/a	30 d[a]	n/a	n/a	n/a	5
	unspec.	0.8 mg/mL	NS	n/a	c	24 h[a]	n/a	n/a	n/a	n/a	n/a	5
	unspec.	1 mg/mL	NS	n/a	c	24 h	14 d	n/a	n/a	n/a	n/a	5
	unspec.	4.8 mg/mL	NS	n/a	c	24 h[a]	28 d[a]	n/a	n/a	n/a	n/a	5
AutoDose (Tandem Medical)	APP	0.85 mg/mL	NS	n/a	c	7 d	30 d	n/a	n/a	n/a	n/a	1
CADD® Cassette (SIMS Deltec)	SC	5.45 mg/mL	D5W	n/a	c	n/a	n/a	30 d	n/a	4 d	2 d[f]	1
Homepump Eclipse®/ Homepump® C-Series (I-Flow Corp.)	unspec.	0.8 mg/mL	NS	n/a	c	24 h	n/a	n/a	n/a	n/a	n/a	7
	unspec.	1 mg/mL	NS, D5W	n/a	c	n/a	n/a	30 d[a]	n/a	n/a	n/a	7
	unspec.	4.8 mg/mL	NS	n/a	c	24 h	28 d	n/a	n/a	n/a	n/a	7

197

Gentamicin Sulfate (cont'd)

Drug	Manufacturer	Concentration	Diluents	Osmolality (mOsm/kg)	pH[c]	Storage Conditions						Refer.
						Temperature			Post-thaw Temp		Body Temp	
						Room	Refrig	Frozen	Room	Refrig		
INFUSOR (Baxter)	SO	0.8–2.4 mg/mL	NS	n/a	c	17 d[e]	17 d[e]	n/a	n/a	n/a	n/a	2
INTERMATE (Baxter)	LY	0.25 mg/mL	W	n/a	c	n/a	10 d	n/a	n/a	n/a	n/a	2
	RS, ES	0.5 mg/mL	NS	n/a	c	48 h	10 d	32 d	24 h	n/a	n/a	2
	LY	0.5–5 mg/mL	NS, D5W	n/a	c	24 h	10 d	30 d	n/a	24 h	n/a	2
COMMERCIAL PREPARATIONS (RTU)												
Flexible Plastic Container (Hospira)	HSP	Various	NS	iso	4–4.5	30 d[b,d]	n/a	n/a	n/a	n/a	n/a	3
Viaflex Bag (Baxter)	BA	Various	NS	iso	4–4.5	30 d[b,d]	n/a	n/a	n/a	n/a	n/a	4

Flush Compatibility: Normal saline.[1] Incompatible with heparin.
Special Considerations: Calculated osmolality of 0.8–1.6 mg/mL in NS or D5W was 285 to 320 mOsm/kg.[1]

Notes

[a] Manufacturer(s) extrapolated data from other sources.
[b] Expiration date per manufacturer's label. Do not extrapolate commercial premix stability data to extemporaneously prepared solutions.
[c] pH of undiluted injection is 3–5.5. pH of commercial solutions in NS is 4–4.5.[1]
[d] Do not use beyond this date after removal of manufacturer's protective overwrap.[3,4]
[e] Stable 17 d at room temperature following 17 d refrigerated.
[f] After 30 d at −20°C and 4 d at 5°C.

References

1. Trissel LA. ASHP's Interactive Handbook on Injectable Drugs. Bethesda, MD: American Society of Health-System Pharmacists. Accessed 2012 Jan.
2. Intermate/Infusor Drug Stability Information. Deerfield, IL: Baxter Healthcare Corporation; October 2008.
3. Medical Communications Department [personal communication]. Lake Forest, IL: Hospira Inc.; April 25, 2008.
4. Gentamicin Sulfate in Sodium Chloride [product labeling]. Deerfield, IL: Baxter Healthcare Corporation; June 2011.
5. Drug Stability Data Using Elastomeric Infusion Systems. B. Braun Medical Production Ltd. (Thailand); August 2011.
6. Rapp RP, Hatton J, Record K. Drug Stability in Plastic Syringes. HealthTek™ and University of KY Lexington; Repro-Med Systems Inc.; 1998.
7. Stability Data for Drugs Using Homepump Disposable Elastomeric Infusion Systems. Lake Forest, CA: I-Flow Corporation; October 2009.

Glycopyrrolate

	Drug Manufacturer	Concentration	Diluents	Osmolality (mOsm/kg)	pH	Temperature			Post-thaw Temp		Body Temp	Refer.
						Room	Refrig	Frozen	Room	Refrig		
CONTAINER												
Polyvinyl (PVC)	LEI	0.025 mg/mL	NS	n/a	n/a	30 d^a,b	30 d^a,b	n/a	n/a	n/a	9 d	1
Syringes, Polypropylene	LEI	0.025 mg/mL	NS	n/a	n/a	30 d^a,b	30 d^a,b	n/a	n/a	n/a	16 d	1
	RB	0.2 mg/mL	undiluted	n/a	2.0–3.0	90 d	90 d	n/a	n/a	n/a	n/a	1
UNSPECIFIED CONTAINER TYPE												
Unspecified	RB	0.0008 mg/mL	D5W, NS, D5½S	n/a	n/a	48 h^c	n/a	n/a	n/a	n/a	n/a	1

Storage Conditions

Flush Compatibility: Normal saline.[1]

Special Considerations: Because of the low pH of glycopyrrolate, admixture with alkaline drugs or solutions that result in an admixed pH above 6.0 will result in glycopyrrolate decomposition through hydrolysis.[1]

Notes

[a]With buprenorphine (Reckitt and Colmann, England) 0.084 mg/mL and haloperidol (Janssen, Belgium) 0.104 mg/mL.
[b]Protected from light.
[c]At glycopyrrolate stability pH range of 2.0 to 6.0.

Reference

1. Trissel LA. ASHP's Interactive Handbook on Injectable Drugs. Bethesda, MD: American Society of Health-System Pharmacists. Accessed 2012 May.

Granisetron Hydrochloride

Drug Manufacturer	Concentration	Diluents	Osmolality (mOsm/kg)	pH[c]	Storage Conditions						Refer.
					Temperature			Post-thaw Temp		Body Temp	
					Room	Refrig	Frozen	Room	Refrig		
CONTAINER											
Polyvinyl Chloride (PVC)											
SKB	0.008–0.53 mg/mL[g]	D5W, NS	n/a	c	35 d	35 d	n/a	n/a	n/a	n/a	7
SKB	0.01, 0.04 mg/mL[b]	D5W, NS	n/a	c	14 d[d]	14 d[d]	n/a	n/a	n/a	n/a	1, 2
SKB	0.024 mg/mL	NS	n/a	c	n/a	15 d	n/a	n/a	n/a	n/a	3
BE	0.056 mg/mL	D5W, NS	n/a	c	n/a	n/a	30 d	n/a	7 d[a]	n/a	1
Syringes, Polypropylene											
SKB	0.05, 0.07, 0.1 mg/mL	D5W, NS	n/a	c	14 d	14 d	n/a	n/a	n/a	n/a	1
BE	0.15 mg/mL	D5W, NS	n/a	c	n/a	n/a	30 d	n/a	7 d[a]	n/a	1
BE	0.15 mg/mL	W	n/a	c	3 d	7 d[e]	30 d[f]	n/a	7 d	n/a	1
SKB	1 mg/mL	undiluted	n/a	c	15 d[d]	15 d	n/a	n/a	n/a	n/a	1, 3
OTHER INFUSION CONTAINERS											
AccuFlo™/ AccuFlux™/ AccuRX® (B. Braun)											
unspec.	0.02 mg/mL	D5W	n/a	c	n/a	14 d	n/a	n/a	n/a	n/a	6, 8
unspec.	0.02 mg/mL	NS	n/a	c	n/a	7 d	n/a	n/a	n/a	n/a	6, 8
Homepump®/ Homepump Eclipse® (I-Flow Corp.)											
SKB	0.02 mg/mL	D5W	n/a	c	n/a	14 d	n/a	n/a	n/a	n/a	4, 6
SKB	0.02 mg/mL	NS	n/a	c	n/a	7 d	n/a	n/a	n/a	n/a	4, 6

Flush Compatibility: Heparin lock flush and normal saline.[1]
Special Considerations: Protect intact vials from freezing and light.[5]

Notes

[a]30 d frozen followed by 7 d refrigerated followed by 3 d at 20°C.
[b]With 0.09 or 0.66 mg/mL dexamethasone sodium phosphate (AMR).
[c]pH of undiluted product (0.1, 1 mg/mL) is 4–6.[5]
[d]Protected from light.
[e]7 d at 4°C followed by 3 d at 20°C.
[f]30 d at −20°C followed by 7 d at 4°C and then 3 d at 20°C.
[g]With and without dexamethasone (SAB) 0.05–0.35 mg/mL.

continued on next page

Granisetron Hydrochloride (cont'd)

References

1. Trissel LA. ASHP's Interactive Handbook on Injectable Drugs. Bethesda, MD: American Society of Health-System Pharmacists. Accessed 2012 Aug.

2. Chin A, Moon YSK, Chung KC, et al. Stability of granisetron hydrochloride with dexamethasone sodium phosphate for 14 days. *Am J Health-Syst Pharm.* 1996; 53:1174–6.

3. Hourcade F, Sautou-Miranda V, Normand B, et al. Compatibility of granisetron towards glass and plastics and its stability under various storage conditions. *Int J Pharm (AMST).* 1997; 154:95–102.

4. *Stability Data for Drugs Using Homepump Disposable Elastomeric Infusion Systems.* Lake Forest, CA: I-Flow Corporation; October 2009.

5. Kytril[R] [package insert]. South San Francisco, CA: Genentech USA; April 2011.

6. Chung KC, Chin A, Gill MA. Stability of granisetron hydrochloride in a disposable elastomeric infusion device. *Am J Health-Syst Pharm.* 1995; 52:1541–3.

7. Walker SE, Law S. Stability and compatibility of granisetron alone and in combination with dexamethasone in 0.9% sodium chloride and 5% dextrose in water solutions. *Can J Hosp Pharm.* 2002; 55:27–38.

8. *Drug Stability Data Using Elastomeric Infusion Systems.* B. Braun Medical Production Ltd. (Thailand); August 2011.

Haloperidol Lactate

Container	Drug Manufacturer	Concentration	Diluents	Osmolality (mOsm/kg)	pH[d]	Temperature			Post-thaw Temp		Body Temp	Refer.
						Room	Refrig	Frozen	Room	Refrig		
CONTAINER												
Polyvinyl Chloride (PVC)	MN	0.1 mg/mL	D5W	n/a	d	38 d	n/a	n/a	n/a	n/a	n/a	1
Syringes, Polypropylene	JN	0.104 mg/mL	NS	n/a	d	30 d[b]	30 d[b]	n/a	n/a	n/a	16 d	1, 3
	EST[e]	0.208 mg/mL[f]	NS	n/a	n/a	15 d[g]	15 d[g]	n/a	n/a	n/a	n/a	1, 4
OTHER INFUSION CONTAINERS												
Glass Vials	MN	0.1–0.75 mg/mL	NS	n/a	d	7 d[a]	n/a	n/a	n/a	n/a	n/a	1
	MN	0.1–3 mg/mL	D5W	n/a	d	7 d[a]	n/a	n/a	n/a	n/a	n/a	1
PVC Cassette (SIMS Deltec)	ON	0.104 mg/mL[b]	NS	n/a	d	30 d[b]	30 d[b]	n/a	n/a	n/a	9 d	1, 3
	unspec.	0.2 mg/mL[c]	unspec.	n/a	d	7 d	n/a	n/a	n/a	n/a	n/a	2
Unspec. Infusion Pump	EST[e]	0.208–0.624 mg/mL[h]	NS	n/a	4.7–5.62	15 d[g]	n/a	n/a	n/a	n/a	n/a	5

Flush Compatibility: Normal saline. Incompatible with heparin lock flush.[1]
Special Considerations: n/a

Notes

[a]Visual testing only.
[b]With buprenorphine (Reckitt and Colemann, England) 0.084 mg/mL and glycopyrrolate (Leiras, Finland) 0.025 mg/mL.
[c]With morphine sulfate 15 mg/mL.
[d]pH of undiluted solution is 3.0–3.8.[1]
[e]Esteve, Spain.
[f]With tramadol HCl (Grunenthal, Germany) 8.33, 16.67, 33.33 mg/mL.
[g]Protected from light.
[h]With tramadol HCl (Grunenthal, Germany) 8.33 mg/mL and hyoscine N-butylbromide 3.3–6.67 mg/mL (BI, Spain).

References

1. Trissel LA. ASHP's Interactive Handbook on Injectable Drugs. Bethesda, MD: American Society of Health-System Pharmacists. Accessed 2012 Feb.
2. Swanson G, Smith J, Bulich R, et al. Patient-controlled analgesia for chronic cancer pain in the ambulatory setting: a report of 117 patients. J Clin Oncol. 1989; 7(12):1903–8.
3. Jäppinen A, Kokki H, Naaranlahti TJ, et al. Stability of buprenorphine, haloperidol, and glycopyrrolate mixture in a 0.9% sodium chloride solution. Pharm World Sci. 1999; 21(6):272–4.
4. Negro S, Martin A, Azuara ML, et al. Stability of tramadol and haloperidol for continuous subcutaneous infusion at home. J Pain Symptom Manage. 2005; 30(2):192–9.
5. Negro S, Martin A, Azuara ML, et al. Compatibility and stability of ternary admixtures of tramadol, haloperidol, and hyoscine N-butylbromide: retrospective clinical evaluation. J Palliat Med. 2010; 13(3):273–7.

Heparin Sodium

	Drug Manufacturer	Concentration	Diluents	Osmolality (mOsm/kg)	pH[j]	Temperature Room	Temperature Refrig	Temperature Frozen	Post-thaw Temp Room	Post-thaw Temp Refrig	Body Temp	Refer.
CONTAINER												
Ethyvinyl Acetate (EVA)	unspec.	10 units/mL	NS	n/a	j	16 d	30 d	n/a	n/a	n/a	2 d[f]	6
Polyvinyl Chloride (PVC)	unspec.	5,000 units/mL	undiluted	n/a	5–8	10 d	7 d	n/a	n/a	n/a	n/a	4
Syringes, Plastic	unspec.	1 unit/mL[b]	n/a	n/a	j	n/a	n/a	n/a	n/a	n/a	52 w	1
Syringes, Polypropylene	unspec.	500 units/mL	NS	n/a	j	3 w	3 w	n/a	n/a	n/a	n/a	1
	ES	1,000 units/mL	undiluted	384	5–8	n/a	n/a	n/a	n/a	n/a	30 d[e]	1
	SCN	40,000 units/mL	undiluted	n/a	5–8	n/a	n/a	n/a	n/a	n/a	30 d[e]	1
OTHER INFUSION CONTAINERS												
AutoDose (Tandem Medical)	unspec.	10 units/mL	NS	n/a	j	16 d	30 d	n/a	n/a	n/a	2 d[f]	6
DEHP-free Plastic Bags (Secure Medical)	FUJ	5 units/mL	NS	n/a	j	n/a	28 d	n/a	n/a	n/a	n/a	3
INFUSOR (Baxter)	DIO	3,248 units/mL[c]	NS	n/a	j	7 d	14 d[k]	n/a	n/a	n/a	n/a	2
Unspecified	DB	1 unit/mL	D5W[g]	n/a	j	7 d	n/a	n/a	n/a	n/a	n/a	1
	DB	1 unit/mL	NS	n/a	j	12 m	n/a	n/a	n/a	n/a	n/a	1
	LY	5 units/mL	NS	n/a	j	n/a	28 d	n/a	n/a	n/a	n/a	1
	DB	10 units/mL	D5W[g]	n/a	j	12 m	n/a	n/a	n/a	n/a	n/a	1
	DB	10 units/mL	NS	n/a	j	12 m	12 m	n/a	n/a	n/a	n/a	1
	AH	35 units/mL	NS	n/a	j	24 h[i]	14 d[l]	n/a	n/a	n/a	n/a	1

continued on next page

Heparin Sodium (cont'd)

Drug Manufacturer	Concentration	Diluents	Osmolality (mOsm/kg)	pH[j]	Storage Conditions						Refer.
					Temperature			**Post-thaw Temp**		**Body Temp**	
					Room	Refrig	Frozen	Room	Refrig		
COMMERCIAL PREPARATIONS (RTU)											
Excel Container (B. Braun) BRN	2 units/mL	NS	n/a	j	h	n/a	n/a	n/a	n/a	n/a	7
BRN	40, 50, 100 units/mL	D5W	n/a	j	h	n/a	n/a	n/a	n/a	n/a	7
Flexible Plastic Bag (Abbott) AB	various	D5W	n/a	j	d	n/a	n/a	n/a	n/a	n/a	5

Flush Compatibility: Heparin lock flush and normal saline.[1]
Special Considerations: n/a

Notes

aDo not freeze; when adding to large volume parenteral solutions, assure thorough admixture to prevent pooling of heparin and dilutional overdosing.
bPolyethylene syringes with polypropylene plungers (Inject, Braun). Plastic syringes with rubber plungers exhibited possible leaching of rubber components.
cConcentration reported by MFR as 20 mg/mL, heparin 162.4 units/mg.
dExpiration date per manufacturer's label. Manufacturer recommends using the commercial product within 7 d of removal of the overwrap.
eAt near-body temperature of 30°C; little loss by HPLC analysis; activity not evaluated.
fTested at 40°C.
gEvaluations of heparin stability in dextrose solutions have revealed conflicting information in the literature. Authors have recommended heparin sodium addition to dextrose solutions immediately prior to administration.
hExpiration date per manufacturer's label.
iStable an additional 14 d at 4°C.
jpH of undiluted injection and lock flush is adjusted to 5–7.5.[1]
kMay be followed by 7 d at room temperature.
lPreceded by 24 h at room temperature.

References

1. Trissel LA. ASHP's Interactive Handbook on Injectable Drugs. Bethesda, MD: American Society of Health-System Pharmacists. Accessed 2012 Jan.
2. Intermate/Infusor Drug Stability Information. Deerfield, IL: Baxter Healthcare Corporation; October 2008.
3. Hensrud DD, Burritt MF, Hall LG. Stability of heparin anticoagulant activity over time in parenteral nutrition solutions. J Parent Enteral Nutr. 1996; 20(3):219–21.
4. Pharmacia Deltec CADD Ambulatory Infusion Pump Systems. Stability Data in Pharmacia Deltec Medication Cassette Reservoirs. St Paul, MN: Pharmacia Deltec; 1992.
5. Janet R. Rubin, RN, BSN [manufacturer's letter]. Lake Forest, IL: Abbott Hospital Products Division; November 12, 1999.
6. AutoDose Stability Reference. San Diego, CA: Tandem Medical Inc.; 2002.
7. Product catalog. Bethlehem, PA: B. Braun Medical; December 2007.

Hydralazine Hydrochloride

Hydralazine Hydrochloride[a]

CONTAINER	Drug Manufacturer	Concentration	Diluents	Osmolality (mOsm/kg)	pH[e]	Storage Conditions Temperature Room	Refrig	Frozen	Post-thaw Temp Room	Refrig	Body Temp	Refer.
Polyvinyl Chloride (PVC)	SI	0.027 mg/mL	NS	n/a	e	1 w[b]	n/a	n/a	n/a	n/a	n/a	1
	AMR	0.2 mg/mL	NS	n/a	4.1–4.9	2 d	n/a	n/a	n/a	n/a	n/a	1
	unspec.	0.35 mg/mL	NS	n/a	e	52 d	n/a	n/a	n/a	n/a	n/a	1
Syringes, Polypropylene	SI	0.027 mg/mL[c]	NS	n/a	e	24 h[d]	n/a	n/a	n/a	n/a	n/a	1

Flush Compatibility: Heparin lock flush and normal saline.[1]

Special Considerations: Hydralazine is not stable in D5W.[1]

Notes

[a]Hydralazine reacts with various metals. Contact with metal parts (e.g. stainless steel needles) should be minimized.

[b]10% loss due to sorption in Travenol 0.9% sodium chloride PVC bags. No loss over 7 h when infused through PVC tubing with a cellulose propionate burette chamber.

[c]Syringes with polyethylene plungers.

[d]Protected from light.

[e]pH of undiluted product is 3.4–4.4.[1]

Reference

1. Trissel LA. ASHP's Interactive Handbook on Injectable Drugs. Bethesda, MD: American Society of Health-System Pharmacists. Accessed 2012 May.

Hydrocortisone Sodium Succinate

	Drug Manufacturer	Concentration	Diluents	Osmolality (mOsm/kg)	pH[a]	Storage Conditions						
						Temperature			Post-thaw Temp		Body Temp	Refer.
						Room	Refrig	Frozen	Room	Refrig		
CONTAINER												
Polyolefin	PH	1 mg/mL	NS	d	a	6 d[c]	48 d	n/a	n/a	n/a	n/a	3
Polyvinyl Chloride (PVC)	UP	0.009 mg/mL	NS	d	a	1 w	n/a	n/a	n/a	n/a	n/a	1
	PH	1 mg/mL	NS	d	a	7 d[c]	41 d	n/a	n/a	n/a	n/a	3
Syringes, Polypropylene	UP	10 mg/mL	NS	d	a	7 d	21 d	n/a	n/a	n/a	n/a	1, 2
	PH	50 mg/mL	W	d	a	6 d	81 d	n/a	n/a	n/a	n/a	1, 3
OTHER INFUSION CONTAINERS												
Glass Vial	UP	125 mg/mL	W, NS[b]	d	a	n/a	n/a	4 w	n/a	n/a	n/a	1

Flush Compatibility: Heparin lock flush and normal saline.[1]
Special Considerations: n/a

Notes

[a]pH of reconstituted solution is 7–8.[1]
[b]Reconstituted vial.
[c]8 d, if protected from light.
[d]A 50 mg/mL solution (AB) is 260–292 mOsm/kg.[1]

References

1. Trissel LA. ASHP's Interactive Handbook on Injectable Drugs. Bethesda, MD: American Society of Health-System Pharmacists. Accessed 2012 Jul.
2. Das Gupta V, Ling J. Stability of hydrocortisone sodium succinate after reconstitution in 0.9% sodium chloride injection and storage in polypropylene syringes for pediatric use. Int J Pharm Compound. 2000; 4(5):396–7.
3. Rigge DC, Jones MF. Shelf lives of aseptically prepared medicines - stability of hydrocortisone sodium succinate in PVC and non-PVC bags and in polypropylene syringes. J Pharm Biomed Anal. 2005; Jun 15 38(2):332–6.

Hydromorphone Hydrochloride^a

Drug Manufacturer	Concentration	Diluents	Osmolality (mOsm/kg)	pH^f	Temperature			Post-thaw Temp		Body Temp	Refer.
					Room	Refrig	Frozen	Room	Refrig		
CONTAINER											
Polyvinyl Chloride (PVC)											
SZ	0.2 mg/mL	NS	n/a	f	7 d^i	n/a	n/a	n/a	n/a	n/a	4
KN	1, 5 mg/mL	NS, D5W	n/a	f	42 d	42 d	n/a	n/a	n/a	n/a	1
KN	20, 100 mg/mL	NS	n/a	f	72 h^b	n/a	n/a	n/a	n/a	n/a	1
Syringes, Plastic											
SZ	0.2 mg/mL	NS	n/a	f	7 d^i	n/a	n/a	n/a	n/a	n/a	4
Syringes, Polypropylene											
SAB	0.02, 0.04 mg/mL	NS^g	n/a	f	91 d^b	91 d^a	n/a	n/a	n/a	n/a	3
KN	0.1 mg/mL	NS	n/a	f	30 d	n/a	n/a	n/a	n/a	n/a	1
d	1.5–80 mg/mL	NS	n/a	f	60 d	60 d^a	n/a	n/a	n/a	n/a	1
KN	10 mg/mL	undiluted	n/a	f	30 d	n/a	n/a	n/a	n/a	n/a	1
OTHER INFUSION CONTAINERS											
Brown Glass Vials											
SZ	0.2 mg/mL	NS	n/a	f	7 d^i	n/a	n/a	n/a	n/a	n/a	4
INFUSOR (Baxter)											
KN	1 mg/mL	D5W, NS	n/a	f	7 d	32 d^c	n/a	n/a	n/a	n/a	2
KN	3–10 mg/mL	D5W	n/a	f	7 d^i	n/a	n/a	n/a	n/a	5 d^i	2
Synchromed® Implanted Pump (Medtronic)											
KN	2, 10 mg/mL	undiluted	n/a	f	n/a	n/a	n/a	n/a	n/a	16 w^{e,h}	1

Flush Compatibility: Normal saline and heparin lock flush.[1]
Special Considerations: n/a

Notes

^{a}Protect from light.
^{b}Under fluorescent light.
^{c}32 d refrigerated, followed by 3 d at room temperature.
^{d}Compounded using hydromorphone hydrochloride powder.
^{e}No adverse effects on pump were noted.
^{f}pH range of undiluted product is 4–5.5.[1]

continued on next page

Hydromorphone Hydrochloride (cont'd)

gWith bupivacaine 2.5 mg/mL.
hStored at 37°C.
iWith ketamine (SZ) 0.2, 0.6, and 1 mg/mL.
j7 d at room temperature, followed by 5 d at 33°C.

References

1. Trissel LA. ASHP's Interactive Handbook on Injectable Drugs. Bethesda, MD: American Society of Health-System Pharmacists. Accessed 2012 Aug.
2. Intermate/Infusor Drug Stability Information. Deerfield, IL: Baxter Healthcare Corporation; October 2008.
3. Donnelly RF. Physical compatibility and chemical stability of bupivacaine and hydromorphone in polypropylene syringes. Can J Hosp Pharm. 2004; 57:230–5.
4. Ensom MHH, DeCarie D, Leung K, et al. Stability of hydromorphone-ketamine solutions in glass bottles, plastic syringes, and IV bags for pediatric use. Can J Hosp Pharm. 2009; 62(2):112–8.

Hydroxyzine Hydrochloride

	Drug Manufacturer	Concentration	Diluents	Osmolality (mOsm/kg)	pH[e]	Temperature			Post-thaw Temp		Body Temp	Refer.
						Room	Refrig	Frozen	Room	Refrig		
CONTAINER												
Syringes, Plastic	PF	12.5 mg/mL[b]	b	n/a	n/a	12 m[c]	12 m[c]	n/a	n/a	n/a	n/a	1
	PF	20 mg/mL[a]	a	n/a	n/a	10 d	10 d	n/a	n/a	n/a	n/a	1
	NF	50 mg/mL[c,d]	d	n/a	e	10 d	10 d	n/a	n/a	n/a	n/a	1
OTHER INFUSION CONTAINERS												
Syringes, Glass	PF	12.5 mg/mL[b]	b	n/a	n/a	12 m[c]	12 m[c]	n/a	n/a	n/a	n/a	1

(Storage Conditions)

Flush Compatibility: Normal saline. Incompatible with heparin lock flush.[1]
Special Considerations: n/a

Notes

[a]With atropine sulfate 0.16 mg/mL (Wyeth) and meperidine HCl 20 mg/mL (Winthrop).
[b]With chlorpromazine HCl 6.25 mg/mL (Elkins-Sinn) and meperidine HCl 25 mg/mL (Winthrop).
[c]Protected from light.
[d]With atropine sulfate USP 1 mg/mL.
[e]pH of undiluted solution is 3.5–6.[1]

Reference

1. Trissel LA. ASHP's Interactive Handbook on Injectable Drugs. Bethesda, MD: American Society of Health-System Pharmacists. Accessed 2012 Jul.

Ibuprofen

CONTAINER	Drug Manufacturer	Concentration	Diluents	Osmolality (mOsm/kg)	pH	Storage Conditions						
						Temperature			Post-thaw Temp			Refer.
						Room	Refrig	Frozen	Room	Refrig	Body Temp	
Polyvinyl Chloride (PVC)	CUP	≤ 4 mg/mL	NS, D5W, LR	n/a	a	24 h	7 d	n/a	n/a	n/a	n/a	1, 2

Flush Compatibility: Normal saline.[1,2]
Special Considerations: Caldolor® contains arginine; vial stopper is latex free. Dilute to a final concentration of 4 mg/mL or less prior to infusion.[1,2] Do not confuse this preparation with ibuprofen lysine injection, which has different physicochemical properties and clinical indications.[3]

Note
[a]pH of 100 mg/mL (undiluted) is approximately 7.4.[1]

References

1. Caldolor® [prescribing information]. Nashville, TN: Cumberland Pharmaceuticals Inc.; June 2009.
2. Professional Affairs, Cumberland Pharmaceuticals Inc. [written correspondence]. Nashville, TN: Cumberland Pharmaceuticals Inc.; January 18, 2012.
3. Cada DJ, Levien T, Baker DE. Ibuprofen lysine injection. Hosp Pharm. 2006; 41(10):970–8.

Ifosfamide

Storage Conditions

Container	Drug Manufacturer	Concentration	Diluents	Osmolality (mOsm/kg)	pH[f]	Temperature Room	Temperature Refrig	Temperature Frozen	Post-thaw Temp Room	Post-thaw Temp Refrig	Body Temp	Refer.
CONTAINER												
Polyvinyl Chloride (PVC)	FL	10 mg/mL	NS	n/a	f	8 d	8 d[d]	n/a	n/a	n/a	n/a	2, 4
Syringes, Plastic	unspec.	50 mg/mL[a,g]	NS	n/a	f	28 d	28 d	n/a	n/a	n/a	n/a	1, 4
OTHER INFUSION CONTAINERS												
CADD® Cassette (Pharmacia Deltec)	FL	20, 40, 80 mg/mL	NS	n/a	f	n/a	n/a	n/a	n/a	n/a	8 d[h]	2, 4
	FL	80 mg/mL	W	n/a	f	n/a	n/a	n/a	n/a	n/a	8 d	4
Glass Vials	BI	83.3 mg/mL[b]	NS	n/a	f	9 d[c]	n/a	n/a	n/a	n/a	9 d[c,d]	3, 4
Graseby™ 9000 Cassette (Graseby Medical)	AM	20 mg/mL[e]	W[e]	n/a	f	n/a	14 d[d]	n/a	n/a	n/a	7 d[d]	4, 5
INFUSOR (Baxter)	AM	0.8–100 mg/mL[i]	NS	n/a	n/a	n/a	7 d[k]	n/a	n/a	n/a	2 d[k]	6
	AM, BI	35–70 mg/mL[i]	W	n/a	n/a	10 d	n/a	n/a	n/a	n/a	n/a	6
	AM, BI	70 mg/mL[i]	NS	n/a	n/a	10 d	n/a	n/a	n/a	n/a	n/a	6
Unspecified	unspec.	0.6, 16 mg/mL	D5W, NS, D5LR, D5S, LR, 1/2S	n/a	n/a	7 d	6 w	n/a	n/a	n/a	n/a	4
	BMS	50 mg/mL	W, BWFI	n/a	f	7 d	6 w	n/a	n/a	n/a	n/a	4

Flush Compatibility: Normal saline.[4]

Special Considerations: Do not use a filter to administer this medication.

Notes

[a]With mesna 40 mg/mL.

[b]With mesna 79 mg/mL or ifosfamide alone. Mesna stability not tested.

[c]Solution stored in daylight at temperature range of 18–24°C, another solution also stored in dark at 27°C.

continued on next page

Ifosfamide (cont'd)

d Protected from light.
e With mesna (AM) 20 mg/mL.
f pH of solution is ~6.0.[1]
g With epirubicin 1 mg/mL.
h At 35°C.
i With mesna (AM) 0.4–100 mg/mL.
j Do not reconstitute ifosfamide with BWFI containing benzyl alcohol.
k 7 d refrigerated, followed by 2 d at 33°C.

References

1. Adams PS, Haines-Nutt RF, Bradford E, et al. Pharmaceutical aspects of home infusion therapy for cancer patients. *Pharm J*. 1987; 238:476–8.
2. Munoz M, Girona V, Pujol M, et al. Stability of ifosfamide in 0.9% sodium chloride solution or water for injection in a portable iv pump cassette. *Am J Hosp Pharm*. 1992; 49:1137–9.
3. Radford JA, Margison JM, Swindell R, et al. The stability of ifosfamide in aqueous solution and its suitability for continuous 7-day infusion by ambulatory pump. *J Cancer Res Clin Oncol*. 1991; 117(Suppl 4):5154–6.
4. Trissel LA. ASHP's Interactive Handbook on Injectable Drugs. Bethesda, MD: American Society of Health-System Pharmacists. Accessed 2012 Aug.
5. Priston MJ, Sewell GJ. Stability of three cytotoxic drug infusions in the Graseby 9000 ambulatory infusion pump. *J Oncol Pharm Practice*. 1998; 4:143–9.
6. Intermate/Infusor Drug Stability Information. Deerfield, IL: Baxter Healthcare Corporation; October 2008.

Imipenem–Cilastatin Sodium

| Drug Manufacturer | Concentration | Diluents | Osmolality (mOsm/kg) | pH[a] | Storage Conditions | | | | | | Refer. |
| | | | | | Temperature | | | Post-thaw Temp | | Body Temp | |
					Room	Refrig	Frozen	Room	Refrig		
CONTAINER											
Ethyvinyl Acetate (EVA) APO	2.5, 5 mg/mL	NS	b	a	8 h	72 h	n/a	n/a	n/a	n/a	1
Polyvinyl Chloride (PVC) ME	2.5 mg/mL	D5W	b	a	6 h	37 h	n/a	n/a	n/a	n/a	1
ME	2.5 mg/mL	NS	b	a	15 h	103 h	n/a	n/a	n/a	n/a	1
OTHER INFUSION CONTAINERS											
AccuFlo™/ AccuFlux™/ AccuRX® (B. Braun) unspec.	5 mg/mL	NS	b	a	10 h	48 h	n/a	n/a	n/a	n/a	4
AutoDose (Tandem Medical) unspec.	2.5, 5 mg/mL	NS	b	a	8 h	72 h	n/a	n/a	n/a	n/a	1
Homepump®/ Homepump Eclipse® (I-Flow Corp.) unspec.	5 mg/mL	NS	b	a	n/a	24 h	n/a	n/a	n/a	n/a	2
INTERMATE (Baxter) MSD	2.5 mg/mL	D5W	b	a	10 h	24 h[c]	n/a	n/a	n/a	n/a	3
MSD	2.5 mg/mL	NS	b	a	18 h	48 h[d]	n/a	n/a	n/a	n/a	3
MSD	2.5 mg/mL	NS	b	a	18 h	24 h[e]	n/a	n/a	n/a	n/a	3
MSD	5 mg/mL	D5W	b	a	8 h	n/a	n/a	n/a	n/a	n/a	3
MSD	5 mg/mL	NS	b	a	13 h	24 h[c]	n/a	n/a	n/a	n/a	3

continued on next page

Flush Compatibility: Normal saline.[1]
Special Considerations: Manufacturer suggests for vials: reconstitute vial with 10-mL diluent, shake well, and transfer resulting suspension to infusion solution container. Repeat with additional 10 mL of diluent to ensure complete transfer of vials contents to the infusion solution. Agitate resulting mixture until clear.[1] Maximum solubility is 5 mg/mL at room temperature. Solubility is lower at lower temperatures.[5]
If an admixed dose is refrigerated prior to administration, shake vigorously upon removal from refrigerator and equilibrate to room temperature. Shake again just prior to administration.[5]

213

Imipenem–Cilastatin Sodium (cont'd)

Notes

[a]pH of the IV product is buffered to 6.5–8.5.[1]

[b]When reconstituted and diluted as directed by the manufacturer, the osmolality of the mixture approximates that of the diluent.[1]

[c]Followed by 9 h at room temperature.

[d]Followed by 10 h at room temperature.

[e]Followed by 13 h at room temperature.

References

1. Trissel LA. ASHP's Interactive Handbook on Injectable Drugs. Bethesda, MD: American Society of Health-System Pharmacists. Accessed 2012 Jan.
2. Stability Data for Drugs Using Homepump Disposable Elastomeric Infusion Systems. Lake Forest, CA: I-Flow Corporation; October 2009.
3. Intermate/Infusor Drug Stability Information. Deerfield, IL: Baxter Healthcare Corporation; October 2008.
4. Drug Stability Data Using Elastomeric Infusion Systems. B. Braun Medical Production Ltd. (Thailand); August 2011.
5. Medical Services [personal communication]. North Wales, PA: Merck & Co. Inc.; January 2008.

Immune Globulin (Human)

Container	Drug Manufacturer	Concentration	Diluents	Osmolality (mOsm/kg)	pH	Temperature Room	Temperature Refrig	Temperature Frozen	Post-thaw Temp Room	Post-thaw Temp Refrig	Body Temp	Refer.
Ethyvinyl Acetate (EVA)	OCT[g]	5%	RTU	310–380	5.1–6	n/a	10 d[n]	n/a	n/a	n/a	n/a	6, 7
	BA[d]	5%, 10%	W[k,l]	636, 1250[4]	6.8±0.4	3 d[n]	14 d[n]	n/a	n/a	n/a	n/a	12
	BA[c]	10%	RTU[m]	240–300[3]	4.6–5.1	n/a	14 d[n]	n/a	n/a	n/a	n/a	10
Glass	CSL[a]	3%	W, D5W, NS[k,l]	192, 444, 498	6.6±0.2	n/a	24 h[n]	n/a	n/a	n/a	n/a	2
	BA[d]	5%, 10%	W[k,l]	636, 1250	6.8±0.4	2 h[o]	24 h[n]	n/a	n/a	n/a	n/a	4
	BA[s]	5%, 10%	W[k,l]	636, 1250	6.8±0.4	2 h[o]	24 h[n]	n/a	n/a	n/a	n/a	19
	CSL[a]	6%	W, D5W, NS[k,l]	384, 636, 690	6.6±0.2	n/a	24 h[n]	n/a	n/a	n/a	n/a	2
	CSL[a]	9%	W, D5W, NS[k,l]	576, 828, 862	6.6±0.2	n/a	24 h[n]	n/a	n/a	n/a	n/a	2
	TAL[f]	10%	RTU[m]	258	4–4.5	8 h[n]	8 h[n]	n/a	n/a	n/a	n/a	5
	KED[t]	10%	RTU, D5W[m]	258	4–4.5	8 h[n]	8 h[n]	n/a	n/a	n/a	n/a	20
	CSL[a]	12%	W, D5W, NS[k,l]	768, 1020, 1074	6.6±0.2	n/a	24 h[n]	n/a	n/a	n/a	n/a	2
PVC	BA[c]	5%, 10%	D5W, RTU[m]	240–300	4.6–5.1	n/a	24 h[n]	n/a	n/a	n/a	n/a	3
	BA[d]	5%, 10%	W[k,l]	636, 1250	6.8±0.4	2 h[o]	24 h[n]	n/a	n/a	n/a	n/a	4
	BA[s]	5%, 10%	W[k,l]	636, 1250	6.8±0.4	2 h[o]	24 h[n]	n/a	n/a	n/a	n/a	19
	GRI[b]	5%, 10%	RTU[p]	204–350	5–6	3–4 h	48 h[n]	n/a	n/a	n/a	n/a	13, 16, 18
OTHER INFUSION CONTAINERS												
Gribag-PVC (Grifols)	GRI	5%	RTU[p]	204–350	5–6	10 d[n]	10 d[n]	n/a	n/a	n/a	n/a	17
INTRAVIA Flexible Container (Baxter)	BA[d]	5%, 10%	W[k,l]	636, 1250[4]	6.8±0.4	3 d[n]	14 d[n]	n/a	n/a	n/a	n/a	12
	BA[c]	10%	RTU[m]	240–300[3]	4.6–5.1	n/a	14 d[n]	n/a	n/a	n/a	n/a	10

continued on next page

Immune Globulin (Human) (cont'd)

Drug Manufacturer	Concentration	Diluents	Osmolality (mOsm/kg)	pH	Storage Conditions						Refer.
					Temperature			Post-thaw Temp		Body Temp	
					Room	Refrig	Frozen	Room	Refrig		
Plastic Infusion Container (Unspec.)											
CSL[a]	3%	W, D5W, NS[k,l]	192, 444, 498	6.6±0.2	n/a	24 h[n]	n/a	n/a	n/a	n/a	2
CSL[a]	6%	W, D5W, NS[k,l]	384, 636, 690	6.6±0.2	n/a	24 h[n]	n/a	n/a	n/a	n/a	2
CSL[a]	9%	W, D5W, NS[k,l]	576, 828, 862	6.6±0.2	n/a	24 h[n]	n/a	n/a	n/a	n/a	2
CSL[a]	12%	W, D5W, NS[k,l]	768, 1020, 1074	6.6±0.2	n/a	24 h[n]	n/a	n/a	n/a	n/a	2
Sterile Infusion Bags (Unspec.)											
BPL[h]	5%	RTU	460–500	4.6–5.1	2 h[n]	2 h[n]	n/a	n/a	n/a	n/a	9
TAL[f]	10%	RTU, D5W[m]	258	4–4.5	8 h[n]	8 h[n]	n/a	n/a	n/a	n/a	5
KED[t]	10%	RTU, D5W[m]	258	4–4.5	8 h[n]	8 h[n]	n/a	n/a	n/a	n/a	20
Unspecified Container											
GRI[b]	5%, 10%	RTU[p]	204–350	5–6	3–4 h[o]	n/a	n/a	n/a	n/a	n/a	13, 16, 18
CSL[e]	10%	RTU[i]	240–440	4.6–5	q	n/a	n/a	n/a	n/a	n/a	14
CSL[j,r]	16%	RTU	n/a	6.4–7.2	q	n/a	n/a	n/a	n/a	n/a	15
CSL[u]	20%	RTU	380	4.6–5.2	n/a	n/a	n/a	n/a	n/a	n/a	21

Flush Compatibility: D5W, normal saline unless noted as incompatible with sodium chloride diluents.[1]

Special Considerations: Unless stated otherwise, Immune globulin (Ig) product manufacturers recommend immediate use (e.g., less than 3 h) when opened or prepared outside an ISO Class 5 environment and/or stored at room temperature. These labeled statements are primarily based on sterility concerns and the potential for Ig solutions to support microbial growth. Some organizations conduct extended sterility studies to support extended dating of IgIV solutions prepared in an ISO Class 5 environment. One published study demonstrated no bacterial or yeast growth over a 7-d period at 3 °C.[8] The optimal pH for IgIV in solution is 4.0–4.5; preparations with higher (e.g., physiologic) pH contain stabilizing agents.[11] Due to the difference in stabilizers and Ig production methods, clinicians should use the data that is specific to the brand of Ig product. Do not freeze Ig products or preparations. Ig solutions should be at room temperature prior to administration.

Notes

[a]Carimune NF®.
[b]Flebogamma® DIF.
[c]Gammagard Liquid®.
[d]Gammagard SD®.

continued on next page

Immune Globulin (Human) (cont'd)

ePrivigen®.
fGamunex C®.
gOctagam®.
hGammaplex®.
iMay dilute with D5W if necessary.
jVivaglobin® Immune Globulin Subcutaneous (Human). For subcutaneous infusion only. Not for intravenous use.
kManufacturer of lyophilized Ig product provides diluent (W) for initial reconstitution and/or infusion. Diluent should be at room temperature prior to reconstitution.
lTo avoid excessive foaming, swirl—do not shake—to dissolve.
mIncompatible with sodium chloride (saline) diluents.
nPrepared in ISO Class 5 (hood) environment.
oPrepared outside of a laminar flow hood.
pDilution with IV fluids is not recommended.
qManufacturer recommends use as soon as vial is entered.
rNo longer sold in the U.S.
sGammagard S/D® Low IgA.
tGammaked.®
uHizentra.®

References

1. Trissel LA. ASHP's Interactive Handbook on Injectable Drugs. Bethesda, MD. American Society of Health-System Pharmacists. Accessed 2012 Jul.
2. Carimune NF® (Immune Globulin Intravenous Human) [prescribing information]. Kankakee, IL: ZLB Behring; October 2010.
3. Gammagard Liquid® (Immune Globulin Intravenous Human) 10% [prescribing information]. Westlake Village, CA: Baxter Healthcare; July 2011.
4. Gammagard S/D® (Immune Globulin Intravenous Human) [prescribing information]. Westlake Village, CA: Baxter Healthcare; December 2009.
5. Gamunex® (Immune Globulin Intravenous Human) [prescribing information]. Research Triangle Park, NC: Talecris Biotherapeutics; October 2010.
6. Octagam® (Immune Globulint Intravenous Human) [prescribing information]. Centreville, VA: Octapharma USA Inc; September 2009.
7. Buchacher A. Short-term stability of Octagam in EVA-bags. Unpublished information. Medical Affairs, Centreville, VA: Octapharma; November 2004.
8. Pfeifer RW, Siegel J, Ayers LW. Assessment of microbial growth in intravenous immune globulin preparations. Am J Hosp Pharm. 1994; 51;1676–9.
9. Gammaplex (Immune Globulin Intravenous Human) 5% [prescribing information]. Hertfordshire, UK: Bio Products Laboratory; September 2009.
10. Gammagard Liquid [written correspondence]. Medical Affairs, Westlake Village, CA: Baxter Bioscience; April 21, 2008.
11. Shah S. Pharmacy considerations for the use of IGIV therapy. Am J Health-Syst Pharm. 2005; 62(suppl 3):S5–11.
12. Gammagard SD [written correspondence]. Medical Affairs, Westlake Village, CA: Baxter Bioscience; April 21, 2008.
13. Flebogamma DIF® (Immune Globulin Intravenous Human) 5% [prescribing information]. Los Angeles, CA: Grifols Biologicals, Inc.; January 2010.
14. Privigen ™ Immune Globulin Intravenous (Human) [product information]. Kankakee, IL: CSL Behring; February 2011.
15. Vivaglobulin® Immune Globulin Subcutaneous (Human) [US package insert]. Kankakee, IL: CSL Behring; April 2010.
16. Pearson S. Flebogamma® Stability Information [written correspondence]. Medical Information, Los Angeles, CA: Grifols Biologicals Inc; April 21, 2008.
17. Lopez M, Costa M, Jorquerea HI. Compatibility study of two intravenous immunoglobulin preparations with plastic containers. Poster presented at: FOCIS 5th Annual Meeting; May 2005; Boston, MA.
18. Flebogamma DIF® (Immune Globulin Intravenous Human) 10% [prescribing information]. Los Angeles, CA: Grifols Biologicals, Inc.; July 2010.
19. Gammagard S/D® Low IgA (Immune Globulin Intravenous Human) [prescribing information]. Westlake Village, CA: Baxter Healthcare; December 2011.
20. Gammaked® (Immune Globulin Intravenous Human) 10% [prescribing information]. Cambridge, MA: Kedrion Biopharmaceutics; October 2010.
21. Hizentra® (Immune Globulin Subcutaneous Human) 20% [prescribing information]. Kankakee, IL: CSL Behring; October 2011.

Infliximab

Drug Manufacturer	Concentration	Diluents	Osmolality (mOsm/kg)	pH[b]	Storage Conditions						Refer.
					Temperature			Post-thaw Temp		Body Temp	
					Room	Refrig	Frozen	Room	Refrig		
CONTAINER											
Ethyvinyl Acetate (EVA) CEN	0.4, 4 mg/mL	NS	n/a	b	24 h[a]	24 h[a]	n/a	n/a	n/a	n/a	1
Polyvinyl Chloride (PVC) CEN	0.4 mg/mL	NS	n/a	b	n/a	14 d[c]	n/a	n/a	n/a	n/a	4
CEN	0.4, 4 mg/mL	NS	n/a	b	24 h[a]	24 h[a]	n/a	n/a	n/a	n/a	1
OTHER INFUSION CONTAINERS											
Polyolefin CEN	0.4, 4 mg/mL	NS	n/a	b	24 h[a]	24 h[a]	n/a	n/a	n/a	n/a	2

Flush Compatibility: Normal saline[1]
Special Considerations: Do not freeze.

Notes

[a]Product remains physically and biochemically stable for 24 h. Manufacturer recommends use within 3 h to ensure against microbiological contamination.
[b]pH of reconstituted solution 10 mg/mL in W is 7.2.[3]
[c]No loss of biological activity as measured by an indirect ELISA method.

References

1. Lozier K [personal communication]. Malvern, PA: Centocor; October 2001.
2. Sturm E [personal communication]. Malvern, PA: Centocor; August 2002.
3. Remicade® [product information]. Malvern, PA: Centocor Inc; October 2011.
4. Ikeda R, Vermeulen LC, Lau E, et al. Stability of infliximab in polyvinyl chloride bags. Am J Health-Syst Pharm. 2012; 69:1509–12.

Interferon alfa-2b

Interferon alfa-2b[g]

CONTAINER	Drug Manufacturer	Concentration	Diluents	Osmolality (mOsm/kg)	pH[f]	Temperature Room	Temperature Refrig	Temperature Frozen	Post-thaw Temp Room	Post-thaw Temp Refrig	Body Temp	Refer.
Glass Vial	SC	3 to 50 million I.U./mL	W	n/a	6.9–7.5	2 d[d]	30 d	n/a	n/a	n/a	n/a	1
Syringes, Plastic	SC	10 million I.U./mL	W	iso	f	n/a	n/a	56 d[a]	n/a	n/a	n/a	1
	SC	10 million I.U./mL	W	iso	f	n/a	n/a	4 w[b]	n/a	n/a	n/a	1
	SC	10 million I.U./mL	W	iso	f	n/a	n/a	1 y[e]	n/a	n/a	n/a	1
Syringes, Polypropylene	SC	2 million I.U./mL	W	n/a	f	n/a	21 d[c]	n/a	n/a	n/a	n/a	1
	SC	2 million I.U./mL	W	n/a	f	n/a	42 d	n/a	n/a	n/a	n/a	1
	SC	6 million I.U./mL	W	n/a	f	n/a	42 d[c]	n/a	n/a	n/a	n/a	1

Flush Compatibility: Normal saline. Incompatible with dextrose-containing solutions.[1]

Special Considerations: Dilution to 500,000 I.U./mL and packaging in polypropylene syringes is considered unsuitable for interferon alfa-2b.[1]

Notes

[a]Frozen at −20°C.
[b]Frozen at −10°C.
[c]Contains albumin 1 mg/mL.
[d]Reconstituted solutions are stable up to 14 d at 30°C and up to 7 d at 35°C. Two-day stability is based on up to 40°C.
[e]Frozen at −80°C.
[f]pH of reconstituted preparation is 6.9–7.5.[1]
[g]Product is labeled in International Units (I.U.).

Reference

1. Trissel LA. ASHP's Interactive Handbook on Injectable Drugs. Bethesda, MD: American Society of Health-System Pharmacists. Accessed 2012 Jan.

Irinotecan Hydrochloride

CONTAINER	Drug Manufacturer	Concentration	Diluents	Osmolality (mOsm/kg)	pH[c]	Storage Conditions					Body Temp	Refer.
						Temperature			Post-thaw Temp			
						Room	Refrig	Frozen	Room	Refrig		
Polyvinyl Chloride (PVC)	RPR	0.4, 1 mg/mL	NS	n/a	c	7 d	n/a	n/a	n/a	n/a	n/a	1, 2
	RPR	0.4, 1, 2.8 mg/mL	NS, D5W	n/a	c	28 d[a]	28 d[a,b]	n/a	n/a	n/a	n/a	1, 2
	RPR	2 mg/mL	D5W, NS	n/a	c	2 h	4 d[b]	n/a	n/a	n/a	n/a	2
	RPR	2.8 mg/mL	NS	n/a	c	14 d	n/a	n/a	n/a	n/a	n/a	1, 2

Flush Compatibility: Normal saline.[1]
Special Considerations: n/a

Notes

[a]Protected from light.
[b]Refrigerated storage of irinotecan hydrochloride in normal saline is not recommended because of occasional visible precipitation.[2]
[c]pH of undiluted solution is 3–3.8.[2]

References

1. Thiesen J, Kramer I. Physicochemical stability of irinotecan injection concentrate and diluted infusion solutions in PVC bags. *J Oncol Pharm Prac.* 2000; 6:115–21.
2. Trissel LA. ASHP's Interactive Handbook on Injectable Drugs. Bethesda, MD: American Society of Health-System Pharmacists. Accessed 2012 May.

Ketamine Hydrochloride

continued on next page

Container	Drug Manufacturer	Concentration	Diluents	Osmolality (mOsm/kg)	pH	Temperature Room	Temperature Refrig	Temperature Frozen	Post-thaw Temp Room	Post-thaw Temp Refrig	Body Temp	Refer.
CONTAINER												
Polyvinyl Chloride (PVC)	SZ	0.2, 0.6, 1 mg/mL[h]	NS[h]	n/a	[g]	7 d[h]	n/a	n/a	n/a	n/a	n/a	4
	JN	1 mg/mL[i]	NS[i]	n/a	[g]	30 d	30 d	n/a	n/a	n/a	n/a	1
	PD	1 mg/mL[b]	NS[b]	n/a	[g]	6 d	n/a	n/a	n/a	n/a	n/a	1
	PD	1.33 mg/mL[a]	NS[a]	n/a	5.5–7.5	4 d	n/a	n/a	n/a	n/a	n/a	1, 3
	PD	25 mg/mL[c]	NS[c]	n/a	[g]	6 d	n/a	n/a	n/a	n/a	n/a	1
Syringes, Plastic	SZ	0.2, 0.6, 1 mg/mL[h]	NS[h]	n/a	[g]	7 d[h]	n/a	n/a	n/a	n/a	n/a	4
	PD	1 mg/mL[d]	NS[d]	n/a	[g]	6 d	n/a	n/a	n/a	n/a	n/a	1
	PD	10, 25 mg/mL[e]	NS[e]	n/a	[g]	6 d	n/a	n/a	n/a	n/a	n/a	1
Syringes, Polypropylene	unspec.	1 mg/mL	NS	[f]	[g]	12 m	12 m	n/a	n/a	n/a	12 m[i]	1
	AB	10 mg/mL	W	[f]	4.2	30 d	n/a	n/a	n/a	n/a	n/a	1, 2
OTHER INFUSION CONTAINERS												
Medication Cassette (Sims Deltec)	PD	25 mg/mL[c]	NS[c]	n/a	[g]	6 d	n/a	n/a	n/a	n/a	n/a	1

Flush Compatibility: Normal saline.
Special Considerations: Do not administer the 100 mg/mL undiluted.[1] Also compatible with D5W[1], but stability data is unavailable.

Notes

[a] Also contains morphine sulfate (AB) 2 mg/mL.
[b] Also contains morphine sulfate 1 mg/mL.
[c] Also contains morphine sulfate 25 mg/mL.
[d] Also contains morphine sulfate 1 or 10 mg/mL.
[e] Also contains morphine sulfate 1, 10, or 25 mg/mL.
[f] Undiluted 10 mg/mL solution is 300 mOsm/kg and undiluted 50 mg/mL solution is 387 mOsm/kg.[1]
[g] pH of undiluted solution is 3.5–5.5.[1]
[h] With hydromorphone (SZ) 0.2 mg/mL.
[i] With fentanyl (DB) 10 mcg/mL and droperidol (JN) 50 mg/mL.
[j] At 40°C.

221

Ketamine Hydrochloride (cont'd)

Ketamine Hydrochloride (cont'd)

References

1. Trissel LA. ASHP's Interactive Handbook on Injectable Drugs. Bethesda, MD: American Society of Health-System Pharmacists. Accessed 2012 Aug.
2. Gupta VD. Stability of ketamine hydrochloride injection after reconstitution in water for injection and storage in 1-mL tuberculin polypropylene syringes for pediatric use. *Int J Pharmaceutic Compound.* 2002; 6:316–7.
3. Schmid R, Koren G, Klein J, et al. The stability of a ketamine-morphine solution. *Anesth Analg.* 2002; 94:898–900.
4. Ensom MHH, Decarie D, Leung K, et al. Stability of hydromorphone-ketamine solutions in glass bottles, plastic syringes, and IV bags for pediatric use. *Can J Hosp Pharm.* 2009; 62(2):112–8.

Ketorolac Tromethamine

Ketorolac Tromethamine

Drug Manufacturer	Concentration	Diluents	Osmolality (mOsm/kg)	pH[a]	Temperature Room	Refrig	Frozen	Post-thaw Temp Room	Refrig	Body Temp	Refer.
CONTAINER											
Polyolefin RC	0.1, 0.3 mg/mL	D5W	i	a	n/a	n/a	15 d[b]	n/a	35 d[b]	n/a	4
RC	0.2 mg/mL	D5W	i	a	n/a	n/a	3 m	n/a	60 d[c]	n/a	3
Polyvinyl Chloride (PVC) RC	0.3 mg/mL	NS	i	6.1–6.7	35 d	50 d	n/a	n/a	n/a	n/a	2
RC	0.3 mg/mL	D5W	i	6.2–6.6	7 d	50 d	n/a	n/a	n/a	n/a	2
RC	0.3, 0.6 mg/mL	NS, D5W	i	5.66–6.84	21 d	21 d	n/a	n/a	n/a	n/a	1
RC	0.6 mg/mL	D5W	i	a	7 d	50 d	n/a	n/a	n/a	n/a	4
OTHER INFUSION CONTAINERS											
INFUSOR (Baxter) REC	0.5–1.5 mg/mL[e]	NS, D5W	i	a	17 d[h]	n/a	n/a	n/a	n/a	7 d[h]	5
REC	0.5–8 mg/mL	NS, D5W	i	a	n/a	28 d[f]	n/a	n/a	n/a	7 d[f]	5
REC	1.5–8 mg/mL[d]	NS, D5W	i	a	28 d[g]	n/a	n/a	n/a	n/a	7 d[g]	5
REC	1.5–8 mg/mL[e]	NS, D5W	i	a	28 d[g]	n/a	n/a	n/a	n/a	7 d[g]	5

Flush Compatibility: Saline flush.
Special Considerations: Solutions should be protected from light.

Notes
[a] pH of solutions is 6.9–7.9.[4]
[b] Refrigerated 35 d after 15 d frozen at −20°C.
[c] Thawed in a cycle-validated microwave oven.
[d] With morphine HCl 0.1–1.6 mg/mL.
[e] With tramadol HCl 1.6–35 mg/mL.
[f] Stored 28 d at 2–8°C, followed by 7 d at 33°C.
[g] Stored 28 d at 25°C, followed by 7 d at 33°C.
[h] Stored 17 d at 25°C, followed by 7 d at 33°C.
[i] Undiluted solutions (15 mg/mL and 30 mg/mL) are isotonic.[4]

continued on next page

Ketorolac Tromethamine (cont'd)

References

238

1. Shi A, Walker SE, Law S. Stability of ketorolac tromethamine in IV solutions and waste reduction. *Can J Hosp Pharm*. 2000; 53:263–9.
2. Das Gupta V, Maswoswe J. Stability of ketorolac tromethamine in 5% dextrose injection and 0.9% sodium chloride injection. *Int J Pharm Compound*. 1997; 1:206–7.
3. Hecq J, Boitquin LP, Vanbeckbergen DF, et al. Effect of freezing, long-term storage, and microwave thawing on the stability of ketorolac tromethamine. *Ann Pharmacother*. 2005; 39:1654–8.
4. Trissel LA. ASHP's Interactive Handbook on Injectable Drugs. Bethesda, MD: American Society of Health-System Pharmacists. Accessed 2012 May.
5. *Intermate/Infusor Drug Stability Information*. Deerfield, IL: Baxter Healthcare Corporation; October 2008.

Leucovorin Calcium[e]

	Drug Manufacturer	Concentration	Diluents	Osmolality (mOsm/kg)	pH[d]	Temperature			Post-thaw Temp			Refer.
						Room	Refrig	Frozen	Room	Refrig	Body Temp	
CONTAINER												
Polyolefin	WY	1.6 mg/mL	D5W	n/a	d	n/a	n/a	95 d	n/a	30 d	n/a	4
Polyvinyl Chloride (PVC)	LE	0.1, 0.5, 1, 1.5 mg/mL	D5W	n/a	d	4 d[a]	4 d[a]	n/a	n/a	n/a	n/a	3
	LE	1, 1.5 mg/mL	NS	n/a	d	4 d[a]	4 d[a]	n/a	n/a	n/a	n/a	3
OTHER INFUSION CONTAINERS												
AccuFlo™/ AccuFlux™/ AccuRx® (B. Braun)	unspec.	4 mg/mL	NS	n/a	d	7 d	7 d	n/a	n/a	n/a	n/a	1
Glass Bottles	LE	0.1, 0.5, 1, 1.5 mg/mL	D5W, NS	n/a	d	4 d[a]	4 d[a]	n/a	n/a	n/a	n/a	3
	LE	1 mg/mL	NS	n/a	d	7 d[a]	7 d[a]	n/a	n/a	n/a	n/a	3
Homepump®/ Homepump® Eclipse (I-Flow Corp.)	unspec.	4 mg/mL	NS	n/a	d	7 d	7 d	n/a	n/a	n/a	n/a	5
INFUSOR (Baxter)	WY	0.2–2 mg/mL	NS, W, D5W	n/a	d	n/a	2 d	n/a	n/a	n/a	24 h[b]	2
	WY	2 mg/mL	NS, W, D5W	n/a	d	n/a	2 d	n/a	n/a	n/a	7 d[c]	2
	WY	2–20 mg/mL	W	n/a	d	n/a	2 d	n/a	n/a	n/a	7 d[c]	2
Polyolefin Bag (McGaw)	LE	1 mg/mL	NS	n/a	d	7 d[a]	7 d[a]	n/a	n/a	n/a	n/a	3

Storage Conditions

Flush Compatibility: Heparin lock flush.[3]
Special Considerations: n/a

Notes

[a]Protected from light.
[b]2 d refrigerated, followed by 24 h at 33°C.
[c]2 d refrigerated, followed by 7 d at 33°C.

continued on next page

225

Leucovorin Calcium (cont'd)

[d]pH of undiluted solution (10 mg/mL) and reconstituted preparation is 6.5–8.5.[3]
[e]Also known as folinic acid.[1,5]

References

1. Drug Stability Data Using Elastomeric Infusion Systems. B. Braun Medical Production Ltd. (Thailand); August 2011.
2. Intermate/Infusor Drug Stability Information. Deerfield, IL: Baxter Healthcare Corporation; October 2008.
3. Trissel LA. ASHP's Interactive Handbook on Injectable Drugs. Bethesda, MD: American Society of Health-System Pharmacists. Accessed 2012 Aug.
4. Lebitasy M, Hecq JD, Athanassopoulos A, et al. Effect of freeze-thawing on the long-term stability of calcium levofolinate in 5% dextrose stored on polyolefin infusion bags. J Clin Pharm Ther. 2009; 34:423–8.
5. Stability Data for Drugs Using Homepump Disposable Elastomeric Infusion Systems. Lake Forest, CA: I-Flow Corporations; October 2009.

Levofloxacin

Container	Drug Manufacturer	Concentration	Diluents	Osmolality (mOsm/kg)	pH[d]	Storage Conditions						Refer.
						Temperature			Post-thaw Temp		Body Temp	
						Room	Refrig	Frozen	Room	Refrig		
CONTAINER												
Polyvinyl Chloride (PVC)	OMJ	0.5, 5 mg/mL	D5W, NS, D5S	n/a	d	72 h[a]	14 d[a]	26 w[a]	n/a	n/a	n/a	1
OTHER INFUSION CONTAINERS												
AccuFlo™/ AccuFlux™/ AccuRX® (B. Braun)	unspec.	5 mg/mL	D5W, NS	n/a	d	72 h[b]	14 d[b]	6 m	n/a	n/a	n/a	3
Homepump Eclipse®/ Homepump® C-Series (I-Flow Corp.)	unspec.	5 mg/mL	D5W, NS	n/a	4.6–4.7	72 h[b]	14 d[b]	6 m	n/a	n/a	n/a	2
COMMERCIAL PREPARATIONS (RTU)												
PVC Bag (Hospira)	OMN	5 mg/mL	D5W	iso	d	c	n/a	n/a	n/a	n/a	n/a	1

Flush Compatibility: Normal saline.[1] Levofloxacin is incompatible with heparin.[1]

Special Considerations: Protect product from light. For RTU solutions, remove protective foil overwrap prior to administration; store protected from light and freezing; avoid excessive heat.[3] Infuse solution diluted to ≤5 mg/mL over at least 60 min (90 min for doses of 750 mg).[1]

Notes

[a]Protected from light.
[b]Manufacturer(s) extrapolated data from other sources.
[c]Expiration date per manufacturer's label. Do not extrapolate commercial premix stability data to extemporaneously prepared solutions.
[d]pH range of diluted solutions is 3.8–5.8, based on the buffering capacity of the diluent.[1]

References

1. Trissel LA. ASHP's Interactive Handbook on Injectable Drugs. Bethesda, MD: American Society of Health-System Pharmacists. Accessed 2012 Jan.
2. Stability Data for Drugs Using Homepump Disposable Elastomeric Infusion Systems. Lake Forest, CA: I-Flow Corporation; October 2009.
3. Drug Stability Data Using Elastomeric Infusion Systems. B. Braun Medical Production Ltd. (Thailand); August 2011.

Linezolid

Linezolid

COMMERCIAL PREPARATIONS (RTU)

Drug Manufacturer	Concentration	Diluents	Osmolality (mOsm/kg)	pH	Storage Conditions Temperature Room	Storage Conditions Temperature Refrig	Storage Conditions Temperature Frozen	Post-thaw Temp Room	Post-thaw Temp Refrig	Body Temp	Refer.
Latex-Free Plastic Bag PF	2 mg/mL	RTU[a]	iso	4.8[3]	[b,c]	12 m[b,e]	n/a	n/a	n/a	6 m[b,d]	1, 2

Flush Compatibility: Heparin lock flush and normal saline.[3]

Special Considerations: Administer IV over 30 to 120 minutes. Yellow color may intensify over time without affecting stability.[1,3]

Notes

[a]RTU sterile isotonic solution. Inactive ingredients include sodium citrate, citric acid, and dextrose. Do not use the RTU bag in series connections.

[b]Expiration date per manufacturer's label; use within 30 d of foil overwrap removal.

[c]Protected from light.

[d]Stability studies conducted by Pharmacia Upjohn at 40°C.

[e]Stability studies conducted by Pharmacia Upjohn at 2–8°C. Do not freeze.

References

1. Zyvox® [product information]. New York, NY: Pfizer Pharmacia Upjohn; March 2012.
2. Steven Johnson, Pharm. D. [personal communication]. Kalamazoo, MI: Pharmacia & Upjohn; October 2000.
3. Trissel LA. ASHP's Interactive Handbook on Injectable Drugs. Bethesda, MD: American Society of Health-System Pharmacists. Accessed 2012 Jan.

Lorazepam

Container	Drug Manufacturer	Concentration	Diluents	Osmolality (mOsm/kg)	pH	Temperature Room	Temperature Refrig	Temperature Frozen	Post-thaw Temp Room	Post-thaw Temp Refrig	Body Temp	Refer.
CONTAINER												
Polyolefin Bag	WY	0.1 mg/mL	D5W, NS	n/a	n/a	7 d	7 d	n/a	n/a	n/a	72 h	1
	WAY	0.1 mg/mL	D5W	n/a	n/a	n/a	n/a	7 d[d]	n/a	n/a	n/a	1
	AB	1 mg/mL	NS	n/a	n/a	35 d[eg]	35 d[eg]	35 d[eg]	n/a	n/a	5 d[eg]	3
Polyvinyl Chloride (PVC)	WY	0.1 mg/mL[a]	n/a	n/a	n/a	n/a	n/a	n/a	n/a	n/a	n/a	1
Syringes, Polypropylene	WAY	0.2, 0.5, 1 mg/mL[e,h]	D5W, NS	n/a	n/a	48 h[e,h,i]	n/a	n/a	n/a	n/a	n/a	1
	WY	1 mg/mL[e]	D5W, NS	n/a	n/a	28 h[e]	n/a	n/a	n/a	n/a	n/a	1
	WY	2 mg/mL[b]	undiluted	n/a	n/a	n/a	n/a	n/a	n/a	n/a	n/a	1
OTHER INFUSION CONTAINERS												
Glass	WY	1 mg/mL	BWFI	n/a	n/a	n/a	7 d	n/a	n/a	n/a	n/a	1
	WY	1 mg/mL	D5W	n/a	n/a	28 h[e]	n/a	n/a	n/a	n/a	n/a	1
	WY	2 mg/mL	D5W	n/a	n/a	28 h[f]	n/a	n/a	n/a	n/a	n/a	1
Glass Test Tubes	WY	2 mg/mL[c]	n/a	n/a	n/a	3 d	6 d	n/a	n/a	n/a	24 h	1, 2

Flush Compatibility: Heparin lock flush and normal saline.[1]

Special Considerations: Care should be taken to ensure the same initial concentration of lorazepam is used for preparation of compounded products to ensure appropriate stability.

Notes

[a]Significant losses were noted when lorazepam 0.1 mg/mL was stored in PVC containers.

[b]Significant losses were noted when lorazepam 2 mg/mL was stored in polypropylene syringes.

[c]1 mL lorazepam 4 mg/mL was mixed with 1 mL hydromorphone 2 mg/mL, 10 mg/mL, and 40 mg/mL (KN).

[d]Manufacturer does not recommend freezing.

[e]Prepared from 2 mg/mL commercial preparation.

[f]Prepared from 4 mg/mL commercial preparation.

[g]Protected from light.

[h]When prepared from 4 mg/mL commercial preparation, consistently precipitated.

[i]Physically stable over 24 h and chemically stable for 48 h at room temperature.

continued on next page

229

Lorazepam (cont'd)

References

1. Trissel LA. ASHP's Interactive Handbook on Injectable Drugs. Bethesda, MD: American Society of Health-System Pharmacists. Accessed 2012 Aug.

2. Walker SC, Iazzetta J, De Angelis C, et al. Stability and compatibility of combinations of hydromorphone and dimenhydrinate, lorazepam, or prochlorperazine. *Can J Hosp Pharm.* 1993; 46(2):61–5.

3. Norenberg JP, Ahusim LE, Steel TH, et al. Stability of lorazepam in 0.9% sodium chloride stored in polyolefin bags. *Am J Health-Syst Pharm.* 2004; 61:1039–41.

Meperidine Hydrochloride

Meperidine Hydrochloride[g]

Container	Drug Manufacturer	Concentration	Diluents	Osmolality (mOsm/kg)	pH[e]	Temperature Room	Temperature Refrig	Temperature Frozen	Post-thaw Temp Room	Post-thaw Temp Refrig	Body Temp	Refer.
CONTAINER												
Polyvinyl Chloride (PVC)	DB	0.071 mg/mL	NS	n/a	e	7 d	n/a	n/a	n/a	n/a	n/a	1
	WI	1.2 mg/mL	D5W	n/a	e	36 h	n/a	n/a	n/a	n/a	n/a	1
	unspec.	2.5 mg/mL	NS	n/a	e	24 d	n/a	n/a	n/a	n/a	n/a	1
Syringes, Glass	WI	25 mg/mL[b]	b	n/a	e	1 y[c]	1 y[c]	n/a	n/a	n/a	n/a	1
Syringes, Plastic	WY	5, 10 mg/mL	D5W, NS	n/a	e	12 w	12 w[c]	12 w[c]	n/a	n/a	n/a	1, 3
	WI	25 mg/mL[b]	b	n/a	e	1 y[c]	1 y[c]	n/a	n/a	n/a	n/a	1
Syringes, Polypropylene (BD)	AB[d]	0.25, 1, 10, 20, 30 mg/mL	D5W, NS	n/a	e	28 d[c]	28 d[c]	n/a	n/a	n/a	n/a	1
OTHER INFUSION CONTAINERS												
CADD® Cassette (SIMS Deltec)	REN	5, 20 mg/mL	NS	n/a	n/a	21 d[c]	n/a	n/a	n/a	n/a	n/a	5
	unspec.	15 mg/mL	W	n/a	e	9 d	14 d	n/a	n/a	n/a	n/a	4
Infusaid Implantable Pump	WI	10 mg/mL	NS	n/a	e	n/a	n/a	n/a	n/a	n/a	90 d[f]	1
INFUSOR (Baxter)	WI	10–100 mg/mL	D5W, NS	n/a	e	7 d	14 d[a]	n/a	n/a	n/a	n/a	2

Flush Compatibility: Heparin lock flush and normal saline. Flush heparinized scalp veins with W or NS to prevent precipitation when meperidine is infused.[1]

Special Considerations: Undiluted 50-mg/mL solution is 302 mOsm/kg.[1]

Notes

[a]Stable for 4 d at room temperature following 14 d refrigerated.
[b]Solution also contained chlorpromazine HCl 6.25 mg/mL and hydroxyzine HCl 12.5 mg/mL.
[c]Protected from light.
[d]Preservative free (AB) product.
[e]pH of undiluted solution is 3.5–6.[1]

continued on next page

Meperidine Hydrochloride (cont'd)

fStored at 37°C.[1]

gMeperidine is known internationally as pethidine.[5]

References

1. Trissel LA. ASHP's Interactive Handbook on Injectable Drugs. Bethesda, MD: American Society of Health-System Pharmacists. Accessed 2012 Aug.

2. *Intermate/Infusor Drug Stability Information.* Deerfield, IL: Baxter Healthcare Corporation; October 2008.

3. Strong ML, Schaaf LJ, Pankaskie MS, et al. Shelf lives and factors affecting the stability of morphine sulphate and meperidine (pethidine) hydrochloride in plastic syringes for use in patient controlled analgesic devices. *J Clin Pharm Ther.* 1994; 19:361–6.

4. *CADD Ambulatory Infusion Pump System Stability Data.* St. Paul, MN: SIMS Deltec Inc; 1995.

5. Laville I, Mercier L, Chachaty E, et al. Shelf lives of morphine sulphate and pethidine solutions stored in patient-controlled analgesia devices: physicochemical and microbiological stability study. *Pathologie Biologie.* 2005; 53:210–6.

Meropenem

Meropenem

Container	Drug Manufacturer	Concentration	Diluents	Osmolality (mOsm/kg)	pH[h]	Room	Refrig	Frozen	Room	Refrig	Body Temp	Refer.
CONTAINER												
Polyvinyl Chloride (PVC)	ASZ	1 mg/mL	NS	n/a	h	22 h	10 d[f]	33 d	n/a	n/a	n/a	3, 9
	ASZ	1 mg/mL	D5W	n/a	h	4 h[d]	1 d	1 d	n/a	n/a	n/a	3, 9
	ASZ	1–20 mg/mL	D5W	n/a	h	1 h	4 h	n/a	n/a	n/a	n/a	1
	ASZ	1–20 mg/mL	NS	n/a	h	4 h	24 h	n/a	n/a	n/a	n/a	1
	ZEN	4 mg/mL	NS	n/a	h	n/a	7 d	n/a	n/a	n/a	n/a	7, 9
	ZEN	10, 20 mg/mL	NS	n/a	h	n/a	5 d	n/a	n/a	n/a	n/a	7, 9
	ZEN	22 mg/mL[e]	NS	n/a	h	17 h	4 d	11 d	n/a	n/a	n/a	3, 9
	ZEN	22 mg/mL[e]	D5W	n/a	h	8 h[d]	2 d	7 d	n/a	n/a	n/a	3, 9
Syringes, Plastic	ASZ	1–20 mg/mL	W, NS	n/a	h	4 h[a]	48 h[a]	n/a	n/a	n/a	n/a	1, 6
	ASZ	1–20 mg/mL	D5W	n/a	h	2 h[a]	6 h[a]	n/a	n/a	n/a	n/a	1
OTHER INFUSION CONTAINERS												
AccuFlo™/ AccuFlux™/ AccuRX® (B. Braun)	unspec.	5 mg/mL	NS	n/a	h	26 h[i]	4 d[i]	n/a	n/a	n/a	n/a	2
	unspec.	5–10 mg/mL	NS	n/a	h	n/a	4 d[i]	n/a	n/a	n/a	n/a	2
	unspec.	10 mg/mL	NS	n/a	h	20 h[i]	4 d[i]	n/a	n/a	n/a	n/a	2
	unspec.	20 mg/mL	NS	n/a	h	14 h[i]	3 d[i]	n/a	n/a	n/a	n/a	2
Glass	ASZ	2.5–50 mg/mL	NS	n/a	h	2 h	18 h	n/a	n/a	n/a	n/a	1, 9
	ASZ	2.5–50 mg/mL	D5W	n/a	h	1 h	8 h	n/a	n/a	n/a	n/a	1, 9
	ASZ	≤50 mg/mL	W	n/a	h	2 h	12 h	n/a	n/a	n/a	n/a	1
Homepump®/ Homepump Eclipse® (I-Flow Corp.)	ZEN	4 mg/mL	NS	n/a	h	n/a	7 d	n/a	n/a	n/a	n/a	7, 9
	unspec.	5 mg/mL	NS	n/a	h	26 h	4 d	n/a	n/a	n/a	n/a	8
	unspec.	5–10 mg/mL	NS	n/a	h	n/a	4 d	n/a	n/a	n/a	n/a	8
	unspec.	10 mg/mL	NS	n/a	h	20 h	4 d	n/a	n/a	n/a	n/a	8
	ZEN	10, 20 mg/mL	NS	n/a	h	n/a	5 d	n/a	n/a	n/a	n/a	7, 9
	unspec.	20 mg/mL	NS	n/a	h	14 h	3 d	n/a	n/a	n/a	n/a	8

continued on next page

Meropenem (cont'd)

Drug Manufacturer	Concentration	Diluents	Osmolality (mOsm/kg)	pH[h]	Storage Conditions					Body Temp	Refer.
					Temperature			Post-thaw Temp			
					Room	Refrig	Frozen	Room	Refrig		
INTERMATE (Baxter)	5 mg/mL	NS	n/a	h	34 h	96 h[g]	n/a	n/a	n/a	n/a	9
	5 mg/mL	NS	n/a	h	6 h[i]	3 d	n/a	n/a	n/a	n/a	10
	5–40 mg/mL	NS	n/a	h	n/a	24 h	n/a	n/a	n/a	n/a	10
	10 mg/mL	NS	n/a	h	20 h	96 h[g]	n/a	n/a	n/a	n/a	9
Minibag Plus (Baxter)	2.5–20 mg/mL	NS	n/a	h	4 h[k]	24 h[k]	n/a	n/a	n/a	n/a	1
	2.5–20 mg/mL	D5W	n/a	h	1 h[k]	6 h[k]	n/a	n/a	n/a	n/a	1
PVC Cassette (SIMS Deltec)	20, 30 mg/mL	NS	n/a	h	24 h[c]	n/a	n/a	n/a	n/a	n/a	5, 9

Flush Compatibility: Normal saline,[1] heparin,[4,b] Y-site intravenous solutions of NS or D5W with potassium chloride 10 or 40 mmol/L.[3]

Special Considerations: n/a

Notes

[a]Stability also applicable to plastic tubing, drip chambers, and volume control devices.[1,9]

[b]Heparin 1 and 20 units/mL was visually compatible with meropenem 1 and 50 mg/mL.

[c]Attached to a portable infusion pump and stored in a cold pouch whose frozen gel packs were replaced every 8 to 12 h.

[d]Storage at room temperature in D5W may result in greater than 10% loss in 6 h. Use within 2 h of preparation if stored at room temperature.[3]

[e]22 mg/mL nominal concentration of meropenem, based on addition of 2,000 mg vial reconstituted with 40 mL diluent, added to 50 mL bag of diluent.

[f]Actual study data revealed greater than 90% of initial concentration for 10 d. However, the authors recommended storage for up to 7 d refrigerated, then for the product to be stored at room temperature for up to 8 h prior to administration.

[g]Solutions refrigerated for 96 h maintained stability for 6 h at room temperature, but became unacceptable on longer room-temperature storage.[9]

[h]pH of reconstituted solution is 7.3–8.3.[9]

[i]Manufacturer extrapolated data from other source(s).

[j]After refrigerated storage for 6 d.

[k]After activation of vial-bag connector.

continued on next page

Meropenem (cont'd)

References

1. Merrem® [product information]. Wilmington, DE: AstraZeneca; December 2010.
2. *Drug Stability Data Using Elastomeric Infusion Systems.* B. Braun Medical Production Ltd. (Thailand); August 2011.
3. Walker SE, Varrin S, Yannicelli D, et al. Stability of meropenem in saline and dextrose solutions and compatibility with potassium chloride. *Can J Hosp Pharm.* 1998; 51(4):156–68.
4. Patel PR. Compatibility of meropenem with commonly used injectable drugs. *Am J Health-Syst Pharm.* 1996; 53:2853–5.
5. Grant EM, Zhong MK, Ambrose PG, et al. Stability of meropenem in a portable infusion device in a cold pouch. *Am J Health-Syst Pharm.* 2000; 57:992–5.
6. Patel PR, Cook SE. Stability of meropenem in intravenous solutions. *Am J Health-Syst Pharm.* 1997; 54:412–21.
7. Smith DL, Bauer SM, Nicolau DP. Stability of meropenem in polyvinyl chloride bags and an elastomeric infusion device. *Am J Health-Syst Pharm.* 2004; 61:1682–5.
8. *Stability Data for Drugs Using Homepump Disposable Elastomeric Infusion Systems.* Lake Forest, CA: I-Flow Corporation; October 2009.
9. Trissel LA. *ASHP's Interactive Handbook on Injectable Drugs.* Bethesda, MD: American Society of Health-System Pharmacists. Accessed 2012 May.
10. *Intermate/Infusor Drug Stability Information.* Deerfield, IL: Baxter Healthcare Corporation; October 2008.

Mesna

	Drug Manufacturer	Concentration	Diluents	Osmolality (mOsm/kg)	pH[l]	Storage Conditions					Body Temp	Refer.
						Temperature			Post-thaw Temp			
						Room	Refrig	Frozen	Room	Refrig		
CONTAINER												
Syringes, Plastic	unspec.	40 mg/mL[a,b]	NS	n/a	—	28 d	28 d	n/a	n/a	n/a	n/a	1, 5
Syringes, Polypropylene	AST	100 mg/mL	undiluted	n/a	—	9 d[i]	9 d[i]	n/a	n/a	n/a	9 d[h,i]	5
OTHER INFUSION CONTAINERS												
Glass Bottles	AW	3 mg/mL[c]	D5W	n/a	—	48 h[d]	n/a	n/a	n/a	n/a	n/a	2, 5
Graseby™ 9000 PVC Cassette (Graseby Medical)	AST	20 mg/mL[g]	W[g]	n/a	—	n/a	14 d[f]	n/a	n/a	n/a	7 d[f]	3, 5
INFUSOR (Baxter)	AM	0.4–100 mg/mL[e]	NS	n/a	—	n/a	7 d	n/a	n/a	n/a	2 d[m]	4
Polyethylene Bag	AM	0.54 mg/mL[k]	D5W	n/a	—	6 h[k]	48 h[k]	n/a	n/a	n/a	n/a	6
	AM	3.2 mg/mL[j]	D5W	n/a	—	24 h[i]	48 h[i]	n/a	n/a	n/a	n/a	6

Flush Compatibility: Normal saline.[1]
Special Considerations: Do not use a filter to administer this medication.

Notes

[a]Braun syringes used in study.
[b]With ifosfamide 50 mg/mL.
[c]With hydroxyzine hydrochloride 0.5 mg/mL.
[d]Although not specifically stated in article, room temperature was inferred as the storage temperature.
[e]With ifosfamide (AM) 0.8–100 mg/mL.
[f]Solution protected from light.
[g]Solution also contained ifosfamide 20 mg/mL.
[h]Stored at 35°C.
[i]Expel air from syringes to slow the formation of dimesna.
[j]Solution also contained cyclophosphamide 10.8 mg/mL.
[k]Solution also contained cyclophosphamide 1.8 mg/mL.
[l]pH of undiluted solution is 7.5–8.5.[5]
[m]7 d refrigerated, followed by 2 d at 33°C.

continued on next page

Mesna (cont'd)

References

1. Adams PS, Haines-Nutt RF, Bradford E, et al. Pharmaceutical aspects of home infusion therapy for cancer patients. *Pharm J*. 1987; 238:476–8.
2. Marquardt ED. Visual compatibility of hydroxyzine hydrochloride with various antineoplastic agents. *Am J Hosp Pharm*. 1988; 45:2127.
3. Priston MJ, Sewell GJ. Stability of three cytotoxic drug infusions in the Graseby 9000 ambulatory infusion pump. *J Oncol Pharm Practice*. 1998; 4:143–9.
4. *Intermate/Infusor Drug Stability Information*. Deerfield, IL: Baxter Healthcare Corporation; October 2008.
5. Trissel LA. ASHP's Interactive Handbook on Injectable Drugs. Bethesda, MD: American Society of Health-System Pharmacists. Accessed 2012 Aug.
6. Menard C, Bourguignon C, Schlatter J, et al. Stability of cyclophosphamide and mesna admixtures in polyethylene infusion bags. *Ann Pharmacother*. 2003; 37:1789–92.

Methadone Hydrochloride

CONTAINER	Drug Manufacturer	Concentration	Diluents	Osmolality (mOsm/kg)	pH[b]	Storage Conditions							Refer.
						Temperature			Post-thaw Temp			Body Temp	
						Room	Refrig	Frozen	Room	Refrig			
Polyvinyl Chloride (PVC)	LI	1, 2, 5 mg/mL	NS	n/a	b	28 d[a]	n/a	n/a	n/a	n/a		n/a	1

Flush Compatibility: Normal saline.[1]
Special Considerations: n/a

Notes

[a]*Solution stored exposed to light.*
[b]*pH of undiluted solution is 4.5–6.5.*[1]

Reference

1. Trissel LA. ASHP's Interactive Handbook on Injectable Drugs. Bethesda, MD: American Society of Health-System Pharmacists. Accessed 2012 May.

Methotrexate Sodium

Container	Drug Manufacturer	Concentration	Diluents	Osmolality (mOsm/kg)	pH[g]	Temperature Room	Temperature Refrig	Temperature Frozen	Post-thaw Temp Room	Post-thaw Temp Refrig	Body Temp	Refer.
CONTAINER												
Polyvinyl Chloride (PVC)	unspec.	0.1, 1, 20 mg/mL	NS	n/a	g	n/a	n/a	12 w[a]	n/a	n/a	n/a	1
	BEL	0.225, 24 mg/mL	NS, D5W	n/a	g	24 h[b]	30 d[b]	n/a	n/a	n/a	n/a	1, 5
	LE	0.5 mg/mL	D5W	n/a	g	n/a	n/a	30 d[a]	n/a	n/a	n/a	1
	unspec.	1 mg/mL	NS	n/a	g	1 d	n/a	n/a	n/a	n/a	n/a	2
	FA	1.25, 12.5 mg/mL	NS	n/a	g	7 d[b,j]	105 d[b,j]	n/a	n/a	n/a	n/a	1
Syringes, Plastic	LE	2.5 mg/mL	W	n/a	g	7 d	7 d	n/a	n/a	n/a	n/a	1
	LE	50 mg/mL[c]	undiluted	f	8.5	8 m	n/a	n/a	n/a	n/a	n/a	1
	BMS, AD	Various[e]	NS	n/a	g	4 w	90 d	90 d	n/a	n/a	n/a	6
OTHER INFUSION CONTAINERS												
AccuFlo™/ AccuFlux™/ AccuRX® (B. Braun)	unspec.	0.03 mg/mL	D5W	n/a	g	7 d	n/a	n/a	n/a	n/a	n/a	7
	unspec.	1.25–12.5 mg/mL	NS	n/a	g	7 d	105 d	n/a	n/a	n/a	n/a	7
Homepump®/ Homepump Eclipse® (I-Flow Corp.)	unspec.	0.03 mg/mL	D5W	n/a	g	7 d[d]	n/a	n/a	n/a	n/a	n/a	4
	unspec.	1.25–12.5 mg/mL	NS	n/a	g	7 d[d]	105 d[d]	n/a	n/a	n/a	n/a	4
INFUSOR (Baxter)	BMS	1.25 mg/mL	NS	n/a	g	1 d[h]	105 d[h]	n/a	n/a	n/a	n/a	3
	BMS	1.25–12.5 mg/mL	NS	n/a	g	10 d	n/a	n/a	n/a	n/a	n/a	3
	BMS	12.5 mg/mL	NS	n/a	g	4 d[i]	105 d[i]	n/a	n/a	n/a	n/a	3

Flush Compatibility: Heparin lock flush and normal saline.[1]
Special Considerations: Protect from light, especially dilute solutions.

Notes

[a]Solution was thawed by microwave irradiation with no loss of potency.
[b]Protected from light.
[c]Sherwood or Becton Dickinson syringes.

continued on next page

Methotrexate Sodium (cont'd)

[d]Manufacturer(s) extrapolated data from other sources.
[e]Concentrations not specified.
[f]Osmolality of undiluted solution is isotonic.[1]
[g]pH of the undiluted solution is 8.5 (7.5–9).[1]
[h]105 d refrigerated, followed by 1 d at room temperature.
[i]105 d refrigerated, followed by 4 d at room temperature.
[j]105 d refrigerated, followed by 7 d at room temperature.

References

1. Trissel LA. ASHP's Interactive Handbook on Injectable Drugs. Bethesda, MD: American Society of Health-System Pharmacists. Accessed 2012 Aug.
2. Vyas HM, Baptista RJ, Mitrano FP, et al. Drug stability guidelines for a continuous infusion chemotherapy program. Hosp Pharm. 1987; 22:685–7.
3. Intermate/Infusor Drug Stability Information. Deerfield, IL: Baxter Healthcare Corporation; October 2008.
4. Stability Data for Drugs Using Homepump Disposable Elastomeric Infusion Systems. Lake Forest, CA: I-Flow Corporation; October 2009.
5. Benaji B, Dine T, Goudaliez F, et al. Compatibility study of methotrexate with PVC bags after repackaging into two types of infusion admixtures. Int J Pharm. 1994; 105:83–7.
6. Rapp RP, Hatton J, Record K. Drug Stability in Plastic Syringes. HealthTek™ and University of KY Lexington. Chester, NY: Repro-Med Systems Inc.; 1998.
7. Drug Stability Data Using Elastomeric Infusion Systems. B. Braun Medical Production Ltd. (Thailand); August 2011.

Methylprednisolone Sodium Succinate

Container / Drug Manufacturer	Concentration	Diluents	Osmolality (mOsm/kg)	pH[c]	Temperature Room	Temperature Refrig	Temperature Frozen	Post-thaw Temp Room	Post-thaw Temp Refrig	Body Temp	Refer.
CONTAINER											
Ethyvinyl Acetate (EVA) PHU	1, 10 mg/mL	NS	n/a	c	2 d[b]	30 d[b]	n/a	n/a	n/a	n/a	1, 5
Polyvinyl Chloride (PVC) UP	0.25 mg/mL	D5W, NS	n/a	c	7 d	n/a	n/a	n/a	n/a	n/a	3
UP	4.6 mg/mL	NS	n/a	c	n/a	n/a	12 m[a]	n/a	n/a	n/a	1
Syringes, Polypropylene UP	10 mg/mL	NS	301–319	c	7 d	21 d	n/a	n/a	n/a	n/a	1, 4
OTHER INFUSION CONTAINERS											
AccuFlo™/ AccuFlux™/ AccuRX® (B. Braun) unspec.	10 mg/mL	NS	301–319	c	24 h	7 d	n/a	n/a	n/a	n/a	1, 6
AutoDose™ (Tandem Medical) PHU	1, 10 mg/mL	NS	n/a	c	2 d[b]	30 d[b]	n/a	n/a	n/a	n/a	1, 5
Glass UP	0.8, 10, 20, 40 mg/mL	D5W, NS	n/a	c	48 h	n/a	n/a	n/a	n/a	n/a	3
UP	2.5, 5 mg/mL	D5W, NS	n/a	c	7 d	n/a	n/a	n/a	n/a	n/a	3
Glass Vials UP	4 mg/mL	W	n/a	c	24 h	7 d	n/a	n/a	n/a	n/a	1
Homepump®/ Homepump Eclipse® (I-Flow Corp.) unspec.	10 mg/mL	NS	301–319	c	24 h	7 d	n/a	n/a	n/a	n/a	1, 2

Flush Compatibility: Heparin lock flush and normal saline.[1]
Special Considerations: n/a

Notes

[a]Stored at −20°C.
[b]Protect from light.
[c]pH of reconstituted preparation is 7–8.[1]

continued on next page

Methylprednisolone Sodium Succinate (cont'd)

References

1. Trissel LA. ASHP's Interactive Handbook on Injectable Drugs. Bethesda, MD: American Society of Health-System Pharmacists. Accessed 2012 Aug.
2. *Stability Data for Drugs Using Homepump Disposable Elastomeric Infusion Systems.* Lake Forest, CA: I-Flow Corporation; October 2009.
3. Slatter V. Solu-Medrol sterile powder compatibility/stability [manufacturer letter]. Horsham, PA: The Upjohn Company; January 7, 1994.
4. Das Gupta V. Chemical stability of methylprednisolone sodium succinate after reconstitution in 0.9% sodium chloride injection and storage in pclypropylene syringes. *Int J Pharm Compound.* 2001; 5(2):148–50.
5. Trissel LA, Zhang Y. Stability of methylprednisolone sodium succinate in AutoDose Infusion System bags. *J Am Pharm Assoc.* 2002; 42(6):868–70.
6. *Drug Stability Data Using Elastomeric Infusion Systems.* B. Braun Medical Production Ltd. (Thailand); August 2011.

Metoclopramide Hydrochloride

Container	Drug Manufacturer	Concentration	Diluents	Osmolality (mOsm/kg)	pH[k]	Temperature			Post-thaw Temp		Body Temp	Refer.
						Room	Refrig	Frozen	Room	Refrig		
CONTAINER												
Polyvinyl Chloride (PVC)	RB	0.2 mg/mL	D5W	n/a	k	24 h	n/a	2 w	24 h	n/a	n/a	1
	RB	0.2, 3.2 mg/mL	NS	n/a	k	24 h	n/a	4 w	24 h	n/a	n/a	1
	SKB	0.5 mg/mL[a]	NS	n/a	k	35 d	182 d[b]	n/a	n/a	n/a	7 d[b]	1
Syringes, Polypropylene	BA	0.5 mg/mL	NS	n/a	k	21 d[j]	n/a	n/a	n/a	n/a	n/a	2
	AST	0.74 mg/mL	d	n/a	k	n/a	n/a	c	n/a	n/a	10 d[e]	5
	SO	2.5 mg/mL	NS	n/a	k	24 h	24 h	n/a	n/a	n/a	n/a	1
OTHER INFUSION CONTAINERS												
MiniMed Syringe (Travenol)	RB	5 mg/mL[f]	undiluted	280	2.5–6.5	60 d	90 d	c	n/a	n/a	7 d[g]	1
PCA INFUSOR (Baxter)	SKB	0.5 mg/mL[a]	D5W	n/a	k	14 d	98 d	n/a	n/a	n/a	n/a	1
	BE	0.5 mg/mL[l]	D5W	n/a	k	35 d[m]	n/a	n/a	n/a	n/a	7 d[m]	6
	BE	0.5 mg/mL[l]	D5W	n/a	k	n/a	154 d[n]	n/a	n/a	n/a	1 d[n]	6
	BE	0.5 mg/mL[l]	D5W	n/a	k	n/a	42 d[o]	n/a	n/a	n/a	3 d[o]	6
	BE	0.5 mg/mL[l]	D5W	n/a	k	n/a	112 d[p]	n/a	n/a	n/a	2 d[p]	6
	BE	0.5 mg/mL[l]	D5W	n/a	k	n/a	56 d[q]	n/a	n/a	n/a	3 d[q]	6
	BE	0.5 mg/mL[l]	D5W	n/a	k	n/a	140 d[r]	n/a	n/a	n/a	1 d[r]	6
	BE	0.5 mg/mL[l]	D5W	n/a	k	n/a	98 d[s]	n/a	n/a	n/a	2 d[s]	6
	BE	0.5 mg/mL[l]	D5W	n/a	k	35 d[t]	n/a	n/a	n/a	n/a	6 d[t]	6
	BE	0.5 mg/mL[l]	D5W	n/a	k	28 d[u]	n/a	n/a	n/a	n/a	7 d[u]	6
PVC Cassette (Pharmacia Deltec)	unspec.	1 mg/mL[i]	unspec.	n/a	k	7 d	n/a	n/a	n/a	n/a	n/a	4
	DU	4 mg/mL[h]	NS	n/a	k	14 d	14 d	n/a	n/a	n/a	n/a	1, 3

Storage Conditions

continued on next page

243

Flush Compatibility: Heparin lock flush and normal saline.[1]
Special Considerations: n/a

Notes

[a]With morphine sulfate 1 mg/mL (Evans).

[b]182 d refrigerated, followed by 7 d at 32°C.

[c]Do not freeze in syringes.

[d]With fentanyl 0.037 mg/mL (DB) and midazolam 0.55 mg/mL (RC).

[e]Protect from light.

[f]With Luer-Lok tip caps (Burron).

[g]Stored at 32°C to simulate wearing a portable infusion pump close to the body.

[h]Tested in 100 mL NS with 40 mg dexamethasone (AMR), 200 mg diphenhydramine (ES), and 4 mg lorazepam (WY). Stability data pertains to dexamethasone, diphenhydramine, and metoclopramide only.

[i]With morphine 15 mg/mL.

[j]Stored at 25°C; pH remained constant 5.0 during study period.

[k]pH of undiluted solution is 2.5–6.5.[1]

[l]With morphine sulfate 2 mg/mL (Evans).

[m]35 d at 25°C, followed by 7 d at 33°C.

[n]154 d at 2–8°C, followed by 1 d at 33°C.

[o]42 d at 2–8°C, followed by 3 d at 33°C.

[p]112 d at 2–8°C, followed by 2 d at 33°C.

[q]56 d at 2–8°C, followed by 3 d at 33°C.

[r]140 d at 2–8°C, followed by 1 d at 33°C.

[s]98 d at 2–8°C, followed by 2 d at 33°C.

[t]35 d at 25°C, followed by 6 d at 33°C.

[u]28 d at 25°C, followed by 7 d at 33°C.

References

1. Trissel LA. ASHP's Interactive Handbook on Injectable Drugs. Bethesda, MD: American Society of Health-System Pharmacists. Accessed 2012 May.
2. Gupta VD. Chemical stability of metoclopramide hydrochloride injection diluted with 0.9% sodium chloride injection in polypropylene syringes at room temperature. *Int J Pharm Compound.* 2005; 9(1):72–4.
3. Stiles MD, Allen LV, Prince SJ, et al. Stability of dexamethasone sodium phosphate, diphenhydramine hydrochloride, lorazepam, and metoclopramide hydrochloride in portable infusion-pump reservoirs. *Am J Hosp Pharm.* 1994; 51(Feb 15):514–7.
4. Swanson G, Smith J, Bulich R, et al. Patient-controlled analgesia for chronic cancer pain in the ambulatory setting: a report of 117 patients. *J Clin Oncol.* 1989; 7(12):1903–8.
5. Peterson GM, Miller KA, Galloway JG, et al. Compatibility and stability of fentanyl admixtures in polypropylene syringes. *J Clin Pharm Ther.* 1998; 23:67–72.
6. *Intermate/Infusor Drug Stability Information.* Deerfield, IL: Baxter Healthcare Corporation; October 2008.

Metronidazole, Metronidazole Hydrochloride

Container	Drug Manufacturer	Concentration	Diluents	Osmolality (mOsm/kg)	pH[g]	Storage Conditions Temperature Room	Refrig	Frozen	Post-thaw Temp Room	Refrig	Body Temp	Refer.
CONTAINER												
Polyvinyl Chloride (PVC)	MB	30 mcg/mL	NS	n/a	n/a	7 d	n/a	n/a	n/a	n/a	n/a	1
OTHER INFUSION CONTAINERS												
AccuFlo™/AccuFlux™/AccuRX® (B. Braun)	unspec.	5 mg/mL	RTU	iso	5.8	24 h[b]	10 d[a,b]	n/a	n/a	n/a	n/a	3
Homepump®/Homepump Eclipse® (I-Flow Corp.)	unspec.	5 mg/mL	undiluted[a]	iso	5.8	24 h	10 d[a]	n/a	n/a	n/a	n/a	2
COMMERCIAL PREPARATIONS (RTU)												
Premixed Bag (B. Braun)	BRN	5 mg/mL	RTU[e]	iso	5.8	d	n/a	n/a	n/a	n/a	n/a	4
Premixed Flexible Container (Hospira)	HSP	5 mg/mL	RTU[f]	iso	5.8	d	n/a	n/a	n/a	n/a	n/a	5
Viaflex Bag (Baxter)	SE	5 mg/mL	[c]	iso	5.8	d	n/a	n/a	n/a	n/a	n/a	1, 6

Flush Compatibility: Heparin lock flush and normal saline.[1]

Special Considerations: Short-term exposure to normal room light does not adversely affect stability. Direct sunlight should be avoided.[1] Infuse over 1 h. Refrigeration may cause crystals to form; these will redissolve when warmed to room temperature.[1]

Notes

[a] RTU metronidazole solution is susceptible to crystallization when refrigerated. The crystals redissolve on warming to room temperature.

[b] Manufacturer(s) extrapolated data from other sources.

[c] The RTU is a buffered, isotonic solution (310 mOsm/L) containing sodium 14 mEq/100 mL.[6]

[d] Expiration date per manufacturer's label. Do not extrapolate commercial premix stability data to extemporaneously prepared solutions.

continued on next page

Metronidazole, Metronidazole Hydrochloride (cont'd)

[e]The premixed solution is isotonic (297 mOsm/L), buffered, and contains sodium 13.5 mEq/100 mL. The container is a copolymer of ethylene and propylene, and it is latex-free, PVC-free, and DEHP-free.

[f]The premixed solution is isotonic (314 mOsm/L), buffered, and contains sodium 14 mEq/100 mL.

[g]pH of RTU metronidazole is 5.8 (range 4.5–7).[1]

References

1. Trissel LA. ASHP's Interactive Handbook on Injectable Drugs. Bethesda, MD: American Society of Health-System Pharmacists. Accessed 2012 Jan.
2. Stability Data for Drugs Using Homepump Disposable Elastomeric Infusion Systems. Lake Forest, CA: I-Flow Corporation; October 2009.
3. Drug Stability Data Using Elastomeric Infusion Systems. B. Braun Medical Production Ltd. (Thailand); August 2011.
4. Metronidazole 500 mg/container (5 mg/mL) (Metronidazole Injection USP) [product information]. Irvine, CA: B. Braun Medical Inc.; July 2008.
5. Metronidazole 500 mg (5 mg/mL) (Metronidazole Injection USP) [product information]. Lake Forest, IL: Hospira, Inc.; June 2008.
6. Metronidazole Injection USP RTU® in Plastic Container (Viaflex Plus) [product Information]. Deerfield, IL: Baxter Healthcare Corporation; April 2011.

Micafungin Sodium

	Drug Manufacturer	Concentration	Diluents	Osmolality (mOsm/kg)	pH[c]	Temperature Room	Temperature Refrig	Temperature Frozen	Post-thaw Temp Room	Post-thaw Temp Refrig	Body Temp	Refer.
CONTAINER												
IV Bag[a]	ASL	0.125, 1 mg/mL	NS	n/a	c	n/a	7 d[b]	n/a	n/a	n/a	n/a	1
	ASL	0.25, 3 mg/mL	NS, D5W	n/a	c	n/a	3 d[b]	n/a	n/a	n/a	n/a	1
	ASL	0.25, 4 mg/mL	NS, D5W	n/a	c	4 d[b]	n/a	n/a	n/a	n/a	n/a	1
	ASL	1 mg/mL	LR, D5¼S	n/a	c	7 d	7 d	n/a	n/a	n/a	n/a	1
	ASL	e	NS, D5W	n/a	c	24 h[b]	n/a	n/a	n/a	n/a	n/a	2
Vial[d]	ASL	5 mg/mL	NS, D5W	n/a	c	2 d[b]	n/a	n/a	n/a	n/a	n/a	1
	ASL	e	NS	n/a	c	24 h	n/a	n/a	n/a	n/a	n/a	2
OTHER INFUSION CONTAINERS												
Homepump®/ Homepump Eclipse® (I-Flow Corp.)	ASL	0.2, 1 mg/mL	NS, D5W	n/a	c	n/a	10 d[b]	n/a	n/a	n/a	n/a	1

Flush Compatibility: Normal saline. Do not mix with heparin or other drugs.[2]
Special Considerations: Protect diluted solution from light. It is not necessary to cover the IV tubing or the infusion drip chamber.[2]

Notes

[a]Material type of IV bag not specified.[1]
[b]Protected from light.
[c]pH of reconstituted solution in NS is 5–7.[2]
[d]Original product vial.
[e]Reconstituted/diluted per product labeling.[2]

References

1. Unpublished data on file [personal communication]. Deerfield, IL: Medical Information Department, Astellas Pharma US Inc.; February 2008.
2. Mycamine® [package insert]. Deerfield, IL: Astellas Pharma US Inc.; June 2011.

Midazolam

Storage Conditions

Container	Drug Manufacturer	Concentration	Diluents	Osmolality (mOsm/kg)	pH[i]	Temperature Room	Temperature Refrig	Temperature Frozen	Post-thaw Temp Room	Post-thaw Temp Refrig	Body Temp	Refer.
CONTAINER												
Glass	RC	0.5 mg/mL	D5W, NS	k	i	36 d[b]	36 d[b]	n/a	n/a	n/a	36 d[b,d]	2
	RC	3 mg/mL	NS	k	i	n/a	n/a	n/a	n/a	n/a	13 d[f]	2
Polyethylene	RC	0.035 mg/mL	D5W, NS	˅	i	24 h	24 h	n/a	n/a	n/a	n/a	2
Polyolefin	RC	0.5 mg/mL	D5W, NS	k	i	30 d[b]	30 d[b]	n/a	n/a	n/a	n/a	2
Polyvinyl Chloride (PVC)	RC	0.035 mg/mL	D5W, NS	k	i	24 h	24 h	n/a	n/a	n/a	n/a	2
	RC	0.5 mg/mL	NS	k	i	28 d[a,b]	n/a	n/a	n/a	n/a	n/a	1
	RC	1 mg/mL	NS	k	i	49 d[b,c]	49 d[c]	n/a	n/a	n/a	n/a	2
	RC	1 mg/mL[j]	NS	k	i	10 d[b,c]	n/a	n/a	n/a	n/a	n/a	2
Syringe, Polypropylene	RC	1 mg/mL	unspec.	k	i	4 w[b]	n/a	n/a	n/a	n/a	n/a	2
	RC	2 mg/mL	NS	k	i	10 d[e]	10 d	n/a	n/a	n/a	n/a	2
	RC	3 mg/mL	NS	k	i	13 d[g]	n/a	n/a	n/a	n/a	13 d[g]	2
	RC	5 mg/mL	unspec.	385	i	36 d[b]	n/a	n/a	n/a	n/a	n/a	2
OTHER INFUSION CONTAINERS												
Unspecified	RC	0.1, 0.5 mg/mL[h]	D5W, NS	k	i	23 d[h]	23 d[h]	n/a	n/a	n/a	n/a	2

Flush Compatibility: Heparin, normal saline.[2]
Special Considerations: n/a

Notes

[a]Combined with morphine tartrate 1 mg/mL and bupivacaine hydrochloride 4 mg/mL.
[b]Protected from light.
[c]Fluorescent light.
[d]Tested at 40°C.
[e]Tested at 30°C.
[f]Tested at 32°C.
[g]Tested at 20°C and 32°C.
[h]Combined with hydromorphone HCl 2 mg/mL and 20 mg/mL.

continued on next page

Midazolam (cont'd)

ʲpH of undiluted solution (5 mg/mL) is 2.9–3.7. pH of 0.625, 1.25, and 1.67 mg/mL in NS is 3.6, 3.4, and 3.4.[2]
ⁱBenzyl alcohol added to a concentration of 1%.
ᵏOsmolality of undiluted solution (5 mg/mL, RC) is 385 mOsm/kg. Diluted in NS to 0.625, 1.25, and 1.67 mg/mL, osmolality is 274, 262, and 259 mOsm/kg.

References

1. La Forgia SP, Sharley NA, Burgess NG, et al. Stability and compatibility of morphine, midazolam, and bupivacaine combinations for intravenous infusion. *J Pharm Practice Res.* 2002; 32:65–8.
2. Trissel LA. ASHP's Interactive Handbook on Injectable Drugs. Bethesda, MD: American Society of Health-System Pharmacists. Accessed 2012 Aug.

Milrinone Lactate

Drug Manufacturer	Concentration	Diluents	Osmolality (mOsm/kg)	pH[c]	Storage Conditions						Refer.
					Temperature			Post-thaw Temp		Body Temp	
					Room	Refrig	Frozen	Room	Refrig		
CONTAINER											
Polyolefin Containers — SW	400, 600, 800 mcg/mL	NS	n/a	[c]	14 d	14 d	n/a	n/a	n/a	n/a	1, 4
Polyvinyl Chloride (PVC) — WI	200 mcg/mL	NS, D5W	n/a	[c]	14 d	14 d	n/a	n/a	n/a	n/a	1, 2
WI	400 mcg/mL	D5W, LR, NS, 1/2S	n/a	[c]	7 d	n/a	n/a	n/a	n/a	n/a	1, 3
SW	400, 600, 800 mcg/mL	D5W	n/a	[c]	14 d	14 d	n/a	n/a	n/a	n/a	1, 4
COMMERCIAL PREPARATIONS (RTU)											
Flexible Plastic Container (Hospira) — HSP	200 mcg/mL	D5W	n/a	[c]	30 d[b,d]	n/a	n/a	n/a	n/a	n/a	7, 8
Flexible PVC Bag — SAV	200 mcg/mL	D5W[a]	n/a	3.2–4	30 d[b,d]	n/a	n/a	n/a	n/a	n/a	1, 5
INTRAVIA Plastic Container (Baxter) — BA	200 mcg/mL	D5W	n/a	3.5	30 d[b,d]	n/a	n/a	n/a	n/a	n/a	9

Flush Compatibility: Heparin lock flush and normal saline.[1,3]
Special Considerations: n/a

Notes

[a]Solution also contains lactic acid 0.95–1.29 mg/mL.[1,6,7]
[b]Expiration date per manufacturer's label when stored in the protective overwrap under labeled storage conditions.
[c]pH of the ready to use product ranges from 3.2–4.[1,6,7]
[d]Do not use beyond this date after removal of manufacturer's protective overwrap.[5,7,8]

continued on next page

Milrinone Lactate (cont'd)

References

1. Trissel LA. ASHP's Interactive Handbook on Injectable Drugs. Bethesda, MD: American Society of Health-System Pharmacists. Accessed 2012 May.

2. Wong F, Gill MA. Stability of milrinone lactate 200 mcg/mL in 5% dextrose injection and 0.9% sodium chloride injection. *Int J Pharm Compound*. 1998; 2(2):168–9.

3. Akkerman SR, Zhang H, Mullins RE, et al. Stability of milrinone lactate in the presence of 29 critical care drugs and 4 i.v. solutions. *Am J Health-Syst Pharm*. 1999; 56(1):63–8.

4. Nguyen D, Gill MA, Wong F. Stability of milrinone lactate in 5% dextrose injection and 0.9% sodium chloride injection at concentrations of 400, 600, and 800 mcg/mL. *Int J Pharm Compound*. 1998; 2:246–8.

5. Medical Information Specialist [personal communication]. Bridgewater, NJ: Sanofi Aventis; April 25, 2008.

6. Milrinone Lactate Injection [prescribing information]. Bedford, OH: Bedford Laboratories; July 2007.

7. Milrinone Lactate Injection [package insert]. Lake Forest, IL: Hospira Inc.; May 2007.

8. Medical Communications Department [personal communication]. Lake Forest, IL: Hospira Inc.; April 25, 2008.

9. Product Information Center [personal communication]. Round Lake, IL: Baxter Healthcare Corporation; April 1, 2008.

Mitomycin

	Drug Manufacturer	Concentration	Diluents	Osmolality (mOsm/kg)	pH[d]	Temperature			Post-thaw Temp			Refer.
						Room	Refrig	Frozen	Room	Refrig	Body Temp	
CONTAINER												
Polyvinyl Chloride (PVC)	unspec.	0.5 mg/mL	W	n/a	d	14 d	n/a	n/a	n/a	n/a	n/a	1
	KY	0.6 mg/mL	NS	n/a	d	n/a	4 d[c]	n/a	n/a	n/a	n/a	5
	BMS	0.6 mg/mL[a]	NS	n/a	d	n/a	n/a	8 w[a]	n/a	n/a	n/a	2, 5
	BR	20 mcg/mL	LR	n/a	d	6 d	n/a	n/a	n/a	n/a	n/a	4, 5
	BR	40 mcg/mL	LR	n/a	d	n/a	15 d	n/a	n/a	n/a	n/a	4, 5
	BR	40 mcg/mL	NS	n/a	d	n/a	5 d	n/a	n/a	n/a	n/a	4, 5
	LCSA	50 mcg/mL	D5W[b]	n/a	d	15 d	120 d	n/a	n/a	n/a	n/a	3, 5
Syringes, Polypropylene	BMS	0.5 mg/mL	W	n/a	d	11 d[c]	42 d[c]	n/a	n/a	n/a	n/a	5
Unspecified	BR	50 mcg/mL	NS	n/a	d	5 d	n/a	n/a	n/a	n/a	n/a	5
OTHER INFUSION CONTAINERS												
Glass Bottles (McGaw)	BR	20 mcg/mL	LR	n/a	d	6 d	n/a	n/a	n/a	n/a	n/a	4, 5
	BR	40 mcg/mL	LR	n/a	d	n/a	20 d	n/a	n/a	n/a	n/a	4, 5
	BR	40 mcg/mL	NS	n/a	d	n/a	5 d	n/a	n/a	n/a	n/a	4, 5

Flush Compatibility: Heparin lock flush and normal saline.[5]
Special Considerations: n/a

Notes

[a] Buffered and unbuffered solutions were frozen at −30°C for 4 w, then thawed. The unbuffered solutions were refrozen for another 4 w. Freezing at −20°C resulted in a precipitate forming in the solution.
[b] Solutions buffered to achieve a pH of approximately 7.8.
[c] Protect from light.
[d] pH of reconstituted product is 6–8.[1]

References

1. Vyas HM, Baptista RJ, Mitrano FP, et al. Drug stability guidelines for a continuous infusion chemotherapy program. *Hosp Pharm.* 1987; 22:685–7.
2. Stolk LML, Fruijtier A, Umans R. Stability after freezing and thawing of solutions of mitomycin C in plastic minibags for intravesical use. *Pharm Weekbl Sci.* 1986; 8:286–8.
3. Quebbeman EJ, Hoffman NE, Ausman RK, et al. Stability of mitomycin admixtures. *Am J Hosp Pharm.* 1985; 42:1750–4.
4. Dorr RT, Liddil JD. Stability of mitomycin C in different infusion fluids: compatibility with heparin and glucocorticosteroids. *J Oncol Pharm Pract.* 1995; 1:19–24.
5. Trissel LA. ASHP's Interactive Handbook on Injectable Drugs. Bethesda, MD: American Society of Health-System Pharmacists. Accessed 2012 Aug.

Mitoxantrone Hydrochloride

	Drug Manufacturer	Concentration	Diluents	Osmolality (mOsm/kg)	pH[b]	Storage Conditions: Temperature Room	Temperature Refrig	Temperature Frozen	Post-thaw Temp Room	Post-thaw Temp Refrig	Body Temp	Refer.
CONTAINER												
Polyvinyl Chloride (PVC)	LE	0.02–0.5 mg/mL	D5W, NS	n/a	[b]	7 d	7 d	n/a	n/a	n/a	n/a	1
Syringes, Plastic (Monoject)	LE	2 mg/mL	NS	n/a	[b]	42 d	42 d	n/a	n/a	n/a	n/a	1, 3
Syringes, Polypropylene (Braun Omnifix)	unspec.	0.2 mg/mL	NS	n/a	[b]	28 d	28 d	n/a	n/a	n/a	24 h	1, 2
OTHER INFUSION CONTAINERS												
Glass	LE	5, 20–500 mg/mL	D5W, NS	n/a	[b]	48 h	48 h	n/a	n/a	n/a	n/a	1
INFUSOR (Baxter)	LE	0.1–0.5 mg/mL	NS	n/a	[b]	2 d[a]	n/a	n/a	n/a	n/a	5 d[a]	4
	LE	0.2 mg/mL	NS	n/a	[b]	8 d	n/a	n/a	n/a	n/a	n/a	4
	LE	0.7 mg/mL	W	n/a	[b]	8 d	n/a	n/a	n/a	n/a	n/a	4

Flush Compatibility: Normal saline. Heparin may cause precipitation in the same admixture.[1]
Special Considerations: n/a

Notes

[a]*Storage of 2 d at room temperature followed by 5 d at body temp (33°C).*
[b]*pH of undiluted concentrate is 3–4.5.*[1]

References

1. Trissel LA. ASHP's Interactive Handbook on Injectable Drugs. Bethesda, MD: American Society of Health-System Pharmacists. Accessed 2012 Aug.
2. Adams PS, Haines-Nutt RF, Bradford E, et al. Pharmaceutical aspects of home infusion therapy for cancer patients. *Pharm J.* 1987; 238:476–8.
3. Walker SE, Lau DWC, DeAngelis C, et al. Mitoxantrone stability in syringes and glass vials and evaluation of chemical contamination. *Can J Hosp Pharm.* 1991; 44(3):143–51.
4. *Intermate/Infusor Drug Stability Information.* Deerfield, IL: Baxter Healthcare Corporation; October 2008.

Morphine Sulfate[a,b,c]

	Drug Manufacturer	Concentration	Diluents	Osmolality (mOsm/kg)[e]	pH[p]	Storage Conditions: Temperature: Room	Temperature: Refrig	Temperature: Frozen	Post-thaw Temp: Room	Post-thaw Temp: Refrig	Body Temp	Refer.
CONTAINER												
Polypropylene Bag (Mark II Polybag)	AST	20 mcg/mL[o]	NS	e	p	30 d[n,o]	n/a	n/a	n/a	n/a	n/a	1, 7
	AST	20, 100 mcg/mL[m]	NS	e	p	30 d[m,n]	n/a	n/a	n/a	n/a	n/a	1, 7
Polyvinyl Chloride (PVC)	AB, AH	0.04, 0.4 mg/mL	D5W, NS	e	p	7 d	7 d	n/a	n/a	n/a	n/a	1
	LI	1, 2 mg/mL	D5W, NS	e	p	n/a	n/a	14 w	n/a	n/a	n/a	1
	unspec.	2, 15 mg/mL	W	e	p	15 d	15 d	n/a	n/a	n/a	n/a	1
	AH	5 mg/mL	D5W, NS	e	p	30 d	n/a	n/a	n/a	n/a	n/a	1
	AH	10 mg/mL	undiluted	e	p	30 d	n/a	n/a	n/a	n/a	n/a	1
Syringes, Plastic (Plastipak, BD)	LI	1, 5 mg/mL	D5W, NS	e	p	6 w	6 w	6 w	n/a	n/a	n/a	1, 3
Syringes, Polypropylene	unspec.	2 mg/mL	NS	e	p	6 w	n/a	n/a	n/a	n/a	n/a	1
	unspec.	5 mg/mL	NS	e	p	60 d	60 d	n/a	n/a	n/a	48 h[aa]	1
	unspec.	50 mg/mL	W, NS	e	p	60 d	n/a	n/a	n/a	n/a	48 h[aa]	1
OTHER INFUSION CONTAINERS												
AccuFlo™/ AccuFlux™/ AccuRX® (B. Braun)	unspec.	20 mg/mL	NS	e	p	7 d	n/a	n/a	n/a	n/a	n/a	4
Accufuser Plus (Moog)	unspec.	2, 10 mg/mL	unspec.	e	p	40 d	40 d	n/a	n/a	n/a	n/a	1
CADD® Cassette (Pharmacia Deltec)	unspec.	1, 5 mg/mL	NS	e	p	14 d	30 d	n/a	n/a	n/a	n/a	1
	unspec.	1, 10 mg/mL	NS	e	p	n/a	n/a	n/a	n/a	n/a	16[bb,cc]	1
	SAB	10, 25, 50 mg/mL	D5W, NS	e	p	31 d	31 d	n/a	n/a	n/a	n/a	1
	unspec.	15, 25 mg/mL	W	e	p	14 d	30 d	n/a	n/a	n/a	n/a	1

continued on next page

Morphine Sulfate (cont'd)

Drug / Manufacturer	Concentration	Diluents	Osmolality (mOsm/kg)[e]	pH[p]	Temperature			Post-thaw Temp		Body Temp	Refer.
					Room	Refrig	Frozen	Room	Refrig		
Cormed III Bag (Kalex) unspec.	0.5, 15, 30 mg/mL	NS	e	p	n/a	14 d	n/a	n/a	n/a	14 d	1
unspec.	60 mg/mL	NS	e	p	n/a	4 d[d]	n/a	n/a	n/a	14 d	1
Homepump® / Homepump Eclipse® (I-Flow Corp.) unspec.	20 mg/mL	NS	e	p	7 d		n/a	n/a	n/a	n/a	5
INFUSOR (Baxter) STE	0.025 mg/mL[y]	NS	e	p	n/a	120 d[l,y]	n/a	n/a	n/a	7 d[l,y]	2
STE	0.1–1.6 mg/mL[z]	D5W, NS	e	p	28 d[k,z]	n/a	n/a	n/a	n/a	7 d[k,z]	2
BA	1–15 mg/mL	D5W, NS	e	p	70 d	99 d	n/a	n/a	n/a	n/a	2
BA	1–15 mg/mL	D5W, NS	e	p	4 d[q]	14 d[q]	n/a	n/a	n/a	n/a	2
EV	2 mg/mL[s]	D5W, NS	e	p	35 d[r,s]	n/a	n/a	n/a	n/a	7 d[r,s]	2
EV	2 mg/mL[s]	D5W, NS	e	p	n/a	182 d[s,ee]	n/a	n/a	n/a	7 d[s,ee]	2
EV	2 mg/mL[t]	D5W	e	p	35 d[r,t]	n/a	n/a	n/a	n/a	7 d[r,t]	2
EV	2 mg/mL[t]	D5W	e	p	n/a	154 d[t,u]	n/a	n/a	n/a	1 d[t,u]	2
EV	2 mg/mL[t]	D5W	e	p	n/a	42 d[t,v]	n/a	n/a	n/a	3 d[t,v]	2
EV	2 mg/mL[t]	D5W	e	p	n/a	112 d[t,w]	n/a	n/a	n/a	2 d[t,w]	2
EV	2 mg/mL[t]	D5W	e	p	n/a	56 d[t,ff]	n/a	n/a	n/a	3 d[t,ff]	2
EV	2 mg/mL[t]	D5W	e	p	n/a	140 d[t,gg]	n/a	n/a	n/a	1 d[t,gg]	2
EV	2 mg/mL[t]	D5W	e	p	n/a	98 d[t,hh]	n/a	n/a	n/a	2 d[t,hh]	2
EV	2 mg/mL[t]	D5W	e	p	35 d[t,x]	n/a	n/a	n/a	n/a	6 d[t,x]	2
EV	2 mg/mL[t]	D5W	e	p	28 d[t,dd]	n/a	n/a	n/a	n/a	7 d[t,dd]	2
unspec.	2, 15 mg/mL	W	e	p	12 d	12 d	n/a	n/a	n/a	12 d[j]	1
INTERMATE 200 (Baxter) unspec.	2, 15 mg/mL	W	e	p	15 d	15 d	n/a	n/a	n/a	15 d[j]	1

continued on next page

Morphine Sulfate (cont'd)

Drug Product	Drug Manufacturer	Concentration	Diluents	Osmolality (mOsm/kg)[e]	pH[p]	Temperature Room	Temperature Refrig	Temperature Frozen	Post-thaw Temp Room	Post-thaw Temp Refrig	Body Temp	Refer.
PVC/Kalex Cassette (Pharmacia Deltec)	CTF	0.5, 1.5, 2.5 mg/mL	NS	e	p	n/a	n/a	n/a	n/a	n/a	60 d[i]	1
Silicone/Polyester Pump Reservoir (Cordis Europa)	unspec.	5 mg/mL (hyperbaric)	D7W	e	p	n/a	30 d	n/a	n/a	n/a	30 d	1
Synchromed Pump (Medtronic)	unspec.	unspec.	undiluted	e	p	90 d	n/a	n/a	n/a	n/a	90 d	6
	unspec.	50 mg/mL[f]	W[f]	e	p	n/a	n/a	n/a	n/a	n/a	90 d	1
Synchromed EL Pump (Medtronic)	BA	2 mg/mL[g]	unspec.[g]	e	p	n/a	n/a	n/a	n/a	n/a	3 m	1
	BA	20 mg/mL[h]	unspec.[h]	e	p	n/a	n/a	n/a	n/a	n/a	3 m	1
VIP 30 Implantable Pump (Fresenius)	unspec.	10 mg/mL	undiluted	e	p	n/a	n/a	n/a	n/a	n/a	8 w	1

Flush Compatibility: Heparin lock flush and normal saline.[1]
Special Considerations: n/a

Notes

[a]Morphine is light sensitive and should be protected from light with UV-protective coverings; stability data is for light-protected conditions only.
[b]Maximum solubility of morphine sulfate is 62.5 mg/mL. Morphine sulfate concentrations above 10 mg/mL are usually diluted in sterile water for injection (W).
[c]Intraspinal infusion requires the use of preservative-free diluents and drug products.
[d]Refrigeration reduces the solubility, which can result in precipitation.
[e]Osmolality of 7.5 mg/mL (DB) in NS is 236 mOsm/kg.[1]
[f]With bupivacaine HCl 25 mg/mL and clonidine HCl 2 mg/mL.
[g]With clonidine 1.84 mg/mL.
[h]With clonidine (BI) 50 mcg/mL.
[i]Stored at 32°C. Evaporation of ~0.8 mL/w increased morphine concentration by ~1%/w.

continued on next page

Morphine Sulfate (cont'd)

jStored at 31°C.

k28 d at room temperature, followed by 7 d at 33°C.

l120 d refrigerated, followed by 7 d at 33°C.

mSolution also contained ropivacaine (ASZ) 2 mg/mL.

nStorage at 30°C.

oSolution also contained ropivacaine (ASZ) 1 mg/mL.

ppH of undiluted solutions range from 2.5–7.[1]

q14 d refrigerated, followed by 4 d at room temperature.

r35 d at room temperature, followed by 7 d at 33°C.

sWith 0.125 mg/mL droperidol (JN).

tWith 0.5 mg/mL metoclopramide (BE).

u154 d refrigerated, followed by 1 d at 33°C.

v42 d refrigerated, followed by 3 d at 33°C.

w112 d refrigerated, followed by 2 d at 33°C.

x35 d at room temperature, followed by 6 d at 33°C.

yWith 2 mg/mL ropivacaine hydrochloride (AST).

zWith 1.5–8 mg/mL ketorolac (Recordati).

aaStored at 37°C.

bbStored at 32°C.

ccProtect from light.

dd28 d at room temperature, followed by 7 d at 33°C.

ee182 d refrigerated, followed by 7 d at 33°C.

ff56 d refrigerated, followed by 3 d at 33°C.

gg140 d refrigerated, followed by 1 d at 33°C.

hh98 d refrigerated, followed by 2 d at 33°C.

References

1. Trissel LA. ASHP's Interactive Handbook on Injectable Drugs. Bethesda, MD: American Society of Health-System Pharmacists. Accessed 2012 Aug.

2. Intermate/Infusor Drug Stability Information. Deerfield, IL: Baxter Healthcare Corporation; October 2008.

3. Strong ML, Schaaf LJ, Pankaskie MS, et al. Shelf lives and factors affecting the stability of morphine sulphate and meperidine (pethidine) hydrochloride in plastic syringes for use in patient controlled analgesic devices. J Clin Pharm Ther. 1994; 19:361–9.

4. Drug Stability Data Using Elastomeric Infusion Systems. B. Braun Medical Production Ltd. (Thailand); August 2011.

5. Stability Data for Drugs Using Homepump Disposable Elastomeric Infusion Systems. Lake Forest, CA: I-Flow Corporation; October 2009.

6. Synchromed Pump Handbook. Minneapolis, MN: Medtronic Neurological Division; 1993.

7. Svedberg KO, McKenzie EJ, Larrivee-Elkins C. Compatibility of ropivacaine with morphine, sufentanil, fentanyl or clonidine. J Clin Pharm Ther. 2002; 27:39–45.

Nafcillin Sodium

CONTAINER	Drug Manufacturer	Concentration	Diluents	Osmolality (mOsm/kg)	pH[e]	Storage Conditions					Body Temp	Refer.
						Temperature			Post-thaw Temp			
						Room	Refrig	Frozen	Room	Refrig		
Ethyvinyl Acetate (EVA)	APC	10 mg/mL	NS	n/a	e	3 d[c]	14 d	n/a	n/a	n/a	n/a	1, 6
Polyvinyl Chloride (PVC)	WY	20 mg/mL	NS	361	e	3 d[h]	24 d[h]	n/a	n/a	n/a	n/a	1
	WY	20 mg/mL	D5W	334	e	24 h[h]	4 d[h]	30 d	24 h	n/a	n/a	1
	WY	20 mg/mL	D5W	n/a	n/a	7 d[h]	15 d[h]	n/a	n/a	n/a	n/a	1
	MAR	20, 120 mg/mL	W	n/a	e	3 d	14 d	n/a	n/a	n/a	n/a	1
Syringes, Polypropylene	APC	10 mg/mL	NS	n/a	e	7 d	44 d	n/a	n/a	n/a	n/a	1
Syringe (Glass)	WY	250 mg/mL	unspec.	n/a	n/a	n/a	n/a	9 m	n/a	n/a	n/a	1
OTHER INFUSION CONTAINERS												
AccuFlo™/ AccuFlux™/ AccuRX® (B. Braun)	unspec.	10 mg/mL	NS	n/a	n/a	24 h[i]	3 d[i]	n/a	n/a	n/a	n/a	3
AutoDose (Tandem Medical)	APC	10 mg/mL	NS	n/a	e	3 d[c]	14 d	n/a	n/a	n/a	n/a	1, 6
CADD® Cassette (Pharmacia Deltec)	MAR	20, 120 mg/mL	W	n/a	n/a	3 d	14 d	n/a	n/a	n/a	n/a	1
	WY	80 mg/mL	W, NS	n/a	n/a	48 h	24 h[g]	n/a	n/a	n/a	n/a	1
Homepump®/ Homepump Eclipse® (I-Flow Corp.)	unspec.	10 mg/mL	NS	n/a	e	24 h	3 d	n/a	n/a	n/a	n/a	4

continued on next page

258

Nafcillin Sodium (cont'd)

Drug Manufacturer	Concentration	Diluents	Osmolality (mOsm/kg)	pH[e]	Storage Conditions						Refer.
					Temperature			Post-thaw Temp			
					Room	Refrig	Frozen	Room	Refrig	Body Temp	
INFUSOR (Baxter)											
BR	10 mg/mL	D5W	n/a	n/a	3 d[f]	14 d[f]	n/a	n/a	n/a	n/a	2
BR	10–40 mg/mL	D5W	n/a	e	48 h[a]	14 d[a]	n/a	n/a	n/a	n/a	2
INTERMATE (Baxter)											
BR	5 mg/mL	D5W	n/a	n/a	24 h	10 d	30 d	24 h	n/a	n/a	2
BR	5–40 mg/mL	D5W, NS	n/a	e	24 h	10 d	30 d	24 h	n/a	n/a	2
Unspecified											
n/a	250 mg/mL	W	n/a	e	n/a	n/a	3 m	n/a	n/a	n/a	1
COMMERCIAL PREPARATIONS (RTU)											
Galaxy Bag (Baxter)											
SKB	20 mg/mL	D	300	6–8.5	n/a	n/a	b, d	72 h[b]	21 d[b]	n/a	1, 5

Flush Compatibility: Heparin lock flush and normal saline.[1]

Special Considerations: Precipitation was observed after 48 h in a solution incubated at 34° to 36°C, at concentrations ≥40 mg/mL in NS. Clinicians may consider limiting the medication in a pump reservoir container to a 24-h supply.[7]

Notes

[a]14 d refrigerated, followed by 48 h at room temperature.

[b]Expiration date per manufacturer's label. Do not extrapolate commercial premix stability data to extemporaneously compounded solutions.

[c]At 5 d, 90.3% ±1.8% of initial concentration remaining.

[d]Thaw at room temperature or under refrigeration. Do not force thaw. Do not refreeze.

[e]pH of reconstituted preparation is 6–8.5.[1]

[f]14 d refrigerated, followed by 3 d at room temperature.

[g]Followed by 48 h of simulated administration at 30°C.

[h]Concentrations of 2–40 mg/mL lose less than 10% potency in 24 h at room temperature or 96 h refrigerated in D5½S, D5W, NS. Consult specific manufacturer labeling since recommended stability periods vary.

[i]Manufacturer(s) extrapolated data from other sources.

References

1. Trissel LA. ASHP's Interactive Handbook on Injectable Drugs. Bethesda, MD: American Society of Health-System Pharmacists. Accessed 2012 Jul.
2. Intermate/Infusor Drug Stability Information. Deerfield, IL: Baxter Healthcare Corporation; October 2008.
3. Drug Stability Data Using Elastomeric Infusion Systems. B. Braun Medical Production Ltd. (Thailand); August 2011.
4. Stability Data for Drugs Using Homepump Disposable Elastomeric Infusion Systems. Lake Forest, CA: I-Flow Corporation; October 2009.
5. Nafcillin Injection USP in Galaxy® Container (PL 2040 Plastic) [prescribing information]. Deerfield, IL: Baxter Healthcare Corporation; January 2012.
6. Zhang Y, Trissel LA. Stability of ampicillin sodium, nafcillin sodium, and oxacillin sodium in AutoDose Infusion System bags. Int J Pharm Compound. 2002; 6(3):226–9.
7. Chan V. Letters: influence of temperature and drug concentration on nafcillin precipitation. Am J Health-Syst Pharm. 2005; 62:1347–8.

Octreotide Acetate

	Drug Manufacturer	Concentration	Diluents	Osmolality (mOsm/kg)	pH[c]	Storage Conditions					Body Temp	Refer.
						Temperature			Post-thaw Temp			
						Room	Refrig	Frozen	Room	Refrig		
CONTAINER												
Polyvinyl Chloride (PVC)	SZ	1.5 mcg/mL	NS	n/a	c	48 h[a]	n/a	n/a	n/a	n/a	n/a	1
	SZ	5, 50, 250 mcg/mL	NS	n/a	c	96 h[f]	n/a	n/a	n/a	n/a	n/a	1
Syringes, Plastic	SZ	100, 500 mcg/mL[b]	undiluted	n/a	3.9–4.5	n/a	30 d	n/a	n/a	n/a	n/a	1
	SZ	200 mcg/mL[e]	undiluted	n/a	3.9–4.5	1 w[d]	29 d[d]	n/a	n/a	n/a	n/a	1
	SZ	200 mcg/mL[e]	undiluted	n/a	3.9–4.5	1 w[f]	15 d[f]	n/a	n/a	n/a	n/a	1
	SZ	200 mcg/mL[g]	undiluted	n/a	3.9–4.5	8 d[d]	60 d[h]	60 d[h]	n/a	n/a	n/a	1, 2
OTHER INFUSION CONTAINERS												
MiniMed	SZ	unspec.	undiluted	n/a	3.9–4.5	14 d	n/a	n/a	n/a	n/a	14 d[i]	2
Syringe (Baxter)	SZ	100, 500 mcg/mL[b]	undiluted	n/a	3.9–4.5	n/a	30 d	n/a	n/a	n/a	n/a	1

Flush Compatibility: Heparin lock flush and normal saline.[1]
Special Considerations: n/a

Notes

[a]At ambient room light.
[b]In Travenol Minimed and Becton Dickinson polypropylene syringes with natural rubber.
[c]pH of undiluted solution is 3.9–4.5.[1]
[d]Protected from light.
[e]In polypropylene syringes with tip caps (both Becton Dickinson).
[f]Not protected from light.
[g]Undiluted in polypropylene syringes (Terumo) with tip caps.
[h]Light conditions unknown.
[i]At 40°C.

References

1. Trissel LA. ASHP's Interactive Handbook on Injectable Drugs. Bethesda, MD: American Society of Health-System Pharmacists. Accessed 2012 May.
2. Linda DeMarzo, R.Ph., MLS, Medical Information Specialist [manufacturer's letter]. East Hanover, NJ: Novartis; November 12, 1999.

Ondansetron Hydrochloride

Container	Drug Manufacturer	Concentration	Diluents	Osmolality (mOsm/kg)	pH[k]	Temperature Room	Temperature Refrig	Temperature Frozen	Post-thaw Temp Room	Post-thaw Temp Refrig	Body Temp	Refer.
CONTAINER												
Polyvinyl Chloride (PVC)	GL	0.016, 0.08 mg/mL	D5W, NS	n/a	k	7 d[a]	7 d[a]	n/a	n/a	n/a	n/a	1
	GL	0.03, 0.3 mg/mL	D5W, NS	n/a	k	48 h	14 d	3 m	n/a	n/a	n/a	1
	GL	0.08 mg/mL	NS	n/a	k	n/a	120 d	120 d	n/a	n/a	n/a	1
	CER	0.1, 0.2, 0.4, 0.64 mg/mL	NS	n/a	k	48 h[c]	30 d[c]	n/a	n/a	n/a	n/a	1
	CER	0.1, 0.2, 0.4, 0.64 mg/mL[b]	NS	n/a	k	48 h[c]	30 d[c]	n/a	n/a	n/a	n/a	1, 4
	GL	0.15 mg/mL[g]	NS	n/a	k	28 d	28 d	n/a	n/a	n/a	n/a	1, 6
	GL	0.15 mg/mL[g]	D5W	n/a	k	3 d	28 d	n/a	n/a	n/a	n/a	1
	GL	0.75 mg/mL[n]	NS	n/a	k	7 d	28 d	n/a	n/a	n/a	n/a	1
Syringes, Polypropylene	unspec.	0.25, 0.5, 1 mg/mL	D5W, NS	n/a	k	48 h	14 d	90 d	48 h	14 d	n/a	1
	unspec.	2 mg/mL	undiluted	281	k	48 h	14 d	90 d	48 h	14 d	n/a	1
Unspecified	GL	0.024, 0.096 mg/mL	D5W, NS, LR	n/a	k	14 d	14 d[l]	n/a	n/a	n/a	n/a	1
	GL	0.1, 1 mg/mL[d]	NS	n/a	k	31 d	31 d	n/a	n/a	n/a	7 d[e]	1
OTHER INFUSION CONTAINERS												
AccuFlo™/ AccuFlux™/ AccuRX® (B. Braun)	unspec.	0.03–0.3 mg/mL	NS, D5W	n/a	k	n/a	14 d[i]	n/a	n/a	n/a	n/a	7
CADD®-1 Cassette (Pharmacia Deltec)	GL	0.24 mg/mL	NS	n/a	k	n/a	30 d[f]	n/a	n/a	n/a	24 h[f,h]	1
Homepump®/ Homepump Eclipse® (I-Flow Corp.)	GL	0.03, 0.3 mg/mL	D5W, NS	n/a	k	n/a	14 d	n/a	n/a	n/a	n/a	1, 5

continued on next page

261

Ondansetron Hydrochloride (cont'd)

| Drug Manufacturer | Concentration | Diluents | Osmolality (mOsm/kg) | pH[k] | Storage Conditions | | | | | | Refer. |
| | | | | | Temperature | | | Post-thaw Temp | | Body Temp | |
					Room	Refrig	Frozen	Room	Refrig		
INTERMATE (Baxter)	GL	0.1–0.7 mg/mL	D5W, NS	n/a	k	24 h[i]	10 d[i]	n/a	n/a	n/a	12 h[i]	3
Polyester Container (CR3)	CER	0.64 mg/mL[b]	D5W	n/a	k	48 h[c]	30 d[c]	n/a	n/a	n/a	n/a	1, 4
COMMERCIAL PREPARATIONS (RTU)											
INTRAVIA Plastic Container (Baxter)	BA	0.64 mg/mL	NS	iso[m]	3.3–4	n/a	n/a	n/a	n/a	n/a	n/a	2

Flush Compatibility: Heparin lock flush and normal saline.[1]
Special Considerations: n/a

Notes

[a] Exposed to light.
[b] With dexamethasone 0.2 and 0.4 mg/mL (ES).
[c] 30 d refrigerated followed by 48 h at room temperature.
[d] With morphine sulfate (AST) 1 mg/mL, hydromorphone HCl (ES) 0.5 mg/mL, or meperidine HCl (WY) 4 mg/mL.
[e] At 32°C to simulate infusion next to body.
[f] 30 d refrigerated, followed by 24 h at 30°C.
[g] With dexamethasone sodium phosphate (MSD) 0.4 mg/mL.
[h] At 30°C to simulate infusion next to body.
[i] 10 d refrigerated, followed by 24 h at room temperature, followed by 12 h at 33°C.
[j] Manufacturer(s) extrapolated data from other sources.
[k] pH of undiluted solutions is 3.3–4.[1]
[l] 14 d refrigerated, followed by 2 d at room temperature.
[m] Expiration date per manufacturer's label. Do not extrapolate commercial premix stability data to extemporaneously compounded solutions.
[n] With dexamethasone sodium phosphate (MSD) 0.23 mg/mL.

continued on next page

Ondansetron Hydrochloride (cont'd)

References

1. Trissel LA. ASHP's Interactive Handbook on Injectable Drugs. Bethesda, MD: American Society of Health-System Pharmacists. Accessed 2012 Aug.

2. Ondansetron Injection USP in Intravia Plastic Container [product information]. Deerfield, IL: Baxter Healthcare Inc.; April 2010.

3. Intermate/Infusor Drug Stability Information. Deerfield, IL: Baxter Healthcare Corporation; October 2008.

4. Hagan RL, Mallett MS, Fox JL. Stability of ondansetron hydrochloride and dexamethasone sodium phosphate in infusion bags and syringes for 32 days. Am J Health-Syst Pharm. 1996; 53:1431–5.

5. Stability Data for Drugs Using Homepump Disposable Elastomeric Infusion Systems. Lake Forest, CA: I-Flow Corporation; October 2009.

6. Evrard B, Ceccato A, Gaspard O, et al. Stability of ondansetron hydrochloride and dexamethasone sodium phosphate in 0.9% sodium chloride injection and 5% dextrose injection. Am J Health-Syst Pharm. 1997; 54:1065–8.

7. Drug Stability Data Using Elastomeric Infusion Systems. B. Braun Medical Production Ltd. (Thailand); August 2011.

Oprelvekin (Interleukin-11)

	Drug Manufacturer	Concentration	Diluents	Osmolality (mOsm/kg)	pH	Storage Conditions						
						Temperature			Post-thaw Temp		Body Temp	Refer.
						Room	Refrig	Frozen	Room	Refrig		
OTHER INFUSION CONTAINERS												
Glass	WY	5 mg/mL	W	iso	7.0[1]	24 h[a]	24 h[a]	n/a	n/a	n/a	n/a	1, 2
Glass[b,c]	WY	5 mg/mL	W	n/a	7.0[1]	3 h	3 h	n/a	n/a	n/a	n/a	1

Flush Compatibility: n/a

Special Considerations: Unreconstituted product should be stored at 2–8°C. Do not freeze or shake the reconstituted preparation. Avoid excessive or vigorous agitation.[1]

Notes

[a]Product remains physically and biochemically stable for 24 h after reconstitution. Manufacturer recommends use within 3 h to ensure against microbial contamination. Storage in syringes is not recommended.

[b]Original glass vials.

[c]Manufacturer states that storage in the original vial up to 3 d at room temperature 25°C (77°F), 60% relative humidity, should not have an adverse effect on the product in terms of quality, purity, or potency.[2,3]

References

1. Neumega® [product information]. Philadelphia, PA: Wyeth Pharmaceuticals; January 2011.
2. Lewis J [personal communication]. Philadelphia, PA: Global Medical Communications, Wyeth; August 12, 2002.
3. Pfizer Medical Information [personal communication]. New York, NY: Medical Information, Pfizer; January 2012.

Oxacillin Sodium

continued on next page

Container	Drug Manufacturer	Concentration	Diluents	Osmolality (mOsm/kg)	pH[e]	Temperature Room	Temperature Refrig	Temperature Frozen	Post-thaw Temp Room	Post-thaw Temp Refrig	Body Temp	Refer.
CONTAINER												
Ethylvinyl Acetate (EVA)	APC	10 mg/mL	NS	321	7.73	7 d[d]	30 d[d]	n/a	n/a	n/a	n/a	1, 6
Glass	SZ	166.67 mg/mL	W	g	n/a	3 d	7 d	n/a	n/a	n/a	n/a	1, 7
Polyvinyl Chloride (PVC)	BR	1 mg/mL	D5W, NS	n/a	e	n/a	24 h	n/a	n/a	r/a	n/a	1
	BR	10 mg/mL	D5W	295	e	n/a	24 h	30 d	24 h	r/a	n/a	1
Syringes, Plastic	BR	8.33, 16.67, 33.33 mg/mL	NS	311, 345, 414	e	24 h	8 d	30 d	n/a	n/a	n/a	1, 5
	BR	8.33, 16.67, 33.33 mg/mL	D5W	288, 322, 390	e	24 h	8 h	30 d	n/a	n/a	n/a	1, 5
	BR	200 mg/mL[b]	W	g	e	n/a	n/a	3 m	n/a	n/a	n/a	1
OTHER INFUSION CONTAINERS												
AccuFlo™/AccuFlux™/AccuRX® (B. Braun)	unspec.	10–100 mg/mL	NS	g	e	7 d[a]	8 d[a]	30 d[a]	n/a	n/a	n/a	4
	unspec.	10–100 mg/mL	D5W	g	e	2 d[a]	8 d[a]	30 d[a]	n/a	n/a	n/a	4
AutoDose (Tandem Medical)	APC	10 mg/mL	NS	321	7.73	7 d	30 d	n/a	n/a	n/a	n/a	1, 6
ADD-Vantage® (Abbott)	unspec.	unspec.	NS	n/a	e	3 d[h]	n/a	n/a	n/a	n/a	n/a	1
	unspec.	unspec.	D5W	n/a	e	24 h[h]	n/a	n/a	n/a	n/a	n/a	1
CADD® Cassette (SIMS Deltec)[f]	MAR	120 mg/mL	W	n/a	e	3 d	14 d	n/a	n/a	n/a	n/a	1
Homepump Eclipse®/ Homepump® C-Series (I-Flow Corp.)	unspec.	10–30 mg/mL	D5W	n/a	e	n/a	4 d[a]	n/a	n/a	n/a	n/a	8
	unspec.	10–100 mg/mL	NS	n/a	e	4 d[a]	7 d[a]	n/a	n/a	n/a	n/a	8
	unspec.	10–100 mg/mL	D5W	n/a	e	n/a	n/a	30 d	n/a	n/a	n/a	8

Oxacillin Sodium (cont'd)

Drug Manufacturer	Concentration	Diluents	Osmolality (mOsm/kg)	pH[e]	Temperature			Post-thaw Temp		Body Temp	Refer.
					Room	Refrig	Frozen	Room	Refrig		
INTERMATE/ INFUSOR (Baxter)											
BR	10–80 mg/mL	D5W, NS	n/a	e	24 h	10 d	30 d	24 h	n/a	n/a	2
BR	40 mg/mL	W	n/a	n/a	n/a	10 d	n/a	n/a	n/a	n/a	2
Unspecified											
BR	1, 10, 50 mg/mL	D5W, NS	n/a	e	24 h	n/a	n/a	n/a	n/a	n/a	1
unspec.	10–30 mg/mL	D5W	g	e	n/a	4 d	n/a	n/a	n/a	n/a	1, 7
SZ	10–100 mg/mL	W, NS	g	e	4 d	7 d	n/a	n/a	n/a	n/a	1, 7
SZ	10–100 mg/mL	D5W	g	n/a	n/a	n/a	30 d	n/a	n/a	n/a	1, 7
SZ	50–100, 166.67 mg/mL	W	g	n/a	n/a	n/a	30 d	n/a	n/a	n/a	7
unspec.	100 mg/mL[b]	NS, 1/2S	n/a	e	3 d	7 d	n/a	n/a	n/a	n/a	1
SZ	100 mg/mL	NS	g	e	n/a	n/a	30 d	n/a	n/a	n/a	7
COMMERCIAL PREPARATIONS (RTU)											
Galaxy Bag (Baxter)											
BA	20, 40 mg/mL	D	300	6–8.5	n/a	n/a	c	48 h[c]	21 d[c]	n/a	1, 3

Flush Compatibility: Heparin lock flush and normal saline.[1]
Special Considerations: Oxacillin sodium can be extremely irritating to veins at higher concentrations.

Notes

[a]Manufacturer(s) extrapolated data from other sources.
[b]At concentrations used for direct IM or IV injection.[1]
[c]Frozen expiration date per manufacturer's label. Do not extrapolate commercial premix stability data to extemporaneously compounded solutions.
[d]Protected from light.
[e]pH of 10 mg/mL is 7.4–7.94 in D5W and 7.73 in NS.[1]
[f]Portable reservoir is PVC material.
[g]166 mg/mL (BR) in W is 596 mOsm/kg by freezing-point depression and 657 mOsm/kg by vapor pressure. 50 mg/mL (BE) is 381 mOsm/kg in D5W and 396 mOsm/kg in NS.[1]
[h]After activation.

continued on next page

Oxacillin Sodium (cont'd)

References

1. Trissel LA. ASHP's Interactive Handbook on Injectable Drugs. Bethesda, MD: American Society of Health-System Pharmacists. Accessed 2012 Jan.
2. *Intermate/Infusor Drug Stability Information.* Deerfield, IL: Baxter Healthcare Corporation; 2008.
3. Oxacillin Injection, USP in Plastic Container [package insert]. Deerfield, IL: Baxter Healthcare; April 2011.
4. *Drug Stability Data Using Elastomeric Infusion Systems.* B. Braun Medical Production Ltd. (Thailand); August 2011.
5. Rapp RP, Hatton J, Record K. *Drug Stability in Plastic Syringes.* HealthTek™ and University of KY Lexington; Repro-Med Systems Inc.; 1998.
6. Yanping Z, Trissel LA. Stability of ampicillin sodium, nafcillin sodium, and oxacillin sodium in AutoDose infusion system bags. *Int J Pharm Compound.* 2002; 6:(3)226–9.
7. Oxacillin [product information]. Princeton, NJ: Sandoz Inc.; July 2011.
8. *Stability Data for Drugs Using Homepump Disposable Elastomeric Infusion Systems.* Lake Forest, CA: I-Flow Corporation; October 2009.

Oxaliplatin

| CONTAINER | Drug Manufacturer | Concentration | Diluents | Osmolality (mOsm/kg) | pH | Storage Conditions | | | | | | Refer. |
| | | | | | | Temperature | | | Post-thaw Temp | | Body Temp | |
						Room	Refrig	Frozen	Room	Refrig		
Glass Vial[f]	SAV	5 mg/mL[a,e]	W, D5W	n/a	n/a	6 h[b]	24 h[b]	n/a	n/a	n/a	n/a	3
INTERMATE (Baxter)	SW	0.1–1 mg/mL[b,c]	D5W	n/a	n/a	28 d	28 d[d]	n/a	n/a	n/a	n/a	6
Polyethylene	SAV	0.2, 1.3 mg/mL	D5W	n/a	n/a	14 d	14 d	n/a	n/a	n/a	n/a	5
Polyolefin	AVE	0.25 mg/mL	D5W	n/a	n/a	90 d	90 d	n/a	n/a	n/a	n/a	2, 4
	SAV	0.7 mg/mL	D5W	n/a	n/a	30 d	30 d	n/a	n/a	n/a	n/a	1, 2
Polypropylene	SAV	0.2, 1.3 mg/mL	D5W	n/a	n/a	14 d	14 d	n/a	n/a	n/a	n/a	5
Polyvinyl Chloride (PVC)	SAV	0.2, 1.3 mg/mL	D5W	n/a	n/a	14 d	14 d	n/a	n/a	n/a	n/a	5
Unspecified	SAV	3 mg/mL[a]	D5W	n/a	n/a	5 d[b]	n/a	n/a	n/a	n/a	n/a	2
	SAV	unspec.[a]	D5W	n/a	n/a	6 h	24 h	n/a	n/a	n/a	n/a	3

Flush Compatibility: Incompatible with normal saline, heparinized saline flush, alkaline drugs, and chloride-containing solutions. Flush administration line with D5W before and after oxaliplatin administration.[2,3]

Special Considerations: Do not freeze. Do not use needles or sets containing aluminum.[2]

Notes

[a]Total dose must be diluted in 250–500 mL D5W prior to administration.

[b]Protect from light.

[c]Avoid concentrations less than 0.1 mg/mL.

[d]Followed by 9 d at 25°C.

[e]Must be further diluted.

[f]Original vial.

References

1. Andre P, Cisternino S, Roy A, et al. Stability of oxaliplatin in infusion bags containing 5% dextrose injection. Am J Health-Syst Pharm. 2007; 64:1950–4.
2. Trissel LA. ASHP's Interactive Handbook on Injectable Drugs. Bethesda, MD: American Society of Health-System Pharmacists. Accessed 2012 Jul.
3. Eloxatin® [prescribing information]. Bridgewater, CT: Sanofi-Aventis US LLC; December 2011.
4. Junker A, Roy S, Desroches MC, et al. Stability of oxaliplatin solution. Ann Pharmacother. 2009; 43:390–1.
5. Eiden C, Philibert L, Bekhtari K, et al. Physicochemical stability of oxaliplatin in 5% dextrose injection stored in polyvinyl chloride, polyethylene and polypropylene infusion bags. Am J Health-Syst Pharm. 2009; 66:1929–33.
6. Intermate/Infusor Drug Stability Information. Deerfield, IL: Baxter Healthcare Corporation; October 2008.

Oxytocin

| CONTAINER | Drug Manufacturer | Concentration | Diluents | Osmolality (mOsm/kg) | pH[a] | Storage Conditions | | | | | | Refer. |
| | | | | | | Temperature | | | Post-thaw Temp | | Body Temp | |
						Room	Refrig	Frozen	Room	Refrig		
Polyvinyl Chloride (PVC)	APP	0.08 units/mL	NS, D5W	n/a	a	90 d[b]	n/a	n/a	n/a	n/a	n/a	1
	APP	0.08 units/mL	LR	n/a	a	28 d[b]	n/a	n/a	n/a	n/a	n/a	1

Flush Compatibility: Heparin lock flush and normal saline.[1]

Special Considerations: n/a

Notes

[a]*pH of undiluted product is 3–5.*[1]

[b]*Protected from light.*

Reference

1. Trissel LA. ASHP's Interactive Handbook on Injectable Drugs. Bethesda, MD: American Society of Health-System Pharmacists. Accessed 2012 May.

Paclitaxel

Container	Drug Manufacturer	Concentration	Diluents	Osmolality (mOsm/kg)	pH	Room	Refrig	Frozen	Room	Refrig	Body Temp	Refer.
Glass	TE	0.3 mg/mL	NS	n/a	f	3 d	13 d	n/a	n/a	n/a	n/a	1, 6
	TE	0.3 mg/mL	D5W	n/a	f	7 d	20 d	n/a	n/a	n/a	n/a	1, 6
	TE	1.2 mg/mL	NS	n/a	f	5 d	8 d	n/a	n/a	n/a	n/a	1, 6
	TE	1.2 mg/mL	D5W	n/a	f	7 d	10 d	n/a	n/a	n/a	n/a	1, 6
Polyethylene[e] (B. Braun)	TE	0.3 mg/mL	NS	n/a	f	3 d	16 d	n/a	n/a	n/a	n/a	1, 6
	TE	0.3 mg/mL	D5W	n/a	f	3 d	18 d	n/a	n/a	n/a	n/a	1, 6
	BMS	0.4, 1.2 mg/mL	D5W	n/a	a	5 d	5 d	n/a	n/a	n/a	n/a	1
	TE	1.2 mg/mL	NS	n/a	f	3 d	12 d	n/a	n/a	n/a	n/a	1, 6
	TE	1.2 mg/mL	D5W	n/a	f	3 d	12 d	n/a	n/a	n/a	n/a	1, 6
Polyolefin[g] (Baxter)	TE	0.3 mg/mL	NS, D5W	n/a	f	3 d	13 d	n/a	n/a	n/a	3 d[h]	1, 6
	TE	1.2 mg/mL	NS	n/a	f	3 d	9 d	n/a	n/a	n/a	3 d[h]	1, 6
	TE	1.2 mg/mL	D5W	n/a	f	3 d	10 d	n/a	n/a	n/a	3 d[h]	1, 6
Polyolefin (McGaw)	BR	0.1, 1 mg/mL	D5W, NS	n/a	a	3 d	3 d	n/a	n/a	n/a	3 d[b]	1
	MJ	1 mg/mL	D5W[c]	n/a	a	7 d[d]	7 d[d]	n/a	n/a	n/a	7 d[b]	2
OTHER INFUSION CONTAINER												
AccuFlo™/AccuFlux™/AccuRX® (B. Braun)	unspec.	6 mg/mL	NS, D5W	n/a	a	7 d	7 d	n/a	n/a	n/a	n/a	7

(Storage Conditions columns: Temperature = Room, Refrig, Frozen; Post-thaw Temp = Room, Refrig; Body Temp)

continued on next page

Flush Compatibility: Heparin lock flush and normal saline.¹
Special Considerations: Precipitation may be exacerbated by the use of peristaltic pumps. Volumetric pumps may reduce this problem.³,⁴,⁵ Since the mechanism of this irregular precipitation has not been identified, care and vigilance are required throughout the infusion.¹ Precipitation is sporadic and unpredictable. Containers and administration sets should not contain DEHP plasticizer.¹

270

Paclitaxel (cont'd)

Notes

[a]pH of 0.6, 1.2 mg/mL in D5W, NS or D5LR is 4.4–5.6.[1]

[b]At 32°C.

[c]Solution contains 20–25% ethanol.

[d]Author recommends maximum 7 d stability due to unpredictability of precipitation. Studies showed stability up to 14 d.

[e]Ecoflac® low density polyethylene bag. Melsungen, Germany; B Braun Melsungen AG.

[f]pH range for all solutions tested was 3.49–4.16.

[g]Viaflo® polyolefin bag. Berkshire UK: Baxter Healthcare.

[h]Protected from light.

References

1. Trissel LA. ASHP's Interactive Handbook on Injectable Drugs. Bethesda, MD: American Society of Health-System Pharmacists. Accessed 2012 Aug.
2. Trissel LA, Xu Q, Martinez JF. Compounding an extended-stability admixture of paclitaxel for long-term infusion. Int J Pharm Compound. 1997; 1:49–53.
3. Woloschuk DM. Drug precipitation and peristaltic pumps. Am J Hosp Pharm. 1994; 51:1473.
4. Pfeifer RW, Hale KN. Precipitation of paclitaxel during infusion by pump. Am J Hosp Pharm. 1993; 50:2518, 2521.
5. Trissel LA. Pharmaceutical properties of paclitaxel and their effects on preparation and administration. Pharmacotherapy. 1997; 17(5 suppl):133S–139S.
6. Donyai P, Sewell GJ. Physical and chemical stability of paclitaxel infusions in different container types. J Oncol Pharm Practice. 2006; 12:211–22.
7. Drug Stability Data Using Elastomeric Infusion Systems. B. Braun Medical Production Ltd. (Thailand); August 2011.

Pantoprazole Sodium

CONTAINER	Drug Manufacturer	Concentration	Diluents	Osmolality (mOsm/kg)	pH	Storage Conditions						Refer.
						Temperature			Post-thaw Temp			
						Room	Refrig	Frozen	Room	Refrig	Body Temp	
Polyvinyl Chloride (PVC)	NY[a]	0.16–0.8 mg/mL[a]	NS	n/a	h	6 h[a,e]	20 d[a,e]	n/a	n/a	n/a	n/a	2
	NY[a]	0.16–0.8 mg/mL[a]	D5W	n/a	h	8 h[a,f]	11 d[a,f]	n/a	n/a	n/a	n/a	2
	SZ[b]	0.4 mg/mL[b]	D5W	n/a	n/a	2 d[b,d]	14 d[b,d]	n/a	n/a	n/a	n/a	4
	SZ[b]	0.4, 0.8 mg/mL[b]	NS	n/a	n/a	3 d[b,d]	28 d[b,d]	n/a	n/a	n/a	n/a	4
	SZ[b]	0.8 mg/mL[b]	D5W	n/a	n/a	3 d[b,d]	28 d[b,d]	n/a	n/a	n/a	n/a	4
	NY[a]	0.8 mg/mL[a]	NS	n/a	h	28 h[a,g]	10 d[a,g]	n/a	n/a	n/a	n/a	2
Syringes, Polypropylene	SZ[b]	4 mg/mL[b]	NS	n/a	n/a	n/a	28 d[b,d]	n/a	n/a	n/a	n/a	4
	WY[b]	4 mg/mL[b]	NS	n/a	c	4 d[b]	4 d[b]	n/a	n/a	n/a	n/a	3
Unspecified	PH[b]	0.4 mg/mL[b]	NS	n/a	n/a	8 d[b]	n/a	n/a	n/a	n/a	n/a	3
	PH[b]	0.4 mg/mL[b]	D5W	n/a	n/a	4 d[b]	n/a	n/a	n/a	n/a	n/a	3

Flush Compatibility: Normal saline.[1]
Special Considerations: The U.S. formulation of Protonix® I.V. contains EDTA.[1] The Canadian formulation of Panto® I.V. contains EDTA.[5]

Notes

[a]Formulated with EDTA.
[b]Formulated without EDTA.
[c]pH of reconstituted Protonix® I.V.[a] in NS is 9.0–10.5.[1]
[d]Protected from light.
[e]Stored at 4°C for 20 d, followed by 6 h at 23°C.
[f]Stored at 4°C for 11 d, followed by 8 h at 23°C.
[g]Stored at 4°C for 10 d, followed by 28 h at 23°C.
[h]pH of 1% aqueous Panto® I.V.[a] Solution is 10.05; pH of 10% aqueous solution is 10.85.[5]

References

1. Protonix® I.V. [prescribing information]. Philadelphia, PA: Wyeth Pharmaceuticals; May 2012.[a]
2. Walker S, Iazzetta J, Law S. Extended stability of pantoprazole for injection in 0.9% sodium chloride or 5% dextrose at 4°C and 23°C. Can J Hosp Pharm. 2009; 62(2):135–41.[a]
3. Trissel LA. ASHP's Interactive Handbook on Injectable Drugs. Bethesda, MD: American Society of Health-System Pharmacists. Accessed 2012 Aug.
4. Donnelly RF. Stability of pantoprazole sodium in glass vials, polyvinyl chloride minibags, and polypropylene syringes. Can J Hosp Pharm. 2011; 64(3):192–8.[b]
5. Panto® I.V. [product monograph]. Oakville, ON: Nycomed Canada, Inc.; January 2012.[a]

Peginterferon alfa-2a

Peginterferon alfa-2a

Storage Conditions

Container	Drug Manufacturer	Concentration	Diluents	Osmolality (mOsm/kg)	pH	Temperature Room	Temperature Refrig	Temperature Frozen	Post-thaw Temp Room	Post-thaw Temp Refrig	Body Temp	Refer.
Syringes, Plastic (BD)[a]	RC	180 mcg/mL	undiluted	n/a	[c]	n/a	5 w[b]	n/a	n/a	n/a	n/a	1

Flush Compatibility: n/a
Special Considerations: n/a

Notes

[a]*Becton Dickinson tuberculin syringes with Monoject® 27 ga ¹/₂″ needle.*
[b]*Protected from light; stored at 5°C.*
[c]*The pH of the undiluted solution is 5.5–6.5.*[2]

References

1. Christopher Pecci, RN, C. [personal communication]. Nutley, NJ: Roche Pharmaceuticals; November 25, 2002.
2. Pegasys® [product information]. Nutley, NJ: Roche; September 2011.

Pemetrexed Disodium

CONTAINER	Drug Manufacturer	Concentration	Diluents	Osmolality (mOsm/kg)	pH[b]	Storage Conditions						Refer.
						Temperature			Post-thaw Temp		Body Temp	
						Room	Refrig	Frozen	Room	Refrig		
Polyvinyl Chloride (PVC)	LI	2, 10, 20 mg/mL	NS, D5W	n/a	b	48 h	24 h[a]	n/a	n/a	n/a	n/a	1, 3, 4
Syringes, Polypropylene	LI	25 mg/mL	NS	n/a	b	2 d	31 d[c]	n/a	n/a	n/a	n/a	2, 4

Flush Compatibility: Normal saline, heparin.[4]

Special Considerations: Avoid freezing. Incompatible with calcium-containing solutions (e.g., LR).[3]

Notes

[a]Although no loss occurred in 31 d by HPLC, unidentified microparticulates developed when refrigerated or frozen in PVC bags.[3]

[b]The pH of reconstituted product is 6.6–7.8. Further dilution is required.[4]

[c]Protected from light.

References

1. Zhang Y, Trissel LA. Physical and chemical stability of pemetrexed in infusion solutions. *Ann Pharmacotherapy.* 2006; 40:1082–5.
2. Zhang Y, Trissel LA. Physical and chemical stability of pemetrexed solutions in plastic syringes. *Ann Pharmacotherapy.* 2005; 39:2026–8.
3. Zhang Y, Trissel LA. Physical instability of frozen pemetrexed in PVC bags. *Ann Pharmacotherapy.* 2006; 40:1289–92.
4. Trissel LA. ASHP's Interactive Handbook on Injectable Drugs. Bethesda, MD: American Society of Health-System Pharmacists. Accessed 2012 Jun.

Penicillin G Potassium

Container	Drug Manufacturer	Concentration	Diluents	Osmolality (mOsm/kg)	pH[c]	Temperature Room	Temperature Refrig	Temperature Frozen	Post-thaw Temp Room	Post-thaw Temp Refrig	Body Temp	Refer.
CONTAINER												
Polyvinyl Chloride (PVC)	SQ	10,000 units/mL	D5W	n/a	c	n/a	24 h	n/a	n/a	n/a	n/a	1
	SQ	10,000 units/mL	D5W	n/a	c	24 h	24 h	30 d	24 h	n/a	n/a	1
	PD	20,000 units/mL	NS	n/a	c	24 h	25 d[d]	25 d[e]	n/a	n/a	n/a	1
	unspec.	40,000 units/mL	D5W, NS	n/a	c	n/a	n/a	30 d	n/a	n/a	n/a	1
Syringes, Plastic	unspec.	16,667 units/mL	NS, D5W	328, 304	c	24 h	24 h	30 d	n/a	n/a	n/a	6
	unspec.	33,333 units/mL	NS, D5W	378, 355	c	24 h	24 h	30 d	n/a	n/a	n/a	6
Unspecified	unspec.	5,000 units/mL	NS, D5S	n/a	c	n/a	48 h	n/a	n/a	n/a	n/a	1
	unspec.	100,000 units/mL	D5W	501	c	48 h	48 h	n/a	n/a	n/a	n/a	1
	unspec.	100,000 units/mL	NS	527	c	n/a	48 h	n/a	n/a	n/a	n/a	1
OTHER INFUSION CONTAINERS												
AccuFlo™/ AccuFlux™/ AccuRX® (B. Braun)	unspec.	2,000 units/mL	NS	n/a	c	24 h[a]	4 d[a]	n/a	n/a	n/a	n/a	4
	unspec.	10,000 units/mL	D5W	n/a	c	24 h[a]	24 h[a]	30 d[a]	n/a	n/a	n/a	4
CADD® Cassette (SIMS Deltec)	unspec.	100,000 units/mL	D5W	501	c	48 h[a]	48 h[a]	n/a	n/a	n/a	n/a	1, 7
	MAR	100,000 units/mL	W	n/a	c	3 d	n/a	n/a	n/a	n/a	n/a	1, 7
	MAR	200,000 units/mL	W	n/a	c	3 d	14 d	n/a	n/a	n/a	n/a	1, 7
Homepump Eclipse®/ Homepump® C-Series (I-Flow Corp.)	PF	10,000 units/mL	D5W	n/a	c	24 h[a]	24 h[a]	30 d[a]	n/a	n/a	n/a	5
	PF	20,000 units/mL	NS	n/a	c	24 h[a]	4 d[a]	n/a	n/a	n/a	n/a	5
INTERMATE/ INFUSOR (Baxter)	PF	20,000– 60,000 units/mL	D5W	n/a	c	24 h	7 d	n/a	n/a	n/a	n/a	2
	PF	20,000–100,000 units/mL	NS	n/a	c	n/a	n/a	30 d	24 h	n/a	n/a	2
	PF	100,000 units/mL	D5W, NS	n/a	c	24 h	10 d	30 d	24 h	n/a	n/a	2

continued on next page

Penicillin G Potassium (cont'd)

					Storage Conditions						
					Temperature			Post-thaw Temp		Body	
Drug Manufacturer	Concentration	Diluents	Osmolality (mOsm/kg)	pH[c]	Room	Refrig	Frozen	Room	Refrig	Temp	Refer.
COMMERCIAL PREPARATIONS (RTU)											
Galaxy Bag (Baxter)	various	20,000, 40,000, 60,000 units/mL	D	300	5.5–8	n/a	n/a	b	24 h[b]	14 d[b]	n/a	1, 3

Flush Compatibility: Heparin lock flush and normal saline.[1]
Special Considerations: n/a

Notes

[a]Manufacturer(s) extrapolated data from other sources.
[b]Frozen expiration date per manufacturer's label. Do not extrapolate commercial premix stability data to extemporaneously compounded solutions.
[c]pH of reconstituted powder for injection is 6.0–8.5.[1]
[d]Stored at 4°C.
[e]Frozen at −7°C.[1]

References

1. Trissel LA. ASHP's Interactive Handbook on Injectable Drugs. Bethesda, MD: American Society of Health-System Pharmacists. Accessed 2012 Jun.
2. Intermate/Infusor Drug Stability Information. Deerfield, IL: Baxter Healthcare Corporation; 2008.
3. Penicillin G Potassium Injection USP in PL 2040 Plastic Container [package insert]. Deerfield, IL: Baxter Healthcare; March 2012.
4. Drug Stability Data Using Elastomeric Infusion Systems. B. Braun Medical Production Ltd. (Thailand); August 2011.
5. Stability Data for Drugs Using Homepump Disposable Elastomeric Infusion Systems. Lake Forest, CA: I-Flow Corporation; October 2009.
6. Rapp RP, Hatton J, Record K. Drug Stability in Plastic Syringes. Health Tek™ and University of KY Lexington; Repro-Med Systems Inc.; 1998.
7. A Pharmacy Handbook for Use with the CADD-Plus Ambulatory Pump. St. Paul, MN: SIMS Deltec Inc.; 1996.

Penicillin G Sodium

| | Drug Manufacturer | Concentration | Diluents | Osmolality (mOsm/kg) | pH[c] | Storage Conditions | | | | | | |
| | | | | | | Temperature | | | Post-thaw Temp | | Body Temp | Refer. |
						Room	Refrig	Frozen	Room	Refrig		
CONTAINER												
Polyvinyl Chloride (PVC)	GL	20,000 units/mL[a]	NS	n/a	c	n/a	56 d[a]	n/a	n/a	n/a	n/a	1
	GL	20,000, 80,000 units/mL	NS	n/a	c	n/a	48 h	n/a	n/a	n/a	n/a	1
	AY	50,000 units/mL	D5W	394	c	n/a	n/a	39 d	n/a	31 d	n/a	1
	SQ	180,000 units/mL	W	n/a	c	n/a	n/a	30 d	n/a	4 d	24 h[b]	1
OTHER INFUSION CONTAINERS												
CADD° Cassette (Pharmacia Deltec)	unspec.	50,000 units/mL	D5W	394	c	n/a	31 d	39 d	n/a	n/a	n/a	1
	MAR	100,000, 200,000 units/mL	W	n/a	c	3 d	n/a	n/a	n/a	n/a	n/a	1
Glass	unspec.		D5W, NS, W	n/a	c	24 h[d]	3–7 d[e]	n/a	n/a	n/a	n/a	1

Flush Compatibility: Heparin lock flush and normal saline.[1]

Special Considerations: The osmolality of 100,000 units/mL is 502 mOsm/kg in NS and 529 mOsm/kg in D5W.[1]

Notes

[a]Reconstituted with citrate buffer (pH 6.5–7.5). Reconstituting with citrate buffers having pH values of 6.5, 7.0, and 7.5 increases stability.[1]

[b]12–16% penicillin loss after 30 d frozen, followed by 4 d refrigerated, then 24 h at 37°C.

[c]pH of solutions range from 5–7.5.[1]

[d]Diluted in infusion solutions.

[e]After reconstitution.

Reference

1. Trissel LA. ASHP's Interactive Handbook on Injectable Drugs. Bethesda, MD: American Society of Health-System Pharmacists. Accessed 2012 Jan.

Pentamidine Isethionate

Container	Drug Manufacturer	Concentration	Diluents	Osmolality (mOsm/kg)	pH[b]	Temperature Room	Temperature Refrig	Temperature Frozen	Post-thaw Temp Room	Post-thaw Temp Refrig	Body Temp	Refer.
CONTAINER												
Polyvinyl Chloride (PVC)	APP	0.8–29.54 mg/mL	D5W	n/a	n/a	n/a	30 d	90 d[a]	n/a	n/a	n/a	3
	APP	0.842, 29.74 mg/mL	W	n/a	n/a	n/a	n/a	90 d	n/a	n/a	n/a	3
	APP	0.86, 29.14 mg/mL	NS	n/a	n/a	n/a	n/a	90 d	n/a	n/a	n/a	3
	LY	1, 2 mg/mL	D5W, NS	n/a	n/a	48 h	n/a	n/a	n/a	n/a	n/a	1
Syringes, Plastic	APP	0.8–96.65 mg/mL	D5W	c	b	n/a	30 d	120 d	n/a	n/a	n/a	3
	APP	0.933–91 mg/mL	W	c	b	n/a	30 d	120 d	n/a	n/a	n/a	3
	LY	50 mg/mL	NS	285	b	48 h	n/a	n/a	n/a	n/a	n/a	5
OTHER INFUSION CONTAINERS												
Glass Vials	APP	0.7–30.7 mg/mL	NS	n/a	n/a	n/a	n/a	90 d	n/a	n/a	n/a	3
	APP	0.93, 2.9, 93.4 mg/mL	W	c	b	n/a	30 d	90 d	n/a	n/a	n/a	3
	APP	50 mg/mL	W	n/a	n/a	48 h	90 d	90 d	n/a	n/a	n/a	3
	APP	91.9, 97.96 mg/mL	D5W	c	b	n/a	30 d	90 d	n/a	n/a	n/a	3
INTERMATE/ INFUSOR (Baxter)	LY	2 mg/mL	NS	n/a	n/a	24 h	10 d	n/a	n/a	n/a	n/a	2
	LY	2–6 mg/mL	D5W	n/a	n/a	24 h	10 d	30 d	24 h	n/a	n/a	2
	LY	2–6 mg/mL	NS	n/a	n/a	n/a	10 d	30 d	24 h	n/a	n/a	2
	LY	3 mg/mL	W	n/a	n/a	n/a	10 d	n/a	n/a	n/a	n/a	2
Unspecified	FUJ	60–100 mg/mL	W	c	5.4	48 h	n/a	n/a	n/a	n/a	n/a	1

Flush Compatibility: Normal saline.[1]
Special Considerations: Do not use sodium chloride 0.9% to reconstitute as precipitation will occur.[1]
For intravenous administration, give diluted in 50–250 mL D5W and infuse over 60–120 min.[4]
Reconstituted solution should be protected from light. Keep at room temperature (22°C to 30°C) to avoid crystallization.[4]

Notes

[a]Frozen stability was 89.5% of initial concentration after 120 d at 0.8965 mg/mL, 90% or greater of initial concentration at 120 d at 2.444 mg/mL.
[b]pH of reconstituted solutions at 60–100 mg/mL is 5.4 in W and 4.09–4.38 in D5W.[1]
[c]Osmolality of 100 mg/mL is 160 in W and 455 in D5W.[1]

continued on next page

Pentamidine Isethionate (cont'd)

References

1. Trissel LA. ASHP's Interactive Handbook on Injectable Drugs. Bethesda, MD: American Society of Health-System Pharmacists. Accessed 2012 May.

2. *Intermate/Infusor Drug Stability Information*. Deerfield, IL: Baxter Healthcare Corporation; 2008.

3. Yang P [letter]. Melrose Park, IL: American Pharmaceutical Partners; October 10, 2002.

4. Pentam® 300 [prescribing information]. Schaumburg, IL: APP Pharmaceuticals; March 2008.

5. Rapp RP, Hatton J, Record K. *Drug Stability in Plastic Syringes*. HealthTek™ and University of KY Lexington; Repro-Med Systems Inc.; 1998.

Piperacillin Sodium–Tazobactam Sodium

Piperacillin Sodium–Tazobactam Sodium[a]

CONTAINER	Drug Manufacturer	Concentration	Diluents	Osmolality (mOsm/kg)	pH[e]	Temperature			Post-thaw Temp			Refer.
						Room	Refrig	Frozen	Room	Refrig	Body Temp	
Polyvinyl Chloride (PVC)	PF	[g]	D5W, NS, W	n/a	e	24 h[f]	7 d[f]	n/a	n/a	n/a	n/a	6
	LE	80 mg/mL	D5W, NS	n/a	e	n/a	n/a	30 d	n/a	n/a	n/a	1
Syringes, Polypropylene	LE	150, 200 mg/mL	D5W, NS	n/a	e	24 h[f]	7 d[f]	30 d	n/a	7 d	n/a	1, 6
OTHER INFUSION CONTAINERS												
AccuFlo™/ AccuFlux™/ AccuRX (B. Braun)	unspec.	10–80 mg/mL	NS	n/a	e	24 h[h]	28 d[h]	n/a	n/a	n/a	n/a	5
	unspec.	18 mg/mL	D5W	n/a	e	7 d[h]	n/a	n/a	n/a	n/a	n/a	5
	unspec.	40 mg/mL	NS	n/a	e	24 h	7 d	n/a	n/a	n/a	n/a	5
ADD-Vantage (Hospira)	unspec.	unspec.	D5W, NS	n/a	e	24 h[b]	d	d	n/a	n/a	n/a	1
Homepump/ Homepump Eclipse (I-Flow Corp.)	unspec.	10–80 mg/mL	NS	n/a	e	24 h	28 d	n/a	n/a	n/a	n/a	4
	unspec.	18 mg/mL	D5W	n/a	e	7 d	n/a	n/a	n/a	n/a	n/a	4
INTERMATE (Baxter)	LE	10–80 mg/mL	D5W, NS	n/a	e	24 h	7 d	30 d	24 h	n/a	n/a	2
COMMERCIAL PREPARATIONS (RTU)												
Galaxy Bag	WY	45, 67.5 mg/mL	D5W	iso	5.5–6.8	n/a	n/a	c	24 h[c]	14 d[c]	n/a	3

Flush Compatibility: Heparin lock flush and normal saline.[1]

Special Considerations: Administer by intravenous infusion over at least 30 min after dilution to at least 50 mL in a compatible diluent.[1] Zosyn® brand in standard vials, Add-vantage, Galaxy bags, and pharmacy bulk packages was reformulated to include EDTA and sodium citrate, which acts as a buffer. Extended stability studies conducted prior to 2007 evaluated a formulation that did not contain EDTA.[7,8]

Notes

[a]Stated concentrations represent piperacillin content. Stability data applies to both components.

[b]After activation.

[c]Frozen expiration date per manufacturer's label. Do not extrapolate commercial premix stability data to extemporaneously compounded solutions.

continued on next page

Piperacillin Sodium–Tazobactam Sodium (cont'd)

[d]Do not refrigerate or freeze ADD-Vantage® vials.

[e]pH of solutions in vials is 4.5–6.8; pH of frozen premixed solution is 5.5–6.8.[1]

[f]ZOSYN® is chemically stable in glass and plastic containers (plastic syringes, I.V. bags, and tubing) when used with compatible diluents for up to 24 h at room temperature and up to 7 d refrigerated.[6]

[g]Reconstituted per manufacturer labeling; dose diluted in 50–150 mL NS, D5W or up to 50 mL W.[6]

[h]Manufacturer extrapolated data from other sources.

References

1. Trissel LA. ASHP's Interactive Handbook on Injectable Drugs. Bethesda, MD: American Society of Health-System Pharmacists. Accessed 2012 Jul.
2. Intermate/Infusor Drug Stability Information. Deerfield, IL: Baxter Healthcare Corporation; 2008.
3. Zosyn® (Piperacillin and Tazobactam Injection) in Galaxy® Containers (PL2040 Plastic) [product information]. Philadephia, PA: Wyeth Pharmaceuticals Inc.; March 2012.
4. Stability Data for Drugs Using Homepump Disposable Elastomeric Infusion Systems. Lake Forest, CA: I-Flow Corporation; October 2009.
5. Drug Stability Data Using Elastomeric Infusion Systems. B. Braun Medical Production Ltd. (Thailand); August 2011.
6. Zosyn® (Piperacillin and Tazobactam Injection) for Injection, USP [package insert]. Philadephia, PA: Pfizer Injectables; March 2012.
7. Medical Communications Product Information Specialist [personal communication]. Philadephia, PA: Wyeth Pharmaceuticals Inc.; January 2008.
8. Zosyn® Reformulation Information. Available at: http://www.zosyn.com/newformulation.asp. Accessed January 23, 2008.

Prochlorperazine[a]

	Drug Manufacturer	Concentration	Diluents	Osmolality (mOsm/kg)	pH	Storage Conditions						Refer.
						Temperature			Post-thaw Temp			
						Room	Refrig	Frozen	Room	Refrig	Body Temp	
CONTAINER												
Syringes, Plastic	RP	1.5 mg/mL[b]	NS	279	n/a	7 d	n/a	n/a	n/a	n/a	n/a	2
OTHER INFUSION CONTAINERS												
Glass Test Tubes	RP	2.5 mg/mL[c]	[c]	n/a	n/a	7 d	7 d	n/a	n/a	n/a	7 d	3

Flush Compatibility: Heparin lock flush and normal saline.[1]
Special Considerations: Protect from light.[1]

Notes

[a]Monograph contains stability data for mesylate and edisylate; see notes for details.
[b]Prochlorperazine MESYLATE with hydromorphone 0.5 mg/mL (Sabex).
[c]Equal volumes of prochlorperazine MESYLATE 5 mg/mL and hydromorphone 2 mg/mL, 10 mg/mL, or 40 mg/mL (KN).

References

1. Trissel LA. ASHP's Interactive Handbook on Injectable Drugs. Bethesda, MD: American Society of Health-System Pharmacists. Accessed 2012 Jan.
2. Trinkle R. Compatibility of hydromorphone and prochlorperazine, and irritation due to subcutaneous prochlorperazine infusion. *Ann Pharmacother.* 1997; 31:789–90.
3. Walker SE, Iazzetta J, De Angelis C, et al. Stability and compatibility of combinations of hydromorphone and dimenhydrinate, lorazepam or prochlorperazine. *Can J Hosp Pharm.* 1993; 46(2):61–5.

Quinupristin–Dalfopristin

| Drug Manufacturer | Concentration | Diluents | Osmolality (mOsm/kg) | pH | Storage Conditions | | | | | | Refer. |
| | | | | | Temperature | | | Post-thaw Temp | | Body Temp | |
					Room	Refrig	Frozen	Room	Refrig		
CONTAINER											
Unspecified	DSM	various[a]	D5W	n/a	n/a	5 h	54 h	n/a	n/a	n/a	n/a	1, 2
OTHER INFUSION CONTAINERS											
AccuFlo™/ AccuFlux™/ AccuRX® (B. Braun)	unspec.	2 mg/mL	D5W	n/a	n/a	5 h[b]	54 h[b]	n/a	n/a	n/a	n/a	4
Homepump®/ Homepump Eclipse® (I-Flow Corp.)	unspec.	2 mg/mL	D5W	n/a	n/a	5 h[b]	54 h[b]	n/a	n/a	n/a	n/a	3

Flush Compatibility: Not compatible with normal saline or heparin. Flush with D5W before and after administration.[1]

Special Considerations: Reconstituted solution may foam; allow foam to dissipate to a clear solution prior to further dilution.[1] Do not freeze. Infuse intravenously diluted in D5W over 60 min.[1] Dilute in 250 mL D5W; 100 mL may be used for central line infusions. If moderate to severe venous irritation occurs following peripheral administration, consider increasing infusion volume to 500–750 mL, changing the infusion site, or infusion by a central line.[1]

Notes

[a]Concentration of combined agents in 100 to 750 mL of diluent.[1]
[b]Manufacturer extrapolated data from other sources.

References

1. Synercid® IV [product information]. Greenville, NC: DSM Pharmaceuticals; November 2007.
2. Trissel LA. ASHP's Interactive Handbook on Injectable Drugs. Bethesda, MD: American Society of Health-System Pharmacists. Accessed 2012 Jan.
3. Stability Data for Drugs Using Homepump Disposable Elastomeric Infusion Systems. Lake Forest, CA: I-Flow Corporation; October 2009.
4. Drug Stability Data Using Elastomeric Infusion Systems. B. Braun Medical Production Ltd. (Thailand); August 2011.

Ranitidine Hydrochloride

continued on next page

Container	Drug Manufacturer	Concentration	Diluents	Osmolality (mOsm/kg)	pH^f	Storage Conditions						Refer.
						Temperature			Post-thaw Temp			
						Room	Refrig	Frozen	Room	Refrig	Body Temp	
CONTAINER												
Polyolefin	GL	0.441 mg/mL	D5W	n/a	f	n/a	n/a	30 d	n/a	10 d	n/a	1
Polyvinyl Chloride (PVC)	GL	0.05 mg/mL	D5W, D5½S	n/a	f	7 d^e	n/a	n/a	n/a	n/a	n/a	1
	GL	0.05 mg/mL	D10W	n/a	n/a	2 d	n/a	n/a	n/a	n/a	n/a	1
	GL	0.05 mg/mL	NS	n/a	n/a	28 d^e	n/a	n/a	n/a	n/a	n/a	1
	GL	0.05, 2 mg/mL	D5W, NS	n/a	f	48 h^e	n/a	n/a	n/a	n/a	n/a	1
	GL	0.5, 1, 2 mg/mL	D5½S NS, D5W, D10W, D5LR	n/a	f	7 d	30 d	n/a	n/a	n/a	n/a	1
	GL	0.5, 1, 2 mg/mL	D5W, NS D5½S, D10W	n/a	f	n/a	n/a	60 d	7 d	14 d	n/a	1
	GL	0.5, 1, 2 mg/mL	D5W, NS	n/a	f	28 d^e	n/a	30 d	n/a	14 d	n/a	1
	GL	1 mg/mL	D5W, NS	n/a	f	n/a	10 d	n/a	n/a	n/a	n/a	1
	GL	1 mg/mL	D5W, NS	260, 302	f	n/a	92 d	n/a	n/a	n/a	n/a	1
	GL	1 mg/mL	D5W, NS	260, 302	f	18 d	66 d	n/a	n/a	n/a	n/a	1
	GL	1.5 mg/mL	D5W, NS	n/a	f	n/a	7 d^d	30 d^a	n/a	24 h^a	24 h^{a,b,d}	1
	GL	2 mg/mL	D5W, NS	257, 294	f	n/a	n/a	100 d	n/a	n/a	n/a	1
Syringes, Plastic	GL	0.83 mg/mL^i	NS, D5W	282, 258	f	48 h	14 d	3 m	n/a	n/a	n/a	3
Syringes, Polypropylene	GL	2.5 mg/mL	BWFI	n/a	f	72 h	91 d	n/a	n/a	n/a	n/a	1
OTHER INFUSION CONTAINERS												
AccuFlo™/ AccuFlux™/ AccuRX® (B. Braun)	unspec.	0.5–2 mg/mL	D5W, NS	n/a	n/a	7 d^c	30 d^c	30 d^c	n/a	n/a	n/a	4

Ranitidine Hydrochloride (cont'd)

Drug	Manufacturer	Concentration	Diluents	Osmolality (mOsm/kg)	pH[f]	Storage Conditions						
						Temperature			Post-thaw Temp		Body Temp	Refer.
						Room	Refrig	Frozen	Room	Refrig		
Homepump Eclipse[i]/ Homepump® C-Series (I-Flow Corp.)	unspec.	0.5–2 mg/mL	D5W, NS	n/a	[f]	7 d[c]	30 d[c]	60 d[c]	n/a	n/a	n/a	2
Unspecified	GL	0.05, 0.1 mg/mL	NS	n/a	[j]	48 h[e]	n/a	n/a	n/a	n/a	n/a	1
	GL	0.1 mg/mL	NS	n/a	[j]	48 h	24 h[g]	n/a	n/a	n/a	n/a	1
	GSK	unspec.[j]	NS, D5W, D10W, LR	n/a	n/a	48 h	n/a	n/a	n/a	n/a	n/a	5
COMMERCIAL PREPARATIONS (RTU)												
Flexible Container (GSK)	GSK	1 mg/mL	½S	180	6.7–7.3	[h]	[h]	n/a	n/a	n/a	n/a	5

Flush Compatibility: Heparin lock flush and normal saline.[1]
Special Considerations: n/a

Notes

[a] 30 d frozen followed by 24 h at 3°C followed by 24 h at 30°C to simulate use conditions in infusion pump reservoirs.
[b] 24 h at 30°C.
[c] Manufacturer(s) extrapolated data from other sources.
[d] 7 d at 3°C followed by 24 h at 30°C.
[e] Tested under fluorescent light.
[f] pH of undiluted solution is 6.7–7.3.[1,5]
[g] Stored under refrigeration for 24 h followed by 24 h at 25°C with or without protection from light.
[h] Store between 2°C to 25°C. Expiration date per manufacturer's label. Do not extrapolate commercial premix stability data to extemporaneously compounded preparations.
[i] Prepared in 60-mL syringes.
[j] Zantac® injection is stable for 48 h at room temperature when added to or diluted with most commonly used IV solutions including D5W, D10W, LR, NS.[5]

References

1. Trissel LA. ASHP's Interactive Handbook on Injectable Drugs. Bethesda, MD: American Society of Health-System Pharmacists. Accessed 2013 Jan.
2. Stability Data for Drugs Using Homepump Disposable Elastomeric Infusion Systems. Lake Forest, CA: I-Flow Corporation; October 2009.
3. Rapp RP, Hatton J, Record K. Drug Stability in Plastic Syringes. HealthTek™ and University of KY Lexington; Repro-Med Systems Inc.; 1998.
4. Drug Stability Data Using Elastomeric Infusion Systems. B. Braun Medical Production Ltd. (Thailand); August 2011.
5. Zantac® [prescribing information]. Research Triangle Park, NC: GlaxoSmithKline; April 2009.

Rituximab

Storage Conditions

CONTAINER	Drug Manufacturer	Concentration	Diluents	Osmolality (mOsm/kg)	pH[b]	Temperature Room	Temperature Refrig	Temperature Frozen	Post-thaw Temp Room	Post-thaw Temp Refrig	Body Temp	Refer.
Polyethylene Bag	Biogen/GEN	1–4 mg/mL	NS, D5W	n/a	b	24 h[a]	24 h[a]	n/a	n/a	n/a	n/a	1
Polyvinyl Chloride (PVC)	Biogen/GEN	1–4 mg/mL	NS, D5W	n/a	b	24 h[a]	24 h[a]	n/a	n/a	n/a	n/a	1

Flush Compatibility: Normal saline.[1]

Special Considerations: Do not freeze or shake. Protect vials from direct sunlight. Keep vials refrigerated.

Notes

[a]Product labeling states that diluted solutions are chemically stable for 24 h under refrigeration and an additional 24 h at room temperature; however, due to lack of preservatives, refrigerated storage is recommended.

[b]The pH of undiluted product is 6.5.

Reference

1. Rituxan® [prescribing information]. South San Francisco, CA: Genentech USA; April 2011.

Ropivacaine Hydrochloride

continued on next page

	Drug Manufacturer	Concentration	Diluents	Osmolality (mOsm/kg)	pH[d]	Storage Conditions Temperature Room	Refrig	Frozen	Post-thaw Temp Room	Refrig	Body Temp	Refer.
CONTAINER												
Ethyvinyl Acetate (EVA)	ASZ	1.5 mg/mL	NS	f	d	51 d[e]	51 d[e]	n/a	n/a	n/a	n/a	1
Polypropylene Bag	ASZ	1, 2 mg/mL[b]	NS	f	d	n/a	n/a	n/a	n/a	n/a	30 d[c]	1, 2
Polyvinyl Chloride (PVC)	ASZ	1.5 mg/mL	NS	f	d	7 d[e]	7 d[e]	n/a	n/a	n/a	n/a	1
Syringes, Polypropylene	ASZ	1.2 mg/mL[a]	n/a	f	d	30 d	30 d	n/a	n/a	n/a	n/a	1, 3
OTHER INFUSION CONTAINERS												
Glass	ASZ	1.5 mg/mL	NS	f	d	51 d[e]	51 d[e]	n/a	n/a	n/a	n/a	1
INFUSOR (Baxter)	AST	1–10 mg/mL	NS	f	d	n/a	120 d[g]	n/a	n/a	n/a	7 d[g]	4
	AST	2 mg/mL[h]	NS	f	d	n/a	120 d[g]	n/a	n/a	n/a	7 d[g]	4

Flush Compatibility: n/a

Special Considerations: Ropivacaine hydrochloride solubility is reduced above pH of 6.[1] Commercially available solution of ropivacaine hydrochloride is isotonic.[1]

Notes

[a]Solution prepared with 3 mL ropivacaine hydrochloride 2 mg/mL and 2 mL 40 mg/mL methylprednisolone, for a final concentration of 1.2 mg/mL ropivacaine hydrochloride and 16 mg/mL methylprednisolone acetate.

[b]Solutions of ropivaicine hydrochloride 1 and 2 mg/mL tested with morphine sulfate 20 and 100 mcg/mL, sufentanil citrate 0.4 and 4 mcg/mL, fentanyl citrate 1 and 10 mcg/mL, and clonidine hydrochloride 5 and 50 mcg/mL in Mark II Polybags.

[c]Tested at 30°C in the dark.

[d]pH of the undiluted solution is 4–6.5.[1]

[e]Combined with fentanyl citrate 3 mcg/mL.

[f]Undiluted ropivacaine hydrochloride solutions are isotonic.[1,5]

[g]Stored at 2–8°C for 120 d, followed by 7 d at 33°C.

[h]Combined with morphine sulfate (Stellorphine) 0.025 mg/mL.

Ropivacaine Hydrochloride (cont'd)

References

1. Trissel LA. ASHP's Interactive Handbook on Injectable Drugs. Bethesda, MD: American Society of Health-System Pharmacists. Accessed 2012 May.
2. Svedberg KO, McKenzie J, Larrivee-Elkins C, et al. Compatibility of ropivacaine with morphine, sufentanil, fentanyl, or clonidine. *J Clin Pharm Ther.* 2002; 27(1):39–45.
3. Robustelli della Cuna FS, Mella M, Magistrali G. Stability and compatibility of methyprednisolone acetate and ropivacaine hydrocholoride in polypropylene syringes for epidural administration. *Am J Health-Syst Pharm.* 2001; 58(18):1753–6.
4. *Intermate/Infusor Drug Stability Information.* Deerfield, IL: Baxter Healthcare Corporation; October 2008.
5. Naropin® [product insert]. Schaumburg, IL: APP Pharmaceuticals; April 2010.

Sargramostim

					Storage Conditions						
					Temperature			Post-thaw Temp		Body	
Drug Manufacturer	Concentration	Diluents	Osmolality (mOsm/kg)	pH[b]	Room	Refrig	Frozen	Room	Refrig	Temp	Refer.
CONTAINER											
Polyvinyl Chloride (PVC) BAY	2.5, 8, 12 mcg/mL	NS[a]	n/a	[b]	48 h	48 h	n/a	n/a	n/a	n/a	1
Syringes, Plastic BAY	250, 500 mcg/mL	BWFI[d]	n/a	[b]	n/a	14 d	n/a	n/a	n/a	n/a	1, 2
OTHER INFUSION CONTAINERS											
Glass (Vial) BAY	250, 500 mcg/mL	W, BWFI[d]	n/a	[b]	30 d	30 d	n/a	n/a	n/a	n/a	1, 2
BAY	500 mcg/mL	undiluted[d]	n/a	[b]	n/a	20 d[c]	n/a	n/a	n/a	n/a	2, 3

Flush Compatibility: Heparin flush, normal saline.[2]

Special Considerations: Store liquid, reconstituted, and lyophilized product at 2°C to 8°C. Do not freeze. Dilute for intravenous infusions only with NS. Concentrations below 10 mcg/mL require the addition of albumin 1 mg per 1 mL of solution. Do not infuse through an inline membrane filter. Liquid product contains 1.1% benzyl alcohol.[3]

Notes

[a] Concentrations below 10 mcg/mL also contained 1 mg human albumin per 1 mL NS.
[b] pH of liquid product is 6.7–7.7. pH of reconstituted lyophilized product is 7.1–7.7.[3]
[c] Storage under refrigeration after initial vial entry.
[d] Do not administer preparations containing benzyl alcohol (including BWFI) to neonates.[3]

References

1. *Stability and Sterility of Leukine*® [personal communication]. Wayne, NJ: Bayer HealthCare Pharmaceuticals; January 23, 2008.
2. Trissel LA. ASHP's Interactive Handbook on Injectable Drugs. Bethesda, MD: American Society of Health-System Pharmacists. Accessed 2012 Jun.
3. Leukine® [prescribing information]. Cambridge, MA: Genzyme Corporation; July 2009.

Sufentanil Citrate

Sufentanil Citrate[a]

Container	Drug Manufacturer	Concentration	Diluents	Osmolality (mOsm/kg)	pH[m]	Temperature			Post-thaw Temp		Body Temp	Refer.
						Room	Refrig	Frozen	Room	Refrig		
CONTAINER												
Mark II Polybag	AST	0.4 mcg/mL	NS	n/a	m	30 d[i,j,k]	n/a	n/a	n/a	n/a	n/a	1, 6
	AST	4 mcg/mL	NS	n/a	m	30 d[i,j,k]	n/a	n/a	n/a	n/a	n/a	1, 6
Polyvinyl Chloride (PVC)[b]	JN	1 mcg/mL	NS	n/a	m	n/a	n/a	4 m[l]	n/a	70 d[l]	n/a	7
OTHER INFUSION CONTAINERS												
CADD® Cassette (SIMS Deltec)	JN	5 mcg/mL	D5W	n/a	m	n/a	30 d	n/a	n/a	n/a	30 d[c,d]	1, 3
	JN	5 mcg/mL	NS	n/a	m	n/a	21 d	n/a	n/a	n/a	21 d[d]	1, 2
	JN	5 mcg/mL	NS[e]	n/a	m	n/a	n/a	n/a	n/a	n/a	21 d[e,f]	4
	JN	5 mcg/mL[g]	NS	n/a	m	n/a	30 d	n/a	n/a	n/a	30 d[d,h]	3
	JN	20 mcg/mL[f]	f	n/a	m	10 d	10 d	n/a	n/a	n/a	10 d	1, 5
	JC	50 mcg/mL	undiluted	n/a	m	14 d	14 d	n/a	n/a	n/a	n/a	1
Polyethylene Bottle (Eur. Ph.)	JN	5 mcg/mL	NS	n/a	m	n/a	21 d	n/a	n/a	n/a	21 d[d]	1, 2

continued on next page

Flush Compatibility: Normal saline.[1]
Special Considerations: n/a

Notes

a Intraspinal infusion requires the use of preservative-free diluents and drug products.
b Sufentanil adsorbs to PVC containers.
c 5% loss in 7 d.
d Studied at 32°C.
e In citrate-buffered solution at pH 4.6, unbuffered solution lost 30% concentration in 24 h due to adsorption to container.
f Diluted with bupivacaine HCl 5 mg/mL to a final concentration of bupivacaine HCl 3 mg/mL; sufentanil concentration decreases below acceptable limits without bupivacaine additive.
g With bupivacaine HCl 2 mg/mL.
h 10% loss of sufentanil, 5% loss of bupivacaine at 32°C.
i Solution also contained ropivacaine HCl 1 mg/mL or 2 mg/mL.
j Storage at 30°C.

Sufentanil Citrate (cont'd)

[k]Protected from light.
[l]Combined with levobupivacaine 1.25 mg/mL; thawed in a validated cycle microwave prior to refrigerated storage.
[m]pH of the undiluted solution is 3.5–6.[1]

References

1. Trissel LA. ASHP's Interactive Handbook on Injectable Drugs. Bethesda, MD: American Society of Health-System Pharmacists. Accessed 2012 Jun.
2. Roos PH, Glerum JH, Meilink JW. Stability of sufentanil citrate in a portable pump reservoir, a glass container, and a polyethylene container. Pharm Weekly. 1992; 14(4):196–200.
3. Roos PJ, Glerum J, Schroeders MJH. Effect of glucose 5% solution and bupivacaine hydrochloride on absorbance of sufentanil citrate in a portable pump reservoir during storage and simulated infusion by an epidural catheter. Pharm World Sci. 1993; 15(6):269–75.
4. Roos PJ, Glerum JH, Meilink JW, et al. Effect of pH on absorptions of sufentanil citrate in a portable pump reservoir during drug storage and administration under simulated epidural conditions. Pharm World Sci. 1993; 15(3):139–44.
5. Brouwers JRB, Van Doorne H, Meevis RF, et al. Stability of sufentanil citrate and sufentanil citrate/bupivacaine mixture in portable infusion pumps. EHP. 1995; 1(1):12–4.
6. Svedberg KO, McKenzie EJ, Larrivee-Elkins C. Compatibility of ropivacaine with morphine, sufentanil, fentanyl or clonidine. J Clin Pharm Ther. 2002; 27:39–45.
7. Boitquin LP, Hecq JD, Vanbeckbergen DF, et al. Stability of sufentanil citrate with levobupivacaine HCl in NaCl 0.9% infusion after microwave freeze-thaw treatment. Ann Pharmacother. 2004; 38:1836–9.

Telavancin

Drug Manufacturer	Concentration	Diluents	Osmolality (mOsm/kg)	pH[b]	Storage Conditions					Refer.
					Temperature			Post-thaw Temp		Body Temp	
					Room	Refrig	Frozen	Room	Refrig		

CONTAINER

Unspecified	ASL	unspec.[a]	NS, D5W	n/a	n/a	4 h[b]	72 h[b]	n/a	n/a	n/a	n/a	1
Polyvinyl Chloride (PVC)	ASL	0.6, 8 mg/mL	NS, D5W, LR	n/a	n/a	12 h	7 d[c]	n/a	n/a	n/a	n/a	2
Glass Vial	ASL	250, 750 mg/mL	D5W, NS, W	n/a	d	12 h	7 d[c]	n/a	n/a	n/a	n/a	2

OTHER INFUSION CONTAINERS

Homepump°/ Homepump Eclipse° (I-Flow Corp.)	ASL	0.6 mg/mL	NS, D5W, LR	n/a	e	n/a	8 d	n/a	n/a	n/a	n/a	2
	ASL	8 mg/mL	NS, D5W, LR	n/a	f	n/a	8 d	n/a	n/a	n/a	n/a	2
INTERMATE/ INFUSOR (Baxter)	ASL	0.6 mg/mL	NS, D5W, LR	n/a	e	n/a	8 d	n/a	n/a	n/a	n/a	2
	ASL	8 mg/mL	NS, D5W, LR	r/a	f	n/a	8 d	n/a	n/a	n/a	n/a	2

Flush Compatibility: Normal saline.[1,2]

Special Considerations: Store original vials at refrigerated temperature. Excursions to ambient temperature are acceptable; avoid excessive heat. Reconstitute with NS, W, or D5W.[1]

Notes

[a] When mixed according to the package insert.[1]

[b] Product labeling states that total time in vial plus the time in the infusion bag should not exceed 4 h at room temperature and 72 h refrigerated.[1]

[c] Protected from light.[2]

[d] pH of reconstituted solution in vial is 4.0–5.0.[1]

[e] pH diluted to 0.6 mg/mL in NS was 5.1–5.3; in D5W was 4.7–4.8; in LR was 5.6–5.7.[2]

[f] pH diluted to 8 mg/mL in NS or LR was 4.8; in D5W was 4.4–4.6.[2]

References

1. VIBATIV° for injection [prescribing information.] Deerfield, IL: Astellas Pharma Inc.; January 2012.
2. Scientific and Medical Affairs [personal communication]. Deerfield, IL: Medical Communications, Astellas Scientific and Medical Affairs, Inc.; January 10, 2012.

Thiotepa

CONTAINER	Drug Manufacturer	Concentration	Diluents	Osmolality (mOsm/kg)	pH[b]	Storage Conditions						Refer.
						Temperature			Post-thaw Temp		Body Temp	
						Room	Refrig	Frozen	Room	Refrig		
Polyolefin Bag	IMM	5 mg/mL	D5W	c	b	3 d	14 d	n/a	n/a	n/a	n/a	2
Polyvinyl Chloride (PVC)	unspec.	0.25 mg/mL	NS	c	b	7 d	n/a	n/a	n/a	n/a	n/a	1
	IMM	0.5 mg/mL	NS	277	b	n/a	48 h[a]	n/a	n/a	n/a	n/a	2
	IMM	1, 3 mg/mL	NS	269, c	b	24 h	48 h	n/a	n/a	n/a	n/a	2
	IMM	5 mg/mL	D5W	c	b	3 d	14 d	n/a	n/a	n/a	n/a	2
Syringes, Plastic	unspec.	10 mg/mL	W	c	b	24 h	24 h	n/a	n/a	n/a	n/a	2

Flush Compatibility: Heparin lock flush and normal saline.[2]

Special Considerations: n/a

Notes

[a]Stored at 8°C.

[b]pH of reconstituted preparation is 5.5–7.5.[2]

[c]Dilutions of 0.5 and 1 mg/mL in NS are 277 and 269 mOsm/kg. Dilutions of 3 and 5 mg/mL in NS are hypotonic.[2]

References

1. Vyas HM, Baptista RJ, Mitrano FP, et al. Drug stability guidelines for a continuous infusion chemotherapy program. *Hosp Pharm.* 1987; 22:685–7.
2. Trissel LA. ASHP's Interactive Handbook on Injectable Drugs. Bethesda, MD: American Society of Health-System Pharmacists. Accessed 2012 Aug.

Ticarcillin Disodium–Clavulanate Potassium[a]

Drug Manufacturer	Concentration	Diluents	Osmolality (mOsm/kg)	pH[b]	Storage Conditions						Refer.
					Temperature			Post-thaw Temp		Body Temp	
					Room	Refrig	Frozen	Room	Refrig		
CONTAINER											
Unspecified											
GSK	10–100 mg/mL	W	f	b	24 h	4 d	n/a	n/a	n/a	n/a	1
GSK	10–100 mg/mL	D5W	g	b	24 h	3 d	7 d	8 h	n/a	n/a	1
GSK	10–100 mg/mL	NS, LR	h	b	24 h	4 d	30 d	8 h	n/a	n/a	1
Syringes, Plastic											
unspec.	52 mg/mL	NS, D5W	n/a	b	24 h	14 d	30 d	n/a	n/a	n/a	2
OTHER INFUSION CONTAINERS											
AccuFlo™/ AccuFlux™/ AccuRX® (B. Braun)	31 mg/mL	NS	n/a	b	24 h[c]	7 d[c]	n/a	n/a	n/a	n/a	4
Homepump®/ Homepump Eclipse® (I-Flow Corp.)	BE	31 mg/mL	NS	n/a	b	24 h	7 d	n/a	n/a	n/a	n/a	5
INTERMATE (Baxter)											
unspec.	10 mg/mL	NS	n/a	b	24 h[e]	10 d	n/a	n/a	n/a	n/a	6
unspec.	10–150 mg/mL	NS	n/a	b	20 h[e]	10 d	n/a	n/a	n/a	n/a	6
COMMERCIAL PREPARATIONS (RTU)											
Galaxy Bag (Baxter)											
BE	30 mg/mL	W	iso	b	n/a	n/a	d	24 h[d]	7 d[d]	n/a	3

Flush Compatibility: Heparin lock flush and normal saline.[1]
Special Considerations: n/a

Notes

[a]Stated concentrations represent ticarcillin content. Stability data applies to both components.
[b]pH of reconstituted solution is 5.5–7.5.[1]
[c]Manufacturer(s) extrapolated data from other sources.
[d]Frozen expiration per manufacturer's label. Do not extrapolate commercial premix stability data to extemporaneously compounded solutions.
[e]After 10 d refrigerated storage.

continued on next page

Ticarcillin Disodium–Clavulanate Potassium (cont'd)

f86 mg/mL in W is 573 mOsm.[1]
g48 mg/mL in D5W is 562 mOsm.[1]
h43 mg/mL in NS is 546 mOsm.[1]

References

1. Trissel LA. ASHP's Interactive Handbook on Injectable Drugs. Bethesda, MD: American Society of Health-System Pharmacists. Accessed 2012 Jun.
2. Rapp RP, Hatton J, Record K. Drug Stability in Plastic Syringes. HealthTek™ and University of KY Lexington; Repro-Med Systems Inc.; 1998.
3. Timentin® Injection in Galaxy® (PL 2040) Plastic Container [prescribing information]. Research Triangle Park, NC: GlaxoSmithKline; June 2011.
4. Drug Stability Data Using Elastomeric Infusion Systems. B. Braun Medical Production Ltd. (Thailand); August 2011.
5. Stability Data for Drugs Using Homepump Disposable Elastomeric Infusion Systems. Lake Forest, CA: I-Flow Corporation; October 2009.
6. Intermate/Infusor Drug Stability Information. Deerfield, IL: Baxter Healthcare Corporation; October 2008.

Tigecycline

CONTAINER	Drug Manufacturer	Concentration	Diluents	Osmolality (mOsm/kg)	pH	Storage Conditions							Refer.
						Temperature			Post-thaw Temp			Body Temp	
						Room	Refrig	Frozen	Room	Refrig			
IV Bag[a]	WY	0.5 mg/mL[b]	NS, D5W	n/a	n/a	18 h	48 h	n/a	n/a	n/a	n/a	1

Flush Compatibility: Heparin lock solution and normal saline.[2]

Special Considerations: The reconstituted solution should be yellow to orange in color; if not, the solution should be discarded. The reconstituted solution may be stored in the vial for up to 6 h at room temperature, then transferred to the IV bag and administered within 24 h.

Notes

[a]Unspecified type of infusion bag.
[b]Maximum concentration for IV bag should be 1 mg/mL.

References

1. Tygacil* [package insert]. Philadelphia, PA: Wyeth Pharmaceuticals Inc.; January 2011.
2. Trissel LA. ASHP's Interactive Handbook on Injectable Drugs. Bethesda, MD: American Society of Health-System Pharmacists. Accessed 2012 Jan.

Tobramycin Sulfate

Tobramycin Sulfate

continued on next page

Container	Drug Manufacturer	Concentration	Diluents	Osmolality (mOsm/kg)	pH	Temperature			Post-thaw Temp		Body Temp	Refer.
						Room	Refrig	Frozen	Room	Refrig		
CONTAINER												
Ethyvinyl Acetate (EVA)	GNS	0.95 mg/mL	NS	n/a	a	7 d	30 d	n/a	n/a	n/a	n/a	1
Polyvinyl Chloride (PVC)	LI	0.2–1 mg/mL	D5W, NS	n/a	a	48 h	n/a	n/a	n/a	n/a	n/a	1
	LI	3.2 mg/mL	D5W, NS	n/a	a	n/a	n/a	30 d	24 h	n/a	n/a	1
Syringes, Plastic	LI	40 mg/mL	undiluted	n/a	a	60 d	60 d	n/a	n/a	n/a	n/a	1
OTHER INFUSION CONTAINERS												
AccuFlo™/ AccuFlux™/ AccuRX® (B. Braun)	unspec.	0.2 mg/mL	NS	n/a	a	24 h[d]	7 d[d]	n/a	n/a	n/a	n/a	4
	unspec.	0.75 mg/mL	NS	n/a	a	24 h	14 d	n/a	n/a	n/a	n/a	4
	unspec.	0.8 mg/mL	NS	n/a	a	24 h[d]	14 d[d]	n/a	n/a	n/a	n/a	4
	unspec.	1 mg/mL	NS	n/a	a	7 d	7 d	n/a	n/a	n/a	n/a	4
	unspec.[b]	4 mg/mL[b]	NS, W	n/a	n/a	7 d	14 d	n/a	n/a	n/a	n/a	4
	unspec.	5 mg/mL	NS, W	n/a	a	7 d	14 d	n/a	n/a	n/a	n/a	4
AutoDose (Tandem Medical)	GNS	0.8, 0.95 mg/mL	NS	n/a	a	7 d	30 d	n/a	n/a	n/a	n/a	1
CADD® Cassette (SIMS Deltec)	LI	1, 10 mg/mL	NS	n/a	a	3 d	14 d	n/a	n/a	n/a	n/a	1
Homepump Eclipse®/ Homepump® C-Series (I-Flow Corp.)	BMS	0.2 mg/mL	NS	n/a	a	24 h	7 d	n/a	n/a	n/a	n/a	3
	BMS	0.8 mg/mL	NS	n/a	a	24 h	14 d	n/a	n/a	n/a	n/a	3

Storage Conditions

continued on next page

297

Tobramycin Sulfate (cont'd)

Drug Manufacturer	Concentration	Diluents	Osmolality (mOsm/kg)	pH	Storage Conditions					Body Temp	Refer.
					Temperature			Post-thaw Temp			
					Room	Refrig	Frozen	Room	Refrig		
INFUSOR (Baxter) LI	0.8–2.4 mg/mL	NS	n/a	a	21 d[c]	19 d[c]	n/a	n/a	n/a	n/a	2
INTERMATE (Baxter) LI	0.5 mg/mL	NS, D5W	n/a	a	24 h	n/a	n/a	n/a	n/a	n/a	2
LI	0.5 mg/mL	D5W	n/a	a	48 h[e]	7 d	n/a	n/a	n/a	n/a	2
LI	0.5–4.8 mg/mL	NS	n/a	a	24 h	10 d	n/a	n/a	n/a	n/a	2
LI	0.5–4.8 mg/mL	D5W	n/a	a	n/a	10 d	n/a	n/a	n/a	n/a	2
LI	0.5–5 mg/mL	NS	n/a	a	48 h[e]	7 d	n/a	n/a	n/a	n/a	2
LI	0.5–5 mg/mL	D5W	n/a	a	24 h[e]	7 d	n/a	n/a	n/a	n/a	2
LI	4.8 mg/mL	D5W	n/a	a	n/a	n/a	30 d	24 h	n/a	n/a	2

Flush Compatibility: Normal saline. Incompatible with heparin.[1]

Special Considerations: The osmolality of typical dilutions in NS or D5W ranges from 285–319 mOsm/kg.[1]

Notes

[a]pH of the undiluted solution is 3–6.5.[1]

[b]Tobramycin HCl.

[c]19 d refrigerated followed by 21 d at room temperature.

[d]Manufacturer extrapolated data from other source(s).

[e]Following 7 d refrigerated.

References

1. Trissel LA. ASHP's Interactive Handbook on Injectable Drugs. Bethesda, MD: American Society of Health-System Pharmacists. Accessed 2012 Jan.
2. Intermate/Infusor Drug Stability Information. Deerfield, IL: Baxter Healthcare Corporation; October 2008.
3. Stability Data for Drugs Using Homepump Disposable Elastomeric Infusion Systems. Lake Forest, CA: I-Flow Corporation; October 2009.
4. Drug Stability Data Using Elastomeric Infusion Systems. B. Braun Medical Production Ltd. (Thailand); August 2011.

Tocilizumab

Tocilizumab

Drug Manufacturer	Concentration	Diluents	Osmolality (mOsm/kg)	pH	Storage Conditions						Refer.
					Temperature			Post-thaw Temp			
					Room	Refrig	Frozen	Room	Refrig	Body Temp	
CONTAINER											
Unspecified[a]	GEN	unspec.[b]	NS	n/a	[c]	24 h[d]	24 h[d,e]	n/a	n/a	n/a	n/a	1

Flush Compatibility: Normal saline.

Special Considerations: For preparation of final administration solution, withdraw a volume of NS equal to the volume of the dose of tocilizumab, then slowly add the medication to the infusion bag or bottle; mix gently and avoid foaming.[1]

Notes

[a]Diluted solutions are compatible with polypropylene, polyethylene, and polyvinyl chloride infusion bags and polypropylene, polyethylene, and glass infusion bottles.[1]

[b]Follow dilution instructions in 50 mL or 100 mL NS specific to dosing and indication.[1]

[c]pH of undiluted 20 mg/mL solution is about 6.5.[1]

[d]Protected from light.[1]

[e]Allow to reach room temperature prior to infusion.[1]

Reference

1. Actemra® [prescribing information]. South San Francisco, CA: Genentech; April 2011.

299

Topotecan Hydrochloride

Container	Drug Manufacturer	Concentration	Diluents	Osmolality (mOsm/kg)	pH[d]	Storage Conditions						Refer.
						Temperature			Post-thaw Temp		Body Temp	
						Room	Refrig	Frozen	Room	Refrig		
CONTAINER												
Polyolefin	SKB	50 mcg/mL	D5W, NS	n/a	d	24 h	7 d[a]	n/a	n/a	n/a	n/a	2, 4
Polyvinyl Chloride (PVC)	SKB	10, 25, 50 mcg/mL	D5W, NS	n/a	d	28 d[a]	28 d[a]	n/a	n/a	n/a	n/a	3, 4
	unspec.	10–500 mcg/mL	D5W, NS	n/a	d	4 d	n/a	n/a	n/a	n/a	n/a	4
	SKB	25, 50 mcg/mL	D5W, NS	n/a	d	24 h	7 d[a]	n/a	n/a	n/a	n/a	2, 4
OTHER INFUSION CONTAINERS												
Glass Bottles (McGaw)	SKB	25, 50 mcg/mL	NS, D5W	n/a	d	24 h	7 d[a]	n/a	n/a	n/a	n/a	2, 4
Glass Vials	SKB	1,000 mcg/mL	W	n/a	d	28 d[a]	28 d[a]	n/a	n/a	n/a	28 d[c]	1, 4
INFUSOR LV-2 (Baxter)	SKB	10, 25, 50 mcg/mL	D5W, NS	n/a	d	28 d[a]	28 d[a]	n/a	n/a	n/a	5 d[a,b]	3, 4

Flush Compatibility: Normal saline.[4]
Special Considerations: Manufacturer recommends use immediately after reconstitution because the product contains no antibacterial preservative.[4]

Notes

[a]Protected from light.
[b]5 d following storage at room temperature.
[c]Stored at 30°C.
[d]pH of reconstituted product is 2.5–3.5.[4]

References

1. Patel K, Craig SB, McBride MG, et al. Microbial inhibitory properties and stability of topotecan hydrochloride injection. *Am J Health-Syst Pharm.* 1998; 55:1584–7.
2. Craig SB, Bhatt UH, Patel K. Stability and compatibility of topotecan hydrochloride for injection with common infusion solutions and containers. *J Pharm Biomed Anal.* 1997; 16:199–205.
3. Kramer I, Thiesen J. Stability of topotecan infusion solutions in polyvinyl chloride bags and elastomeric portable infusion devices. *J Oncol Pharm Practice.* 1999; 5:75–82.
4. Trissel LA. ASHP's Interactive Handbook on Injectable Drugs. Bethesda, MD: American Society of Health-System Pharmacists. Accessed 2012 Jun.

Trastuzumab

CONTAINER	Drug Manufacturer	Concentration	Diluents	Osmolality (mOsm/kg)	pH[d]	Temperature			Post-thaw Temp		Body Temp	Refer.
						Room	Refrig	Frozen	Room	Refrig		
Glass Vial	GEN	21 mg/mL	W[b]	n/a	6	n/a	28 d[b]	c	n/a	n/a	n/a	1
Polyethylene Bag	GEN	unspec.[a]	NS	n/a	d	n/a	24 h	c	n/a	n/a	n/a	1
Polyvinyl Chloride (PVC)	GEN	unspec.[a]	NS	n/a	d	n/a	24 h	c	n/a	n/a	n/a	1

(Storage Conditions)

Flush Compatibility: Saline.[1]

Special Considerations: Do not mix with dextrose 5% solution. Do not administer undiluted solutions; do not administer IV push or bolus.[1] Do not mix with other medications,[1] including heparin.

Notes

[a]Concentrations will vary; calculated dosage should be added to 250 mL NS IV bag.
[b]Bacteriostatic Water for Injection. If reconstituted with unpreserved W, use immediately and discard unused portion.
[c]Do not freeze reconstituted or diluted solutions.[1]
[d]pH of product reconstituted with W or BWFI to 21 mg/mL is about 6.[1]

Reference

1. Herceptin® [package insert]. South San Francisco, CA: Genentech Inc.; October 2010.

Treprostinil

Storage Conditions

Container	Drug Manufacturer	Concentration	Diluents	Osmolality (mOsm/kg)	pH[c]	Temperature Room	Temperature Refrig	Temperature Frozen	Post-thaw Temp Room	Post-thaw Temp Refrig	Body Temp	Refer.
CONTAINER												
Polyvinyl Chloride (PVC)	UTC	0.004 mg/mL	W, NS	n/a	[c]	n/a	n/a	n/a	n/a	n/a	48 h	1, 4
	UTC	0.02 mg/mL	D5W	n/a	[c]	n/a	n/a	n/a	n/a	n/a	48 h	1, 4
	UTC	0.13 mg/mL	W, NS, D5W	n/a	[c]	n/a	n/a	n/a	n/a	n/a	48 h	1, 4
	UTC	1, 2.5, 5, 10 mg/mL	undiluted	n/a	6–7.2[1]	n/a	n/a	n/a	n/a	n/a	72 h	2
Syringes, Polypropylene	UTC	≥0.004 mg/mL	W, NS	n/a	[c]	n/a	n/a	n/a	n/a	n/a	48 h	2
	UTC	1, 2.5, 5, 10 mg/mL	undiluted	n/a	6–7.2[1]	n/a	n/a	n/a	n/a	n/a	72 h	2
OTHER INFUSION CONTAINERS												
MiniMed Plastic Syringe Pump Reservoir	UTC	1, 2.5, 5, 10 mg/mL	undiluted	n/a	6–7.2[1]	60 d	60 d[b]	60 d[b]	n/a	n/a	60 d[b]	1, 3
Sims Deltec Cassette	UTC	0.004 mg/mL, 0.13 mg/mL	NS	n/a	[c]	n/a	n/a	n/a	n/a	n/a	48 h[a]	1
	UTC	0.02 mg, 0.13 mg/mL	D5W	n/a	[c]	n/a	n/a	n/a	n/a	n/a	48 h[a]	1
Syringes, Glass	UTC	1, 2.5, 5, 10 mg/mL	undiluted	n/a	6–7.2[1]	n/a	n/a	n/a	n/a	n/a	72 h	2

Flush Compatibility: n/a

Special Considerations: Infusion should not be interrupted.

Notes

[a]Tested at 40°C.

[b]Samples stored in refrigerator, freezer, and incubator were protected from light.

[c]pH of undiluted solution is 6–7.2.[1]

References

1. Trissel LA. ASHP's Interactive Handbook on Injectable Drugs. Bethesda, MD: American Society of Health-System Pharmacists. Accessed 2012 Jan.
2. Remodulin® [product information]. Research Triangle Park, NC: United Therapeutics Corp.; February 2011.
3. Xu QA, Trissel LA, Pham L. Physical and chemical stability of treprostinil sodium injection packaged in plastic syringe pump reservoirs. Int J Pharm Compound. 2004; 8(3):230.
4. Phares KR, Weiser WE, Miller SP, et al. Stability and preservative effectiveness of treprostinil sodium after dilution in common intravenous diluents. Am J Health-Syst Pharm. 2003; 60(May 1):916.

Valproate Sodium

Storage Conditions

Container	Drug Manufacturer	Concentration	Diluents	Osmolality (mOsm/kg)	pH[a]	Temperature Room	Temperature Refrig	Temperature Frozen	Post-thaw Temp Room	Post-thaw Temp Refrig	Body Temp	Refer.
CONTAINER												
Polyethylene (Polyolefin)	SW	1.6 mg/mL	D5W, NS, LR	n/a	a	6 d	n/a	n/a	n/a	n/a	n/a	2
Polyvinyl Chloride (PVC)	SW	1.6 mg/mL	D5W, LR, NS	n/a	a	6 d	n/a	n/a	n/a	n/a	n/a	2
	AB	unspec.	D5W, NS, LR	n/a	a	24 h	n/a	n/a	n/a	n/a	n/a	1
OTHER INFUSION CONTAINERS												
Glass	AB	unspec.	D5W, NS, LR	n/a	a	24 h	n/a	n/a	n/a	n/a	n/a	1
	SW	1.6 mg/mL	D5W, NS, LR	n/a	a	6 d	n/a	n/a	n/a	n/a	n/a	2

Flush Compatibility: Normal saline.[1,2]

Special Considerations: Administer IV over at least 60 min with maximum rate of 20 mg/min, diluted in at least 50 mL of a compatible solution.[1,2]

Note

[a]pH of undiluted solution is 7.6.[2]

References

1. Depacon® [prescribing information]. North Chicago, IL: Abbott Laboratories; November 2009.
2. Trissel LA. ASHP's Interactive Handbook on Injectable Drugs. Bethesda, MD: American Society of Health-System Pharmacists. Accessed 2012 May.

Vancomycin Hydrochloride

continued on next page

Storage Conditions

Container	Drug Manufacturer	Concentration	Diluents	Osmolality (mOsm/kg)	pH[e]	Temperature Room	Temperature Refrig	Temperature Frozen	Post-thaw Temp Room	Post-thaw Temp Refrig	Body Temp	Refer.
CONTAINER												
Ethyvinyl Acetate (EVA)	APP	10 mg/mL	NS	n/a	e	7 d	30 d	n/a	n/a	n/a	n/a	1
Glass	LI	5 mg/mL	D5W, NS	249, 291	e	17 d	63 d	n/a	n/a	n/a	n/a	1
Polyvinyl Chloride (PVC)	LI	5 mg/mL	D5W, NS	249, 291	e	17 d	n/a	n/a	n/a	n/a	n/a	1
	LI	5, 10 mg/mL	D5W	n/a	e	n/a	58 d	n/a	n/a	n/a	n/a	1
Syringes, Plastic	unspec.	8.33 mg/mL	NS, D5W	287, 264	e	24 h	17 d	17 d	n/a	n/a	n/a	5
	LI	10 mg/mL	D5W, NS, W	n/a	e	29 d[a]	84 d	n/a	n/a	n/a	n/a	1
	unspec.	16.67 mg/mL	NS, D5W	297, 274	e	24 h	17 d	17 d	n/a	n/a	n/a	5
Syringes, Polypropylene	unspec.	5 mg/mL	D5W, NS	n/a	e	14 d	6 m[b]	n/a	n/a	n/a	n/a	1
OTHER INFUSION CONTAINERS												
AccuFlo™/ AccuFlux™/ AccuRX® (B. Braun)	unspec.	4 mg/mL	NS	n/a	e	24 h[d]	14 d[d]	n/a	n/a	n/a	n/a	4
	unspec.	5 mg/mL	NS	n/a	e	24 h	14 d	n/a	n/a	n/a	n/a	4
	unspec.	5 mg/mL	D5W	n/a	e	17 d[d]	63 d[d]	n/a	n/a	n/a	n/a	4
	unspec.	5–15 mg/mL	NS	n/a	e	24 h[d]	28 d[d]	n/a	n/a	n/a	n/a	4
AutoDose (Tandem Medical)	APP	10 mg/mL	NS	n/a	e	7 d	30 d	n/a	n/a	n/a	n/a	1
CADD® Cassette (SIMS Deltec)	AB	20, 40 mg/mL	D5W	n/a	e	4 d	30 d	n/a	n/a	n/a	n/a	1
Homepump Eclipse®/ Homepump® C-Series (I-Flow Corp.)	unspec.	5 mg/mL	D5W	249[1]	e	17 h[d]	63 d[d]	n/a	n/a	n/a	n/a	3
	unspec.	5 mg/mL	NS	n/a	e	24 h	14 d	n/a	n/a	n/a	n/a	3
	unspec.	5, 10, 15 mg/mL	NS	n/a	e	24 h	28 d	n/a	n/a	n/a	n/a	3

Vancomycin Hydrochloride (cont'd)

Drug Manufacturer	Concentration	Diluents	Osmolality (mOsm/kg)	pH[e]	Storage Conditions						Refer.
					Temperature			Post-thaw Temp			
					Room	Refrig	Frozen	Room	Refrig	Body Temp	
INFUSOR (Baxter)											
LI	10–20 mg/mL	D5W	n/a	e	3 d[f]	17 d	n/a	n/a	n/a	n/a	2
INTERMATE (Baxter)											
LI	10–20 mg/mL	NS, D5W	n/a	e	24 h	10 d	30 d	24 h	n/a	n/a	2
LI	10–20 mg/mL	D5W	n/a	e	n/a	n/a	31 d	24 h	n/a	n/a	2
LI	15 mg/mL	W	n/a	e	n/a	10 d	n/a	n/a	n/a	n/a	2
COMMERCIAL PREPARATIONS (RTU)											
Galaxy Bag (Baxter)											
LI	5 mg/mL	D	iso	3–5	n/a	n/a	c	72 h[c]	30 d[c]	n/a	6

Flush Compatibility: Normal saline. Incompatible with heparin.[1]

Special Considerations: Administer higher concentrations via a central line to avoid irritation; administration durations >90 min may be required if Redman syndrome develops.

Notes

[a]Chemical degradation was dependent on the diluent. This is the shortest time in which the drug degraded 10%.

[b]Stable for 48 h warmed to room temperature after refrigeration.

[c]Frozen expiration date per manufacturer's label. Do not extrapolate commercial premix stability data to extemporaneously compounded solutions. Thaw at room temperature or under refrigeration. Do not force thaw. Do not refreeze.

[d]Manufacturers extrapolated data from other sources.

[e]pH of the undiluted solution is 3.8–6. pH of reconstituted preparation in W or NS is 3.9. pH of a 5% solution in W is 2.5–4.5.[1]

[f]Following 17 d refrigerated storage.

References

1. Trissel LA. ASHP's Interactive Handbook on Injectable Drugs. Bethesda, MD: American Society of Health-System Pharmacists. Accessed 2012 Jan.
2. Intermate/Infusor Drug Stability Information. Deerfield, IL: Baxter Healthcare Corporation; 2008.
3. Stability Data for Drugs Using Homepump Disposable Elastomeric Infusion Systems. Lake Forest, CA: I-Flow Corporation; October 2009.
4. Drug Stability Data Using Elastomeric Infusion Systems. B. Braun Medical Production Ltd. (Thailand); August 2011.
5. Rapp RP, Hatton J, Record K. Drug Stability in Plastic Syringes. HealthTek™ and University of KY Lexington. Chester, NY: Repro-Med Systems Inc.; 1998.
6. Vancomycin injection USP in Galaxy Plastic Container [package insert]. Deerfield, IL: Baxter Healthcare; February 2008.

VinBLAStine Sulfate

Container	Drug Manufacturer	Concentration	Diluents	Osmolality (mOsm/kg)	pH[b]	Temperature Room	Temperature Refrig	Temperature Frozen	Post-thaw Temp Room	Post-thaw Temp Refrig	Body Temp	Refer.
CONTAINER												
Polyvinyl Chloride (PVC)	LI	0.1 mg/mL	NS, D5W	n/a	b	n/a	7 d[a]	n/a	n/a	n/a	n/a	6
	LI	0.15 mg/mL	NS	n/a	b	8 d	n/a	n/a	n/a	n/a	n/a	1
Syringes, Plastic	LI	1 mg/mL	W	n/a	b	30 d	30 d	n/a	n/a	n/a	n/a	2
Syringes, Polypropylene	LI	1 mg/mL	NS	n/a	b	30 d[a]	n/a	n/a	n/a	n/a	n/a	3, 6
	DB	1 mg/mL	unspec.	n/a	b	23 d[a]	31 d[a]	n/a	n/a	n/a	n/a	6
OTHER INFUSION CONTAINERS												
Glass Vials	LI	1 mg/mL	W	n/a	b	n/a	21 d[a]	4 w	n/a	n/a	n/a	4
INFUSOR (Baxter)	LI	0.015 mg/mL	NS	n/a	b	n/a	77 d[c]	n/a	n/a	n/a	2 d[c]	5
Polypropylene Test Tubes	LI	20 mcg/mL	D5W, NS, LR	n/a	b	21 d[a]	n/a	4 w	n/a	n/a	n/a	4, 6

Flush Compatibility: Heparin lock flush and normal saline.[6]

Special Considerations: Affix special warning sticker to individual dosage container stating **"Fatal if given intrathecally. For intravenous use only."**[6]

Notes

[a]Protected from light.

[b]pH of reconstituted solution is 3.5–5; pH of undiluted preserved solution (1 mg/mL) is 3–5.5.[6]

[c]77 d refrigerated, followed by 2 d at 33°C.

References

1. Vyas HM, Baptista RJ, Mitrano FP, et al. Drug stability guidelines for a continuous infusion chemotherapy program. *Hosp Pharm.* 1987; 22:685–7.
2. Weir PJ, Ireland DS. Chemical stability of cytarabine and vinblastine injections. *Br J Pharm Pract.* 1990; 12:53–4, 60.
3. Girona V, Prat J, Pujol M, et al. Stability of vinblastine sulphate in 0.9% sodium chloride in polypropylene syringes. *Boll Chim Farmaceutico.* 1996; 135:413–4.
4. Beijnen JH, Vendrig DEMM, Underberg WJM. Stability of vinca alkaloid anticancer drugs in three commonly used infusion fluids. *J Parent Sci Technol.* 1989; 43:84–7.
5. *Intermate/Infusor Drug Stability Information.* Deerfield, IL: Baxter Healthcare Corporation; October 2008.
6. Trissel LA. ASHP's Interactive Handbook on Injectable Drugs. Bethesda, MD: American Society of Health-System Pharmacists. Accessed 2012 Aug.

VinCRIStine Sulfate

Container		Drug Manufacturer	Concentration	Diluents	Osmolality (mOsm/kg)	pH[i]	Storage Conditions						Refer.
							Temperature			Post-thaw Temp		Body Temp	
							Room	Refrig	Frozen	Room	Refrig		
CONTAINER													
Polyolefin Bags		LI	5 mcg/mL[g]	NS	n/a	i	n/a	124 h	n/a	n/a	n/a	124 h[f]	6, 8
		LI	10 mcg/mL[j]	NS	n/a	i	n/a	124 h	n/a	n/a	n/a	124 h[f]	6, 8
		LI	16 mcg/mL[d]	NS	n/a	i	n/a	124 h	n/a	n/a	n/a	124 h[f]	6, 8
Polyvinyl Chloride (PVC)		LI	10, 20, 40, 60, 80, 120 mcg/mL	NS	n/a	i	2 d[e]	7 d[e]	n/a	n/a	n/a	n/a	6, 7
		LI	20 mcg/mL	NS, D5W	n/a	i	n/a	7 d[c]	n/a	n/a	n/a	n/a	5, 6
		LI	36 mcg/mL[a]	NS	n/a	i	n/a	7 d[b]	n/a	n/a	n/a	4 d[b]	1, 6
Syringes, Polypropylene (BD)		LI	25, 50, 100, 150 mcg/mL	NS	n/a	i	2 d[e]	7 d[e]	n/a	n/a	n/a	n/a	6, 7
OTHER INFUSION CONTAINERS													
Graseby™ PVC 9000 Cassette (Graseby Medical)		FA	200 mcg/mL[h]	W[h]	n/a	i	n/a	14 d	4 w	n/a	n/a	7 d	4, 6
INFUSOR (Baxter)		LI	36 mcg/mL[a]	NS	n/a	i	n/a	7 d[b]	n/a	n/a	n/a	4 d[b]	6
		LI	40–200 mcg/mL	NS	n/a	i	10 d	n/a	n/a	n/a	n/a	n/a	3
		LI	200 mcg/mL	NS	n/a	i	n/a	29 d	n/a	n/a	n/a	n/a	3
Polypropylene Test Tubes		LI	20 mcg/mL	D5W, NS, LR	n/a	i	21 d[c]	21 d[c]	4 w	n/a	n/a	n/a	2, 6
Unspec. Implanted Pump		LI	33 mcg/mL[k]	NS, D2.5½S	n/a	i	14 d	n/a	n/a	n/a	n/a	14 d[l]	6

Flush Compatibility: Heparin lock flush and normal saline.[6]

Special Considerations: Affix special warning sticker to individual dosage container stating **"Fatal if given intrathecally. For intravenous use only."**[6]

continued on next page

VinCRIStine Sulfate (cont'd)

Notes

[a]With doxorubicin (NP) 1.67 mg/mL.

[b]Stored for 7 d at 4°C, followed by 4 d at 35°C.

[c]Solutions protected from light.

[d]With doxorubicin (PHU) 400 mcg/mL and etoposide phosphate (BMS) 2000 mcg/mL.

[e]Stored at 4°C for 7 d, followed by 2 d at room temperature.

[f]At 35–40°C.

[g]With doxorubicin (PHU) 120 mcg/mL and etoposide phosphate (BMS) 600 mcg/mL.

[h]With doxorubicin (PHU) 2 mg/mL.

[i]pH of undiluted solution (1000 mcg/mL) is 3.5–5.5.[6]

[j]With doxorubicin (PHU) 240 mcg/mL and etoposide phosphate (BMS) 1200 mcg/mL.

[k]With doxorubicin (FA) 1.4 mg/mL.

[l]At 30 and 37°C.

References

1. Nyhammar EK, Johansson SG, Seiving BE. Stability of doxorubicin hydrochloride and vincristine sulfate in two portable infusion-pump reservoirs. *Am J Health-Syst Pharm.* 1996; 53:1171–3.

2. Beijnen JH, Vendrig DEMM, Underberg WJM. Stability of vinca alkaloid anticancer drugs in three commonly used infusion fluids. *J Parent Sci Technol.* 1989; 43:84–7.

3. Intermate/Infusor Drug Stability Information. Deerfield, IL: Baxter Healthcare Corporation; October 2008.

4. Priston MJ, Sewell GJ. Stability of three cytotoxic drug infusions in the Graseby 900 ambulatory infusion pump. *J Oncol Pharm Practice.* 1998; 4(3):143–9.

5. Dine T, Luyckx M, Cazin JC, et al. Stability and compatibility studies of vinblastine, vincristine, vindesine and vinorelbine with PVC infusion bags. *Int J Pharm.* 1991; 77:279–85.

6. Trissel LA. ASHP's Interactive Handbook on Injectable Drugs. Bethesda, MD: American Society of Health-System Pharmacists. Accessed 2012 Aug.

7. Trissel LA, Zhang Y, Cohen MR. The stability of diluted vincristine sulfate used as a deterrent to inadvertent intrathecal injection. *Hosp Pharm.* 2001; 36:740–5.

8. Yuan P, Grimes GJ, Shankman SE, et al. Compatibility and stability of vincristine sulfate, doxorubicin hydrochloride, and etoposide phosphate in 0.9% sodium chloride injection. *Am J Health-Syst Pharm.* 2001; 58:594–8.

Vinorelbine Tartrate

Container	Drug Manufacturer	Concentration	Diluents	Osmolality (mOsm/kg)	pH[c]	Storage Conditions Temperature Room	Refrig	Frozen	Post-thaw Temp Room	Refrig	Body Temp	Refer.
CONTAINER												
Polyethylene[b]	PIF	0.385 mg/mL	NS	n/a	c	7 d	n/a	n/a	n/a	n/a	n/a	1
Polyvinyl Chloride (PVC)	PIF	0.385 mg/mL	NS	n/a	c	7 d	n/a	n/a	n/a	n/a	n/a	1
	PIF	0.5 mg/mL	D5W	n/a	c	n/a	7 d[a]	n/a	n/a	n/a	n/a	1, 2
	PIF	0.5 mg/mL	NS	n/a	c	n/a	3 d[a]	n/a	n/a	n/a	n/a	1, 2
	GW	0.5, 2 mg/mL	D5W, NS	n/a	c	5 d	n/a	n/a	n/a	n/a	n/a	1
OTHER INFUSION CONTAINERS												
Glass	PIF	0.385 mg/mL	NS	n/a	c	7 d	n/a	n/a	n/a	n/a	n/a	1
INTERMATE (Baxter)	PIF	0.1–2 mg/mL	D5W, NS	n/a	c	24 h[d]	21 d[d]	n/a	n/a	n/a	n/a	3

Flush Compatibility: Heparin lock flush and normal saline.[1]
Special Considerations: n/a

Notes

[a]Solutions protected from light.
[b]Low density polyethylene (Ecoflac®), B. Braun Melsungen AG container.
[c]pH of undiluted solution is 3.5.[1]
[d]21 d refrigerated, followed by 24 h at room temperature.

References

1. Trissel LA. ASHP's Interactive Handbook on Injectable Drugs. Bethesda, MD: American Society of Health-System Pharmacists. Accessed 2012 Aug.
2. Dine T, Luyckx M, Cazin JC, et al. Stability and compatibility studies of vinblastine, vincristine, vindesine and vinorelbine with PVC infusion bags. Int J Pharm. 1991; 77:279–85.
3. Intermate/Infusor Drug Stability Information. Deerfield, IL: Baxter Healthcare Corporation; October 2008.

Voriconazole

Storage Conditions

CONTAINER	Drug Manufacturer	Concentration	Diluents	Osmolality (mOsm/kg)	pH	Temperature Room	Temperature Refrig	Temperature Frozen	Post-thaw Temp Room	Post-thaw Temp Refrig	Body Temp	Refer.
Polyolefin Bag	PF	2 mg/mL	NS	n/a	n/a	8 d[c]	8 d[c]	n/a	n/a	n/a	n/a	1
	PF	2 mg/mL	NS	n/a	n/a	n/a	32 d	n/a	n/a	n/a	n/a	1
	PF	2 mg/mL	D5W	n/a	n/a	5 d[c]	6 d[c]	n/a	n/a	n/a	n/a	1
Polyvinyl Chloride (PVC)	PF	0.5 mg/mL	NS	n/a	n/a	<2 d[b-d]	11 d[a,c]	n/a	n/a	n/a	n/a	2
	PF	0.5 mg/mL	D5W	n/a	n/a	<2 d[b-d]	9 d[a,c]	n/a	n/a	n/a	n/a	2
	PF	4 mg/mL	D5W	n/a	n/a	n/a	15 d	n/a	n/a	n/a	n/a	1
Unspecified	PF	0.5–5 mg/mL	NS, LR, D5LR, D5½S, D5W, ½S, D5S	n/a	n/a	24 h[b]	24 h[b]	n/a	n/a	n/a	n/a	3

Flush Compatibility: Saline.

Special Considerations: Reconstitute via with 19 mL W to 10 mg/mL, then dilute to a concentration of 5 mg/mL or less infusion solution. Infuse over 1–2 h at a maximum rate of 3 mg/kg/h. Do not use vial if vacuum does not draw in diluent. Do not dilute with sodium bicarbonate 4.2% infusion.[3]

Notes

[a]There was evidence of drug sorption by PVC bags at the end of the stability study.
[b]Manufacturer recommends using immediately or within 24 h if refrigerated.[3]
[c]Protected from light.
[d]Based on analysis at time 0 and 2 d interval post preparation.

References

1. Trissel LA. ASHP's Interactive Handbook on Injectable Drugs. Bethesda, MD: American Society of Health-System Pharmacists. Accessed 2012 Jan.
2. Adams A, Morimoto L, Meneghini L, et al. Treatment of invasive fungal infections: stability of voriconazole infusion solutions in PVC bags. *The Brazilian Journal of Infectious Diseases* 2008; 12(5):400–4.
3. Vfend® [prescribing information]. New York, NY: Pfizer USA; November 2011.

Ziconotide Acetate[a]

	Drug Manufacturer	Concentration	Diluents	Osmolality (mOsm/kg)	pH	Temperature			Post-thaw Temp		Body Temp	Refer.
						Room	Refrig	Frozen	Room	Refrig		
CONTAINER												
Syringes, Plastic	ELN	25 mcg/mL	d	n/a	n/a	n/a	28 d[d]	n/a	n/a	n/a	n/a	1
	ELN	25 mcg/mL	e	n/a	n/a	n/a	25 d[e]	n/a	n/a	n/a	n/a	1
	ELN	25 mcg/mL	f	n/a	n/a	n/a	17 d[f]	n/a	n/a	n/a	n/a	1
Unspecified	ELN	unspec.	NS[b]	n/a	c	n/a	24 h	n/a	n/a	n/a	n/a	2
Vial, Plastic	ELN	25 mcg/mL	h	n/a	5.8[h]	n/a	30 d	n/a	n/a	n/a	30 d	4
	ELN	25 mcg/mL	j	n/a	6.0[j]	n/a	30 d	n/a	n/a	n/a	n/a	4
OTHER INFUSION CONTAINERS												
Synchromed[®] II Implantable Pump (Medtronic)	ELN	25 mcg/mL	g	n/a	n/a	n/a	n/a	n/a	n/a	n/a	22 d	1
	ELN	25 mcg/mL	d	n/a	n/a	n/a	n/a	n/a	n/a	n/a	28 d	1
	ELN	25 mcg/mL	i	n/a	n/a	n/a	n/a	n/a	n/a	n/a	26 d	1
	ELN	25 mcg/mL	e	n/a	n/a	n/a	n/a	n/a	n/a	n/a	19 d	1
	ELN	25 mcg/mL	k	n/a	n/a	n/a	n/a	n/a	n/a	n/a	34 d	1
	ELN	25 mcg/mL	l	n/a	n/a	n/a	n/a	n/a	n/a	n/a	19 d	1
	ELN	25 mcg/mL	f	n/a	n/a	n/a	n/a	n/a	n/a	n/a	8 d	1
	ELN	25 mcg/mL	m	n/a	n/a	n/a	n/a	n/a	n/a	n/a	33 d	1
	ELN	25 mcg/mL	h	n/a	5.8[h]	n/a	n/a	n/a	n/a	n/a	12 d	4
	ELN	25 mcg/mL	j	n/a	6.0[j]	n/a	n/a	n/a	n/a	n/a	20 d	4

Flush Compatibility: Normal saline.[1]

Special Considerations: Refrigerate diluted and undiluted product. Protect from light and freezing.[2]

Use ziconotide 25 mcg/mL (undiluted) for initial priming and first fill of drug-naïve (new) Synchromed® pumps; refill new pump within 14 d due to initial drug sorption; subsequent refills with undiluted drug should be at least every 84 d, or with diluted drug at least every 40 d.[1,2,3]

Use ziconotide 5 mg/mL in preservative-free NS for initial fill of CADD-Micro® external microinfusion device. Follow manufacturer specifications for device fills and refills.[1,2]

Due to implanted reservoir volumes and rate limitations associated with intrathecal (IT) infusion devices, polytherapy (combinations of medications) is not uncommon; practitioners should be experienced with pharmacology, physicochemical parameters, and sterility requirements when preparing and administering IT infusions.

continued on next page

Ziconotide Acetate (cont'd)

Notes

[a]For intrathecal use only with SynchroMed® EL, SynchroMed II Infusion Systems (Medtronic), and CADD-Micro Ambulatory Infusion Pump (Smiths Medical MD).[2]

[b]Preservative-free NS.

[c]pH of undiluted solution is 4.0–5.0.[2]

[d]With clonidine HCl (dissolved powder) 2 mg/mL.

[e]With hydromorphone HCl (dissolved powder) 35 mg/mL.

[f]With morphine sulfate (dissolved powder) 35 mg/mL.

[g]With bupivacaine HCl (dissolved powder) 5 mg/mL.

[h]With commercial Lioresal Intrathecal® baclofen 1.5 mg/mL.

[i]With fentanyl citrate (dissolved powder) 1 mg/mL.

[j]With baclofen (dissolved powder) 2 mg/mL.

[k]With morphine sulfate (dissolved powder) 10 mg/mL.

[l]With morphine sulfate (powder) 20 mg/mL.

[m]With sufentanil citrate (powder) 1 mg/mL.

References

1. Trissel LA. ASHP's Interactive Handbook on Injectable Drugs. Bethesda, MD: American Society of Health-System Pharmacists. Accessed 2012 May.
2. Prialt® [package insert]. Philadelphia, PA: Azur Pharma International; May 2010.
3. Shields DE, Liu W, Gunning K, et al. Statistical evaluation of the chemical stability of ziconotide solutions during simulated intrathecal administration. Journal of Pain and Symptom Management 2008; 36(1):e4–e6.
4. Shields D, Montenegro N, Aclan J. Chemical stability of admixtures combining ziconotide with baclofen during simulated intrathecal administration. Neuromodulation 2007; 10(s1):12–7.

Zidovudine[a]

Drug Manufacturer	Concentration	Diluents	Osmolality (mOsm/kg)	pH[b]	Storage Conditions						Refer.
					Temperature			Post-thaw Temp		Body Temp	
					Room	Refrig	Frozen	Room	Refrig		
CONTAINER											
Polyvinyl Chloride (PVC) BW	4 mg/mL	D5W, NS	n/a	b	8 d	8 d	n/a	n/a	n/a	n/a	1
OTHER INFUSION CONTAINERS											
INTERMATE/ INFUSOR (Baxter) WEL	4 mg/mL	D5W, NS	n/a	b	8 d	8 d	n/a	n/a	n/a	n/a	2

Flush Compatibility: Heparin lock flush and normal saline.[1]

Special Considerations: Dilute in D5W to a concentration no greater than 4 mg/mL.[1] Administer intravenously over 1 h.[1]

Notes

[a]Manufacturer recommends that zidovudine diluted in D5W or NS be used within 8 h at room temperature or 24 h if refrigerated, as there is no preservative in the formulation. The drug is chemically stable for longer periods.[1]

[b]pH of undiluted solution is 5.5.[1]

References

1. Trissel LA. ASHP's Interactive Handbook on Injectable Drugs. Bethesda, MD: American Society of Health-System Pharmacists. Accessed 2012 Jan.
2. Intermate/Infusor Drug Stability Information. Deerfield, IL: Baxter Healthcare Corporation; October 2008.

Zoledronic Acid

	Drug Manufacturer	Concentration	Diluents	Osmolality (mOsm/kg)	pH[d]	Storage Conditions					Body Temp	Refer.
						Temperature			Post-thaw Temp			
						Room	Refrig	Frozen	Room	Refrig		
CONTAINER												
Polyethylene Bag	NVS	0.03–0.04 mg/mL	NS, D5W	n/a	n/a	a	24 h	n/a	n/a	n/a	n/a	1, 2
Polypropylene Bag	NVS	0.03–0.04 mg/mL	NS, D5W	n/a	n/a	a	24 h	n/a	n/a	n/a	n/a	1, 2
Polyvinyl Chloride (PVC)	NVS	0.03–0.04 mg/mL	NS, D5W	n/a	n/a	a	24 h	n/a	n/a	n/a	n/a	1, 2
OTHER INFUSION CONTAINERS												
INTERMATE/INFUSOR (Baxter)	NVS	0.04 mg/mL	D5W	n/a	n/a	24 h	n/a	n/a	n/a	n/a	24 h[e]	5
COMMERCIAL PREPARATIONS (RTU)												
Glass	NVS	0.05 mg/mL	RTU[b]	n/a	6.0–7.0	c	24 h[c]	n/a	n/a	n/a	n/a	3, 4

Flush Compatibility: Normal saline.[1,3]

Special Considerations: Infuse in a separate line from all other medication. Do not mix with calcium or other divalent cation-containing solutions (e.g., LR.)[1,2,4] Administer solutions at room temperature.[1,3]

Notes

[a]Manufacturer recommends immediate use after dilution if not refrigerated; time between reconstitution, dilution, refrigerated storage, and end of administration must not exceed 24 h.[1,2]

[b]Each 100 mL of RTU Reclast® brand of zoledronic acid solution contains 4,950 mg mannitol and 30 mg sodium citrate.[3]

[c]Expiration date per manufacturer's label. After opening, may be refrigerated for 24 h prior to administration.[3]

[d]pH of 0.7% solution in W is 2.0.[1,3]

[e]24 h at 33°C following 24 h at 25°C.

References

1. Zometa® [prescribing information]. East Hanover, NJ: Novartis Pharmaceuticals; June 2011.
2. Medical Information, Communication, and Education [personal communication]. East Hanover, NJ: Novartis Pharmaceuticals; February 29, 2008.
3. Reclast® [prescribing information]. East Hanover, NJ: Novartis Pharmaceuticals; August 2011.
4. Reclast® [material safety data sheet]. East Hanover, NJ: Novartis Pharmaceuticals; August 2007.
5. Intermate/Infusor Drug Stability Information. Deerfield, IL: Baxter Healthcare Corporation; October 2008.

Part III

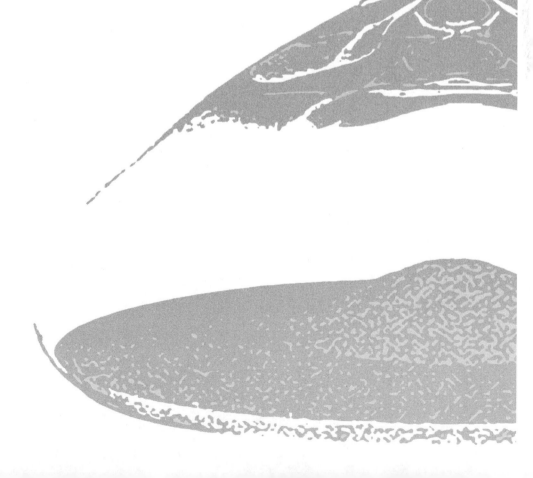

Appendix A

Manufacturer and Compendium Abbreviations

AAB	Apoteket AB
AB	Abbott
ACT	Actelion
AD	Adria
AH	Allen & Hanburys
AM	Astra Medica
AMG	Amgen
AMR	American Regent
APC	Apothecon
APO	Apotex
APP	American Pharmaceutical Partners
AS	Arnar-Stone
ASH	Ash-Stevens
ASL	Astellas
AST	Astra
ASM	AstraMedica
ASZ	AstraZeneca
AVE	Aventis
AW	Asta Werke
AY	Ayerst
BA	Baxter
BAY	Bayer
BB	B & B Pharmaceuticals
BD	Becton, Dickinson and Company
BE	Beecham
BED	Bedford
BEL	R. Bellon
BI	Boehringer Ingelheim
BMS	Bristol-Myers Squibb
BPL	Bio Products Laboratories
BR	Bristol
BRN	B Braun
BW	Burroughs Wellcome
BX	Berlex
CAD	Cadence
CE	Carlo Erba
CEN	Centocor
CER	Cerenex
CET	Cetus
CG	Ciba Geigy
CGC	Ciba Geigy Canada, LTD
CHI	Chiron
CI	Ciba
CPF	Coop. Pharmaceutique Francaise
CSL	CSL Behring
CTF	Centafarm
CUB	Cubist Pharmaceutical
CUP	Cumberland Pharmaceuticals

CUR	Curomed
DB	David Bull Laboratories
DI	Dista
DIO	Diosynth
DSM	DSM Pharmaceuticals
DU	DuPont
EL	Enzon, Inc.
ELN	Elan Pharmaceuticals
ES	Elkins-Sinn
EST	Esteve
EV	Evans
FA	Farmitalia
FAU	Faulding
FL	Funk Labs
FOR	Forest
FUJ	Fujisawa
GEN	Genentech
GG	Geigy
GIL	Gilead
GL	Glaxo
GNS	Gensia
GRI	Grifols Biologicals
GSK	GlaxoSmithKline
GW	Glaxo Wellcome
HC	Hillcross
HMR	Hoechst Marion Roussel
HO	Hoechst-Roussel
HSP	Hospira
ICN	ICN Pharmaceuticals
IMM	Immunex
JC	Janssen-Cilag
JN	Janssen
KED	Kedrion Biopharmaceutics
KN	Knoll
KY	Kyowa
LCSA	Laboratoire Choay Societe Anonyme
LE	Lederle
LEI	Leiras, Finland
LI	Lilly
LUN	Lundbeck
LY	Lyphomed
LZ	Labaz Laboratories
MAR	Marsam
MB	May & Baker
ME	Merck
MG	McGaw
MI	Miles
MIL	Millennium
MJ	Mead Johnson
MN	McNeil
MON	Monarch

MSD	Merck Sharp & Dohme
NF	National Formulary
NNO	Novo-Nordisk
NOV	Novo
NP	Nycomed-Pharma
NVS	Novartis
NY	Nycomed
OB	Ortho Biotech
OCT	Octapharma
OMJ	OMJ Pharmaceuticals
OMN	Ortho McNeil Pharmaceuticals
ON	Orion
OR	Organon
ORT	Ortho
PAD	Paddock
PD	Parke-Davis
PF	Pfizer
PH	Pharmacia
PHU	Pharmacia-Upjohn
PIF	Pierre-Fabre
PX	Pharmax
QU	Quad
RB	Robins
RC	Roche
REC	Recordati
REN	Renaudin
ROX	Roxane Labs
RP	Rhône-Poulenc
RPR	Rhône-Poulenc-Rorer
RR	Roerig
RS	Roussel
SAB	Sabex
SAV	Sanofi-Aventis
SC	Schering
SCN	Schein
SE	Searle
SEQ	Sequus
SGT	Sarget
SH	Spectrum Healthcare
SI	Sigma
SIT	Sigma Tau
SKB	SmithKline Beecham
SKF	Smith Kline & French
SO	SoloPak
SQ	Squibb
SS	Sanofi Synthelabo
STE	Stella
STU	Stuart
SW	Sanofi Winthrop
SY	Syntex
SZ	Sandoz

TAL	Talecris
TE	Teva
TLP	Therabel Lucien Pharma
UN	Unknown
UP	Upjohn
UTC	United Therapeutics
WAS	Wasserman
WAY	Wyeth-Ayerst
WEL	Wellcome
WI	Winthrop
WL	Warner Lambert
WY	Wyeth
XGN	X-Gen
ZEN	Zeneca
ZNS	Zeneus Pharma

Glossary of Terms

Beyond-Use Date: The expiration date assigned by the pharmacist and placed on the prescription label. This date is based on the pharmacist's knowledge of chemical stability, use of a validated sterile preparation compounding process, and anticipated conditions for delivery, storage, and administration.

Controlled Room Temperature: Maintained thermostatically between 20°C–25°C; mean kinetic temperate ≤25°C; some excursions between 15°C–30°C; spikes above 40°C if product manufacturer instruction permits.

Extended Stability: The maximum time period in which 90 percent or greater of a labeled active ingredient is measurable in the solution and container specified, under the stated storage conditions. An exception applies to coagulation factors, which are considered stable when at least 80% of the factor activity is retained.

Inference: The decision to assume that when drugs with well-established stabilities in common container materials, such as PVC and glass, are repeatedly determined to exhibit the same stabilities in containers made of a newer material, such as EVA (with no adverse influence of the container on the stabilities of those drugs being found), then additional drugs of similar compositions will also exhibit stabilities unaltered by this newer container material.

Interpolation: The practice of assuming that data, which demonstrates drug stability at a higher concentration and a lower concentration, supports stability and a concentration in-between the two.

Preparation: A compounded sterile preparation (CSP) that is a sterile drug or nutrient prepared in a licensed pharmacy or other health care related facility pursuant to the order of a licensed prescriber, which may or may not contain sterile products.

Product: A commercially manufactured sterile drug or nutrient that has been evaluated for safety and efficacy by the U.S. Food and Drug Administration (FDA). Products are accompanied by full prescribing information, which is commonly known as the FDA-approved manufacturer's labeling or product package insert.

Stability: The length of time that the preparation retains the labeled potency of the active ingredient(s) under the labeled storage conditions.